Technology and
the Doctor-Patient
Relationship

McFarland Health Topics
Series Editor Elaine A. Moore

Living with Multiple Chemical Sensitivity: Narratives of Coping. Gail McCormick. 2001

Graves' Disease: A Practical Guide. Elaine A. Moore with Lisa Moore. 2001

Autoimmune Diseases and Their Environmental Triggers. Elaine A. Moore. 2002

Hepatitis: Causes, Treatments and Resources. Elaine A. Moore. 2006

Arthritis: A Patient's Guide. Sharon E. Hohler. 2008

The Promise of Low Dose Naltrexone Therapy: Potential Benefits in Cancer, Autoimmune, Neurological and Infectious Disorders. Elaine A. Moore and Samantha Wilkinson. 2009

Living with HIV: A Patient's Guide. Mark Cichocki, RN. 2009

Understanding Multiple Chemical Sensitivity: Causes, Effects, Personal Experiences and Resources. Els Valkenburg. 2010

Type 2 Diabetes: Social and Scientific Origins, Medical Complications and Implications for Patients and Others. Andrew Kagan, M.D. 2010

The Amphetamine Debate: The Use of Adderall, Ritalin and Related Drugs for Behavior Modification, Neuroenhancement and Anti-Aging Purposes. Elaine A. Moore. 2011

CCSVI as the Cause of Multiple Sclerosis: The Science Behind the Controversial Theory. Marie A. Rhodes. 2011

Coping with Post-Traumatic Stress Disorder: A Guide for Families, 2d ed. Cheryl A. Roberts. 2011

Living with Insomnia: A Guide to Causes, Effects and Management, with Personal Accounts. Phyllis L. Brodsky and Allen Brodsky. 2011

Caregiver's Guide: Care for Yourself While You Care for Your Loved Ones. Sharon E. Hohler. 2012

You and Your Doctor: A Guide to a Healing Relationship, with Physicians' Insights. Tania Heller, M.D. 2012

Autogenic Training: A Mind-Body Approach to the Treatment of Chronic Pain Syndrome and Stress-Related Disorders, 2d ed. Micah R. Sadigh. 2012

Advances in Graves' Disease and Other Hyperthyroid Disorders. Elaine A. Moore with Lisa Marie Moore. 2013

Cancer, Autism and Their Epigenetic Roots. K. John Morrow, Jr. 2014

Living with Bipolar Disorder: A Handbook for Patients and Their Families. Karen R. Brock, M.D. 2014

Cannabis Extracts in Medicine: The Promise of Benefits in Seizure Disorders, Cancer and Other Conditions. Jeffrey Dach, M.D., Elaine A. Moore and Justin Kander. 2015

Managing Hypertension: Tools to Improve Health and Prevent Complications. Sandra A. Moulton. 2016

*Mammography and Early Breast Cancer Detection:
How Screening Saves Lives.* Alan B. Hollingsworth, M.D. 2016

*Central Sensitization and Sensitivity Syndromes:
A Handbook for Coping.* Amy Titani. 2017

*Hurting Like Hell, Living with Gusto:
My Battle with Chronic Pain.* Victoria Stopp. 2017

*When Love Meets Dementia: Frontotemporal
Degeneration (FTD) and the Family.* Ada Anbar. 2018

Technology and the Doctor-Patient Relationship.
D.C. Lozar, M.D. 2019

Technology and the Doctor-Patient Relationship

D.C. Lozar, M.D.

McFarland Health Topics
Series Editor Elaine A. Moore

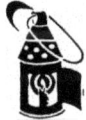

McFarland & Company, Inc., Publishers
Jefferson, North Carolina

ISBN (print) 978-1-4766-7520-6
ISBN (ebook) 978-1-4766-3744-0

Library of Congress and British Library
cataloguing data are available

© 2019 D.C. Lozar, M.D. All rights reserved

No part of this book may be reproduced or transmitted in any form or by any means, electronic or mechanical, including photocopying or recording, or by any information storage and retrieval system, without permission in writing from the publisher.

Front cover images © 2019 Shutterstock

Printed in the United States of America

*McFarland & Company, Inc., Publishers
Box 611, Jefferson, North Carolina 28640*
www.mcfarlandpub.com

To my wonderful wife and amazing son and daughter:
each of you inspires me every single day.

Table of Contents

Author's Note   xii

Preface   1

Introduction   3

One. Buck Rogers Medicine (Utopia)   7
 The Electronic Medical Record 7 • Rebooting Humanity 13 • Challenging Evolutionary Barriers 15 • Augmentation and Wearable 16 • My Thoughts 17 • Reality Check 18

Two. George Orwell Medicine (Dystopia)   20
 We Are a Trade, Not a Business 20 • Censorship—Net Neutrality 25 • Freedom 26 • Universal Health Identifier 27 • My Thoughts 28 • Reality Check 30

Three. Frontier Medicine (Old School)   31
 Cowboy Charlie 31 • Tragedy Loves Ignorance 35 • Hospitals Built on Bedlam 37 • A Doctor's Doctor 39 • Sawbones 41 • Apothecaries 42 • The Nightingale's Song 44 • My Thoughts 45 • Bringing Us Up to Date 47

Four. Beam Me Up, Scotty (Telemedicine)   49
 Unexpected Consequences 49 • Luddites 52 • Taylorism 53 • Dumb and Dumber 55 • My Thoughts 57 • Prescribing Caution 60

Five. The Healing Touch (Origin Story)   61
 Lifting the Hood 61 • The Power of Proximity 63 • The Death of the Physical Exam 65 • Case Studies 65 • Appearance Is More Than Skin Deep 69 • You Can't Arrest Me 70

Six. Go Gently into That Good Night (Death)   72
Waiting for Godot/Death 72 • Accepting Death 74 •
Immortality 76 • Death Is Not Our Enemy 78 •
My Thoughts 79 • A Good Death 81

Seven. Lawyers, Doctors and Lobbyists, Oh My (*Mala Praxis*)   82
Mala Praxis 82 • Sharks in the Water 84 • Bad Medicine 85 •
Money Talks, Doctors Walk 87 • Defending the Castle 88 •
Politics Is a Shell Game 91 • My Thoughts 92 • Case Closed 94

Eight. Medicine Is Dirty (Don't Bring It Home)   96
The Training Gauntlet 96 • Dividing Up the Family 99 • Testing
the Monkey 100 • Cannon Fodder 103 • Quitting Life 106 •
The Sterile Glass Ceiling 107 • Mamas, Don't Let Your Babies
Grow Up to Be Doctors 108 • My Thoughts 109 •
The Not-So-Perfect Match 111 • Technology May Clean Up
Medicine 112

Nine. It's The Money, Stupid (Terminal Economics)   113
How Much Is Your Life Worth? 113 • The Maintenance
of Certification (MOC) Scam 116 • Fraudulent Billing 118 •
Big Pharma, Little Ethics 119 • Unions 120 • My Thoughts 123 •
Prove It 125

Ten. We're Only Human (That's the Point)   127
Trigger Warning 127 • Intersubjective Angst 128 • Dataism
Versus Vitalism 130 • Calculating Compliance 133 •
Epicureanism 134 • My Thoughts 135 • The Invisible World 137

Eleven. The Librarians (Custodians of Health)   139
The Good Librarian 139 • Metaphors Are Magic 141 • You've
Got to Have Heart 141 • Vintage Cars 144 • Minions and
Mood 145 • The Never-Ending Story 147 • It's Only Skin
Deep 148 • The Endocrine Economy 149 • My Thoughts 152 •
Trust Your Librarian 156

Twelve. The Altered Mind of a Physician (Evolution?)   157
Losing Our Minds 157 • Neuroplasticity 159 • There's a Hole
in My Bucket, Dear ELIZA 162 • Deskilled Doctors 164 • Why
Can't I Open the Black Box? 167 • My Thoughts 169 • Paging:
Doctor Watson 171

Thirteen. We Are Not Alone (It's Called a Planet)   173
   Socialized Medicine—It Works for Them 173 • Tiered Health System 174 • Global United Health Care 175 • My Thoughts 178 • What Next? 180

Fourteen. The Brave New World (Is Here)   181
   Invasion of the Doctor Snatchers 181 • Artificial Emotional Intelligence 183 • That Epigenetic Smile 185 • Waiter, There's a Cyborg in My Soup 187 • My Thoughts 189 • Datopia 191

Fifteen. Doctor Tomorrow (What's Next?)   193
   The M in D Is a Terrible Thing to Waste 193 • A Hands-Free Physical Exam 195 • AI-Run Nursing Homes 196 • AI, Dearest 198 • My Final Thoughts 200 • Dr. Laicifitra 202

Addendum   205

Chapter Notes   209

Bibliography   223

Index   241

Author's Note

Please keep in mind as you read this book that all references made to specific patients or case reports are purely "hypothetical" or "representative" composites manufactured from my experience caring for hundreds of thousands of patients and so are essentially pure fabrications (I am a science fiction writer, after all). Specifically, I have taken the liberty of combining personal and clinical experiences, flipping genders (or not), randomly choosing names, and modifying events to create concise educational vignettes that clarify the discussion topic, but which are not biographies of real events. Thus, any resemblance to actual people, living or dead, that the reader finds in my prose is coincidental, unintentional, and the sole product of the reader's imagination. This book does not dispense legal or medical advice nor should anything I've written be used to direct individual patient care or legal choices. Nothing in this book is intended to replace, circumvent, or dissuade a patient or physician from obtaining the services of a licensed, trained physician or lawyer in their state and following that professional's advice. Indeed, I would recommend that the reader seek out these professionals if anything I've written makes them feel as if they need to act in the real world. This is a nonfiction book that weighs the pros and cons of technology as it pertains to the doctor-patient relationship, but the opinions expressed by the author are my own and should not be ascribed to any institution, organization, group, associate, or practice that I have been affiliated with in the past, present, or future.

Additionally, I would like to extend my deep thanks and appreciation to my beta and peer review readers for their thoughts and suggestions.

Preface

Technology and the Doctor-Patient Relationship was written for anyone who has ever considered a career in health care and for any patient who has had an office exam where a provider spent more time doing data entry than listening or examining them. The profession of medicine is an ancient trade that has evolved as one generation of craftspeople passed it down to the next. It is a distinguished, flawed, and astoundingly rewarding vocation, but it may be coming to an end. A brave new world populated by computer algorithms promises our patients better access, safer therapies, and more predictable outcomes. Technology allows us to reduce costs, design more effective and personalized treatments, and diminish fraud and waste. Balanced against these miraculous outcomes is the risk that we, the medical artisans, will forget that our primary responsibility is to our patients and not to a medical template.

As a primary care physician with more than two decades of experience in the trenches, I've practiced in both the analog and digital medical world. I've seen the difference, and I know things are better now and wouldn't want to turn back the clock. However, I worry we are trading too much of our craft's hard-won lessons for the unsubstantiated promises of corporate America.

I laid this book out as a journey, an adventure, if you will, from where I started as an entrenched anti-tech Luddite to the hopeful conclusions I've drawn at the end of this book. Keeping this in mind, readers may discover the problem of technology is approached more pessimistically in the first half of the book while later sections reflect a deeper appreciation of the challenges and benefits of this complex tool. We begin by exploring both a utopian and then a dystopian future before digging into the not-so-romantic reality of old-school medicine. We address the risks of poor communication, the benefits of a hands-on approach, and how critical human empathy is to our patients at the end of their lives. Detailing the legal, financial, and human elements of medicine, including the scams and greed that have tainted the craft, we discuss promising philosophies of practice and a Doctors' Bill of Rights. In the last third of the book, we move fully into that bright new age of health care directed by artificial intelligence, robotic nursing homes, and conclude with why the office visit of the future may be closer and better than we realize.

Introduction

One of my first memories is having a toy stethoscope slung over my neck and hearing that I looked like a doctor. I responded that I was, in fact, going to be a doctor when I grew up. This declaration won me smiles and nods of approval. As my previous aspirations to become either a superhero or space explorer had earned me little more than conciliatory pats on the head, I bit down hard on the idea of becoming a physician and didn't open my eyes again until I'd accomplished the task.

I mention this "origin story" as I feel it mirrors that of many of my colleagues, ones who, like myself, bought into the mystic of the profession without reading the fine print, the romantics and idealists who believed that a medical degree would bestow on them the power to make the world a better place. This Dumbo fallacy—the idea that we need a crow's feather to accomplish a task we are already capable of achieving—is likely a contributing factor to the disillusionment and burnout many experience later in their careers. There are a plethora of other fields including teaching, police and social work, research, and philosophy that depend on the personality traits (patience, critical thinking, empathy, tenacity, and integrity) concentrated within the medical profession. Each of these trades gives back to society, advances our understanding of the human condition, and deserves society's admiration and appreciation. So why become a physician? The honest answer is that I saw the esteem, financial security, autonomy, and presumed intellectual rigor associated with the degree as having a higher value than that of other fields. Yes, the upfront time commitment and personal sacrifice were great, but the remunerations, I told myself, more than evened the playing field.

I was wrong.

I am privileged to practice medicine, to make a small, positive difference in the lives in those who trust me, but my contributions to the universal "good deeds" jar are no more valuable than anyone else's and to presume otherwise is a crime for which I am still serving time.

For I am guilty of having played the game.

You see, the road to a medical degree is strewn with gatekeepers, application readers, and interviewers who ask the same prerequisite questions. I answered that I "loved" to help people, that I wanted to give back, and that I hoped to make a difference. These tenets were what they wanted to hear, what I was supposed to believe, and so I acted the part, not because I honestly felt those things at the time but because I was determined to get the degree—the crow's feather. I did community service, volunteered for summer research projects, and wrote essays about how Aunt Nelly's untimely death inspired me to become a doctor. Here again, I knew the readers shuffling through applications were looking to check off these boxes, and so I was happy to oblige. I'll acknowledge that there are saintly young adults who volunteer their time out of the goodness of their heart and feel fulfilled by their efforts, and to them I say, "age quod agi."[1] However, at the time, I was merely padding my resume.

That's not to say I was wrong or the exception. There is a pragmatic path to achieving a degree in medicine, the dusty certificate we hang on the wall behind our desks, and it has little to do with how we end up practicing medicine in our offices. The system demands certain things, mandatory criteria that it feels produces better graduates, and no one is likely to change the requirements simply by pointing out that the doorkeeper's checkboxes are populated with actions taken for action's sake rather than due to a moral prerogative. Why, then, are budding physicians expected to show that they've done compassionate things, that they can empathize, that they are willing to make personal sacrifices for others? Because these are traits found in those who work in health care. In Immanuel Kant's *Critique of Pure Reason*[2] published in 1781, he explains that the difficulty with this perspective was "a priori" (a conclusion drawn from the results) and found such assumptions lacking when compared to solutions attained by "a priori knowledge" (conclusions attained through direct personal experience). Having graduated from Northwestern Medical School, worked a preliminary year as a surgical resident, completed a residency at the University of Massachusetts in Family Practice, and having spent my career working face-to-face with my patients, I would argue that a degree bestows the privilege and responsibility of our profession, but it does not magically impart the tacit wisdom earned from years of experience. The M.D. is merely the key that opens the door to our real training, and it is the daily practice of helping our patients live fuller lives that gives us license to be compassionate physicians.

Much of what we learn in college and medical school is what Michael Polanyi in his 1958 book *Personal Knowledge*[3] would term explicit knowledge. We are given the patient's vitals, their labs, and a thumbnail history with pertinent physical exam findings, and asked to pick the "one" correct diagnosis or next step. Computers are very good at this type of problem solving, and algorithmic programs are likely to outperform even senior physicians in the next few years. However, when Mrs. Jones shows up complaining of back pain, nausea, chest pain, and irregular bowels after a week of weight loss, I know she's depressed and needs someone to talk to about her husband who passed away a year ago to the day. The perfunctory dance of labs, ECG, and exam are merely the opening volley before we sit down and reminisce about the love of her life. Intuitively knowing she needs to make a human connection rather than receive a diagnosis is called tacit knowledge, and computers stink at it.

So how do we get from the explicit mind-set of the medical student to the tacit knowledge of a seasoned professional? There is no right answer, no simple path, but it does require us to begin a lifelong journey.

In 1949, Joseph Campbell published *The Hero with a Thousand Faces*[4] to detail the sequence of steps he felt successful protagonists needed to complete for their story to capture our imagination. He concisely described this journey as "a hero ventures forth from the world of common day into a region of supernatural wonder: fabulous forces are there encountered, and a decisive victory is won: the hero comes back from this mysterious adventure with the power to bestow boons on his fellow man." Archetypal stories like this are timeless because their plot points mimic truisms in our daily lives. Most start with the protagonist thinking they know what needs to be done only to discover that they failed to understand the scope of the problem. We need our early ambitions to get us into the new world, the real world of medicine, where we learn that we know absolutely nothing. We make mistakes, we find mentors, we question our motives, and we learn that the goal isn't, and should never have been, to get a degree or pass an exam. The stakes in the field are our patients' lives, their suffering and dignity, and, in some cases, our own integrity. When you save someone's life by catching a missed diagnosis, when you deliver a baby, when you take out an appendix, when you help a patient go on living, when you assist another human being to pass painlessly through the veil, and when you listen, really listen, you are learning to be a physician, a healer, and an active member of our austere profession. The lessons we learn after graduation are tragic, inspiring, and impossible to teach in a book or with a lecture; they are tacit knowledge of life. The grades we receive come in the form of homemade cookies, tearful thanks, and our patients' trust that we will do all we can to keep them healthy. You see, we all start out thinking the hero's journey is about us, the doctors, and what we discover is that we are merely supporting characters in the lives of our patients.

And what does a good supporting character do?

We keep our heroes, even the misguided ones, alive by lending them our skills, advice, and whatever clinical tools we have to offer. The question I asked before deciding to write this book was "Given how essential tacit knowledge is to our profession, how much can we depend on a tool built to answer explicit knowledge questions?" Is unfettered technology the panacea we want for our patients? If so, what kind of algorithms are best and what are we willing to give up in exchange for them? Are we, as a society, going to open our eyes years from now and find that the mystic of innovation was yet another Dumbo fallacy and regret buying so many crow feathers from corporate America?

Chapter One

Buck Rogers Medicine (Utopia)

The Electronic Medical Record

Have you ever shown up for an office visit and left feeling like your physician spent more time interacting with their computer than with you? Have you ever called your doctor's office for an appointment only to be asked a series of algorithmic questions that felt like a telemarketer's survey? Have you ever had medication that you've taken for years changed to formulary alternatives without being told? If you bumped into your doctor on the street, would they know your name? Would they be happy to see you? Sadly, the answer to many of these questions reflects how sick the American healthcare system has become. With the advent of electronic medical records (EMRs), diagnostic protocols, large-scale pharmacy conversions, and capitalization of care, many Americans feel their doctors see them as numbers on a screen rather than as fellow humans. Technology has altered how doctors think about, treat, and carry on relationships with patients, and physicians have a professional responsibility to ensure that these changes are ethical, healthy, and sustainable.

In this, we are failing.

In a telling 2017 study published in the *Annals of Family Medicine*,[1] the investigators examined the patient charts of 142 actively practicing family physicians over the course of three years. The results were as shocking as they were predictable with nearly six hours of a physician's 11-hour day being spent performing clerical or administrative work on EMRs. That's roughly half of their professional day allotted to logging data into a digital chart that was meant to improve health care but that instead has become a barrier to access, sustainable work/life balance, and to one-on-one patient interactions. Over the last decade, the EMR has grown from a niggling concept into a ubiquitous parasite that actively competes with the patient for the doctor's attention.

Detractors say that patients understand that this is part of modern medicine and don't mind sacrificing office time with their doctor to achieve the highest standard of care. This is a reasonable assumption until we look at the 2016 article published in the *Journal of the American Medical Association*[2] in which office encounters where the computer was used aggressively were rated significantly lower by patients. In the same year, Medscape[3] asked 15,285 physicians in more than 25 specialties how electronic health records (EHRs, considered a more inclusive abbreviation but for this book EHR and EMR will be used interchangeably) affected practice operations and patient encounters. Per the results, "57% of respondents said that EHRs reduce face-to-face time with patients, and 50% noted a reduction in the number of patients they can see."

However, there must have been evidence that EMRs improve clinical outcomes for the United States to have invested $38 billion in promoting eHealth. Indeed, looking around the world, we find that England spent nearly £13 billion to fuse EMRs into their National Health Service.[4] They must have had a good reason to do so.

I'm afraid not.

A 2011 review in the *Public Library of Science*[5] that looked at all the previously published works about digital health care found "that despite support from policymakers, there was relatively little empirical evidence to substantiate many of the claims made in relation to these technologies." This means that lawmakers in two of the most educated nations of the modern world spent more than $56 billion of their taxpayers' money on something that sounded like a good idea but which had no evidence-based studies to support their expenditures—oops.

Finger's crossed. Maybe it'll all work out.

Fast-forward to 2013 where RAND Health[6] (a research group dedicated to health-care policy research around the world) issued a report in which its author said, "Across a wide range of EHR software products and practice models, physicians reported poor EHR usability, time-consuming data entry, interference with face-to-face patient care, degraded clinical documentation (as a consequence of template-based notes), and inefficient and less fulfilling work content.... These findings suggest that the current state of EHR technology may be insufficient to deliver on the promise of EHRs." Please keep in mind that this is the same RAND Health Group[7] that issued a report in 2005 saying that the U.S. health-care system "could save more than 81 billion annually and improve quality of care" if doctors and hospitals were mandated to go digital.

We were, and yet in 2018, the Centers for Medicare & Medicaid Services[8] forecasted a significant uptick in annual U.S. health-care expenditures to $5.7 trillion in 2026 or 19.7 percent of our GDP—double oops.

So they messed up, mistakes happen. Right? After all, RAND Health calls itself "the nations' most trusted source of objective health policy research."[9] They made an unbiased guess and got it wrong. It's not as if the technology companies that stood to make money from the study's conclusions paid to have the study done.

Oh, but wait, that's exactly what happened. As was so eloquently pointed out in Nicholas Carr's book *The Glass Cage*,[10] Cerner Corporation, General Electric, Hewlett Packard, and Xerox all helped fund the initial RAND study and then gobbled up the billions of dollars the United States paid them in exchange for their medical software—triple oops.

I'll bet the policymakers who pushed the EMRs on Congress hope no one notices the conflict of interest.

They did notice in the United Kingdom, and they were none too happy.

The United Kingdom sued the U.S.-based Computer Science Corporation, one of the four companies that helped implement their country's National Programme for Information Technology and recouped £97.5 million.[11] Maybe we should do the same to the companies that promoted the 2005 RAND study?

But wait. Isn't technology supposed to make things faster? I mean, it may cost a great deal, but if patients are seen faster, it might be worth it. A valid point, and where would speed be most essential? I would suggest the emergency room. Yet a 2013 article published in *The American Journal of Emergency Medicine*[12] found that ER physicians spent 44 percent of their time logging data into their computers instead of doing direct patient care. Instead of having the men and women who are trained to make split-second life-and-death decisions see patients, we're asking them to do clerical work. Is it any wonder the lines are so long?

Okay, that's not ideal. But at least once a patient gets to see a physician they interact with a chipper, well-rested, and empathetic professional. I'm afraid not. According to a 2016 article published in the *Mayo Clinic Proceedings*,[13] 6,560 physicians were surveyed and their complaints of progressive burnout and job dissatisfaction were linked to the EMR and the needless data entry it requires.

But legible charting, thorough documentation of a patient's health, is essential. Coding is vital because it helps physicians take better care of the patient. Maybe this is true in Europe where ICD-10 codes are used for epidemiologic reasons, but in the United States, these same codes are tied to reimbursement. The more codes we keystroke into the patient's chart, the higher the compensation for the visit. Therefore, a single patient may have a code for type II diabetes, type II diabetes with peripheral neuropathy, type II diabetes with retinopathy, type II diabetes with nephropathy, etc. Did you want to complain to the American Medical Association (AMA), the prestigious group of professionals who for years have been advocates of ethical practices and physician rights? Sorry, the old guard has moved on to greener pastures. In her book *An American Sickness*,[14] Elisabeth Rosenthal aptly describes how the AMA owns the Current Procedural Terminology codes used to bill and how it demands royalties and licensing fees for its use. No longer run by stolid doctors, the AMA's board now includes stakeholders and business professionals whose exorbitant salaries are in no way diminished by the volume of data the physicians in the field must input. Case in point: according to CEO Update,[15] Dr. James Madara, the AMA's current CEO, reported earning $1,883,047 on his 2016 taxes. That's 33 times the median household income in the United States.[16] Do you think he might be a bit biased toward maintaining the status quo?

"Anyone? Bueller. Anyone? Bueller."[17]

Okay. So now that we've sold the family cow for a handful of magic beans is there any way to make this digital beanstalk reach the proverbial castle in the clouds they promised us?

Yes.

But to do that we need to understand what's wrong with it.

Theoretically, the EMR is a good idea. The problem, in my opinion, is that it wasn't allowed to evolve naturally in the marketplace. One of the immense benefits of a capitalist market is that products with errors cannot survive. Consumers will stop purchasing them and will write scathing reviews, and the manufacturer will then have to modify their product or abandon it. Neither physicians or patients had the opportunity to push back, to say "try again" to the technology companies, or to choose to stay with paper charts until something so undeniably better was presented that there was a natural, albeit glacial, shift to that new product. Instead, we were forced to adopt a computer-centric program (one in which the human operator helps the computer do its job) instead of an industry-tested, human-centric medical tool (one used to augment and enhance the human's job).

Why?

As part of the 2009 ARRA (American Recovery and Reinvestment Act),[18] all health-care groups were required to adopt and show meaningful use of electronic medical records or suffer reductions in their Medicaid and Medicare reimbursement. The Congressional Budget Office[19] estimates the government will have spent $821 billion between 2009 and 2019 on an act that's purpose was to reverse and blunt the effects of the Great Recession. Nearly $19 billion was earmarked for health information technology to encourage investments and incentive payments.[20] This was a windfall for businesses that were trying to get their versions of an EMR off the ground and for health-care informatics specialists and did succeed in stimulating the economy. It's important to remember that the goal of the act was not to make physicians' lives better or to implement proven health-care tools for patients but to create work (lots of work). Washington may have been less concerned about the practicality of the work done than if it produced jobs, and so was able to ignore the fact that there was no hard evidence to support its presumption that EMR would improve our profession.

Thus, we find ourselves married to a system that conceptually makes sense but one that did not evolve naturally. Worse yet, the programs are now so blended with our care delivery that there is no way for the utilizers, both the physicians and patients, to push back, to say the programs are robbing us of the eye contact, the active listening, the freedom to contemplate a diagnosis and therapy plan. For centuries, we have completed purposeful, efficient, focused histories, physicals, and treatments for our patients. We did our jobs swiftly because there were more people who needed our help, patients who would complain or suffer if we took more time than needed. We stayed late, sacrificed our personal lives, and studied diseases because we took an oath and we believed our efforts made a difference in the lives of others.

Things have changed.

Now, we stay late to plug data into templates so someone can compare disease-of-the-week graphs in administrative meetings. We are no longer reprimanded when we fail to provide proper care to our patients but instead given "guidance" by those who know nothing about the individuals we treat but have found an easy way to "help." If we run behind, we postpone charting until the end of the day so our patients don't have to wait. If someone high up on the technology food chain decides they'd like to look at a new data point, we have to plug it in before the chart closes. It's just a few more clicks they think. No big deal. Really? If it takes me 30 seconds to complete the new task and I see 22 patients a day for five days, that's an hour of my life gone at the end of the week. Pffft. How do I get that back? Do I get paid for it? Does it make any of my patient's lives better? We are part of a profession dedicated to making a difference in the lives of other humans; for this, we took an oath; for this, we are willing to make sacrifices. The problem is, no actively practicing physician believes half the data points we are required to input do more than complete a generic billing template. We are sacrificing our time, our patient's time, to make a computer's algorithm happy. Physicians are humans; we break when we're misused, as was shown in *The Mayo Clinic Proceedings*[21] that looked at over 35,000 doctors between 2011 and 2014 and found more than 50 percent were suffering from burnout. Job dissatisfaction leads to early retirement and discouraging words to bright-eyed teens that ask if they should go into the profession. This is a real problem, as the Association of American Medical Colleges[22] report released in 2015 predicts a shortfall of up to 90,000 physicians by the year 2025 with more than one-third of doctors set to retire in the next decade.

Don't worry; they've built an AI program to replace us.

I'm not kidding. Take a moment to look at the United Kingdom's Babylon Health.[23]

The Future is now.

We complain that we don't want to be data entry monkeys. Maybe this is how it should be done? Maybe we need to let go, stop fighting it, and see where the path we're on might lead?

Not everyone will remember the pulp magazines of the 1920–1930s, but I am an unabashed enthusiast of the dime-store short stories of the time. In my opinion, Buck Rogers embodied the human capacity for adaptation. For those unfamiliar with Anthony's story, after being exposed to radioactive gas in a cave in 1927, he fell into a state of suspended animation for 500 years. He woke in 2419 to have adventures that demanded he apply his 20th-century thinking to a 25th-century world.[24] Buck Rogers resonated with a generation of people who were inspired by rapid technologic growth even as it irrevocably changed their jobs, health, and international security. The author, Philip Francis Nowlan, didn't suggest society abandon technology but rather reminded us that personal relationships and common sense, no matter how antiquated, were more powerful tools to solve society's problems than space-age innovation. In our current climate of technologic upheaval, we would do well to take this maxim to heart. Modern health care is entering a Buck Rogers future in which our understanding of human physiology could create a medical utopia free from pain and suffering. As custodians of the tools needed to cultivate this new world, we have a responsibility to avoid the temptations of greed, self-promotion, and data manipulation that hang like ripe cherries along our path.

Technology is no more to blame for harming our profession or our relationship with our patients than a fire is for burning down a house. Self-indulgence, ignorance, and apathy have inexpertly wielded this revolutionary tool, and now we must pay the price, learn from our mistakes, and repair the damage. Reprogrammed to assist rather than demand, to remind if requested, and to be vulnerable to user (rather than market or administrative) demands, medical technology has the potential to improve and extend our patients' lives while easing the stressors in ours. Let's take a creative moment to consider what the health-care field might look like in a future that is getting closer every day.

Rebooting Humanity

Imagine a future where we finally realize that it is in everyone's best interest—except for those who profited from chronic disease—to treat illnesses aggressively. Consider a world where a global health-care initiative is devised and supported by pooled international funds with the founding principles that free health care, access to immunizations, and preventative care services are fundamental human rights and so not subject to the political pandering of a single government or politician. DNA samples are taken from every person to determine their risks for cancer, metabolic/immunologic errors, or diseases that may respond to gene therapy. Recognizing that many communicable diseases are the result of poverty, ignorance, and lack of access to basic needs such as food and clean water, international efforts are made to wipe out these factors for the welfare of all. Biometric tracking devices track the choices every living human makes so they can be given personalized suggestions and therapy to help them steer clear of risky behavior. Imagine a future where a single world health organization knows basic details about every human on the planet and has the capacity to send resources to those who need it most.

For those who squirm at the thought of having their every action monitored, documented, and archived, I'll ask you to leave your cell phone on the table as you leave the room.

We're already voluntarily doing these things. As I write this, GSMA[25] (the Global System for Mobile Communication) shows that of the 7.6 billion people[26] on the planet more than five billion have cell phones. That's more than 66 percent. How hard would it be to use the information this network collects for the good of all rather than to keep our Facebook profiles up to date?

Human beings are rational animals who wish to live happy, pain-free lives while contributing something positive or memorable to the world to mark their finite existence. Technology is designed to increase real personal connectivity, to register an individual's impact (good or bad) on the global community, and help people achieve a sense of self-worth, of having "done something." Language barriers are overcome with instant real-time translators and culture perspective modulators so that different regions of the world feel less isolated and more dialed into our planetary community. Digital copies of the brain waves of family members are made and stored so that new generations can understand and interact with their ancestors. How better to avoid the mistakes of the past than having our great-great-grandparents tell us what happened from their perspective? As unbelievable as it sounds, the scientific community is already working on this. A project called the Human Connectome Project initially funded by NIH (the National Institute of Health) is actively collecting MRI data (both static and active thought images) from individuals bridging the entire human lifespan. The most recent data, all 76 terabytes of it, concerning 1,206 young adults, reside within AWS (Amazon Web Services) with open access for all.[27] CCF's (Connectome Coordination Facility) underlying goal is to help researchers map the human brain—in much the same way we decoded the human genome—to better identify and treat disease processes. Furthermore, the 2045 Initiative[28]—headed by Russian businessman Dmitri Itskov—is convinced we will be able to download a digital copy of the human mind into an artificial matrix with the anticipation that the program will behave and learn as if the copy were the original brain. Even now, there are groups like eterni.mi[29] where you or your loved ones can set up an avatar that will interact with and respond to their questions as you would have once you are gone.

As complex as our brain is, there are a finite number of connections and potential interactions and so we will eventually map it. We've already done it with worms. In the OpenWorm Project, scientists successfully recorded, analyzed, and programmed every aspect of the nematode Caenorhabditis elegans into a computer chip and placed that digital copy into a Lego robot that behaved precisely as if it were a living worm.[30]

So we've created an artificially intelligent worm. What does that have to do with health care? Everything. A report by Global Market Insights, Inc.,[31] predicts that the health-care artificial intelligence market will be worth more than $10 billion by 2024. They've made a worm. Are doctors next?

If so, patients will no longer need to fear losing their empathetic family physician to retirement, as a digital copy of the provider's mind can be downloaded into the robotic construct assigned to do their physical exam. This does raise some sticky ethical questions such as who owns the physician's digital memories. Do they belong to the patient, to the corporation that programmed the copy, or to the copy itself, as it would be an autonomous, fully-aware consciousness with the same goals and desires as any other human.

There are muddy waters ahead.

Challenging Evolutionary Barriers

Some want even more than the augmented immortality promised by the 2045 Initiative to copy brains, as they realize that the original mind from which the copy was downloaded would be left in an aging body while a digital duplicate walked away with a brand new body. Instead of photocopying our brains, these practical researchers are instead focusing their efforts on finding ways to slow the telomere turnover rate. For those unfamiliar with the concept, the DNA replication needed each time new cells are formed to replace those that die off due to damage or age shortens the replicating agent that allows this replacement. Perhaps the best way to understand this is to think of the telomere as the thread used by a tailor to repair a long tear that never stops coming apart in a dress. Eventually, the tailor runs out of thread and the fabric of life begins to unravel. Finding a way to reduce the number of stitches needed for each repair allows us to mitigate programed cell death. In new research at Stanford and published in *The FASEB Journal*[32] (Federation of American Societies for Experimental Biology), investigators were able to physically lengthen telomeres and thereby increase human cellular division by as much as 40 times.[33] Imagine not aging, even reversing the process; we may soon be able to walk right through the molecular minefield built into our code.

Even without intervention, the human lifespan has improved from approximately 36 years in the 1800s to more than 80 years today.[34] Many would argue that sanitation, immunization, and culture have contributed to this, but there is a lesser-known argument that bares consideration. Consider for a moment that Darwin's theory of evolution suggests a creature only need to live up to the point at which it has reproduced—as the doomed male praying mantis will attest. After procreation has occurred, there is no selective bias to keep the male mantis around other than as a food source for his female counterpart. Delaying the point at which reproduction occurs in a species creates a selection bias for longevity as only those with healthier codes will reach the later set point and be able to pass on their genetic material. This theory was validated in a *Scientific America Article*[35] in which fruit fly reproduction was delayed over ten generations, and the subsequent super-healthy offspring were found to have two to three times longer lifespans. Most recently, a ground-breaking study published in *The Proceedings of the National Academy of Science*[36] showed that delayed paternal age of reproduction in humans was associated with longer telomeres. Between 1970 and 2000, the age at which a woman has her first child has gone up steadily by 2.6 years, begging the question "Are we extending our lifespans by culturally delaying reproduction?"

Longer lives mean more time to experiment, to explore, and to test the boundaries of what it means to be human. Brain-machine interfaces are becoming more prevalent and sophisticated with new products on the launching pad from technology innovators like Elon Musk, DARPA, and Facebook.[37] In the next few years, we will be downloading vital statistics from subdural monitors or neuro implants as part of our transhuman physical exam.

Augmentation and Wearable

The rule of thumb in medical school was that you had three attempts to place an IV or draw blood. If you failed, you called in backup, which usually consisted of a fellow student who was just as inept as yourself. If the task still proved insurmountable, then the "blood nurse" was called. Every hospital has someone who is so talented at finding veins and threading needles through them that they are given whispered respect from both staff and clinicians alike. Unfortunately, this skill may soon go the way of cursive and fire starting. New products (Accuvein,[38] Venoscope, VeinViewer) use lasers to detect the hemoglobin in our veins and then project a roadmap image on the patient's skin. These innovations have improved the accuracy of blood draws, reduced patient pain, and may soon be used for cosmetic surgery in plastic surgery offices.

Pharmaceutical companies are even now using augmented reality to show patients 3D live-action models of how their medications will work in their bodies. Hololens[39] and other augmented reality tools are being used in major teaching hospitals to help students understand and interact with human anatomy. Patients find it easier to exercise if zombies are pursuing them or they are hunting for Pokémon. Surgeons are beginning to use it to help visualize the position of tumors below the skin, so they choose the best approach with which to remove or treat them.[40]

Wearable technology is being used to help physical therapists isolate treatments for stroke victims.[41] Physical therapy is controlled by specially designed exoskeleton devices that analyze a patient's limitations and then develop treatment programs to regain muscle strength and flexibility like the Rapael Smart Glove.[42] Painless blood glucose monitors[43] provide patients and physicians invaluable data about the patient's sugars and thus can help both direct care toward personalized diet, medication, and exercise goals. Monitors that track things like heel strike for runners, fertility, blood pressure, and sleep cycles are all available, and our patients bring this data into our offices and demand to know how to use it to improve their health.[44]

Many doctors scratch their heads, wring their hands, and say they can't believe the data, that they have no way to download the information, and that the patients should forget about high-tech toys.

And this is where we run the risk of extinction.

Our patients feel the data is valid, accurate or not. It is a diary of their health and effort to make improvements. It is a way of showing us that they are interested in the nuances of their body's mechanics, and we should make every effort to encourage them while being honest about our technological inexperience. Hopefully, dialogue about our hesitations while expressing an open mind will find common ground that can benefit both parties.

My Thoughts

One of my predictions for the future focuses on the patient chart. We've recently transitioned from paper to the digital chart and from notes being hidden from patients to open notes where patients are both able to see and give feedback on the clinician's assessment. In my practice, I write everything in front of the patient as we finish up the visit so that I never say anything in the chart that I'm not willing to say to my patient's face. I believe this leads to a more transparent and productive relationship, but it also ameliorates the need for an explanation later if you've written something the patient might find offensive or untrue. Additionally, reviewing the digital chart provides us with talking points and with validation for the plan I've suggested.

I believe we will soon transition from the paper/digital chart into something that looks like a patient avatar, a digital representation of the patient that can be worked on together using the concept of Med-Aikido that we will discuss in more detail in Chapter Eleven. Imagine a 3-D projection of that patient, warts and all, being pulled up in the middle of the exam room and populated with the person's most recent labs, surgical procedures, vitals, and family history/genetic risks. The doctor would be able to unwrap the avatar in real time to show how the patient's new heart valve worked, why their sleep apnea is causing pulmonary hypertension and how this then leads to congestive heart failure, and what their lungs look like after years of smoking.

Then the physician would divide the avatar into two separate patients and advance the program so that one avatar continues with no changes in their lifestyle while the other follows the doctor's advice and is compliant with medications. Showing an extrapolated visual depiction of the patient in three, five, or ten years to illustrate how their unaddressed risk factors are likely to lead to cancer, stroke, or diabetic complications will be a scary and powerful tool that will help invest patients in making changes. Conversely, showing them how well the second "compliant" avatar performs will provide them with incentive to work toward healthy personal goals. The patient avatar program will allow them to change their perspective, to step outside of the excuses and situational stressors that hold most of us hostage and join the physician in creating the best future possible for both the avatar and patient.

Reality Check

Although I've used a bit of creative license to describe a few near-future events, many high-tech tools—previously undreamed of—are readily available for purchase even as we speak. In researching this book, I've learned why so many of us, both patient and physician, are thrilled with the promise of these medical innovations. The potential they represent is inspiring.

However, I remain hesitant.

Perhaps it is because I'm an idealist and grew up watching shows like *M*A*S*H*, *Trapper John, M.D.*, and *Saint Elsewhere*. Perhaps I'm deluded in thinking that there exists an ethereal element to the doctor-patient relationship, an ambiance that grows with time and shared experiences to create a bond that cannot be broken down into pure numbers and graphed. Perhaps my fear that technology has already eroded this link beyond repair is unfounded.

The last reported sighting of a wild dodo bird was in 1662. It was thought to have been the victim of invasive species introduced into its environment by Dutch sailors when they visited the island of Mauritius in the Indian Ocean. This near-mythical bird's story can only be pieced together from drawings and DNA samples. Little is known about its behavior, what potential it might have had for us as a food source, or how it fit into the Galapagos-like ecosystem of its island. Lewis Carroll featured the bird in *Alice in Wonderland* and even adopted Dodo as a nickname due to his tendency to stutter when introducing himself as Mr. Dodgson[45]—his legal surname. Extrapolated data suggests the birds were indigenous to the island's swamp, grew more than three feet in height, lived up to 20 years, and were exceptionally fast, robust, and territorial. Yet, with no living specimen to defend its nobility, most of us think of the dodo as a slow, fat, clueless creature.

I don't want to see the doctor-patient relationship go the way of the dodo, so I'm slowly learning to adapt to my new environment while hoping my journey helps others to do the same. This book was written to promote an informed discussion about how technology is influencing our profession and changing the dynamics of the relationship we have with our patients. Although biased, I will do my best to show both sides as we dig deeper into the aforementioned topics and others. My goal is not for us to return to paper charts and leeches, but to remind everyone that our profession is about one human helping another and these subtleties are exceptionally hard to digitize.

Chapter Two

George Orwell
Medicine (Dystopia)

We Are a Trade, Not a Business

Who doesn't remember Winston Smith sitting at his desk at the Ministry of Truth, diligently censoring words for Big Brother in George Orwell's novel[1] *Nineteen Eighty-Four* released as an iconic film[2] on the year it references? The concept of doublethink—lauded in the book as being one of the virtues of the Party—was the practice of holding two conflicting thoughts in one's mind at the same time. Sadly, this is what modern medicine feels like for a great many doctors: we know that technology improves patient care even as it erodes the bedrock upon which we had previously delivered that care. In our modern era, pining for the "good old days" is akin to committing a thought crime. No one believes you want to go back to the way things were, including yourself, so you should close your trap and keep your head down. Why? Well, if you complain too much a nice man named O'Brien—there's one in every practice—will show up at your office one day to "invite" you to a programming session in room 101.

"Let's start. The first thing you have to do is copy this paragraph from your last note. Good," coaxes Orwell's O'Brien as he leans over your shoulder. "Now, paste it into your new note, auto-populate the physical, and write in a few unique words here at the end to make it seem like you've done something different. Well done. You see. The problem is you just don't understand the system well enough. There are so many wonderful shortcuts like this one. Next, I'm going to show you something fascinating. If you click on your brain while simultaneously holding down Shift-Alt-Delete, watch what happens."

The typical physician's response to this bastardization of the patient's chart is paraphrased by Dr. McCoy of the original *Star Trek*,[3] "Dammit, Jim. I'm a doctor, not an engineer."

Predictably, our modern O'Brien will counter with a phrase stolen from

Star Trek's greatest enemy, the Borg[4]—a collective of drones dedicated to assimilating all into their hive mind—when he explains that our "resistance is futile."

Indeed, the Office of the National Coordinator for Health Technology[5] reports that in 2015 nearly 90 percent of office-based physicians had adopted an EMR. That amount has doubled since 2008, and yet *Medical Economics*[6] reports that almost 70 percent of physicians are unhappy with the functionality of the system. One survey respondent said, "We used to see 32 patients a day with one tech, and now we struggle to see 24 patients a day with four techs, and we provide worse care." In a 2014 survey conducted by the AMA,[7] only 34 percent of physicians were satisfied with their EHR systems, a number that dropped from 61 percent five years ago. The authors of the report said,[8] "From the physicians' perspective, it appears that the significant investment in EHR system(s) over the past few years in the United States is failing to offer significant returns. Far from helping physicians to operate efficiently and have more time to spend with patients, the opposite appears to be the case." Translation: We are frustrated, slower, and concerned. In a significant study done by Robin Chisholm for the School of Informatics, Computing & Engineering at Indiana University in 2014,[9] emergency room physicians were watched to see if using the EMR would, as was suspected, reduce medical error versus using a paper chart. Surprisingly, there was no documented change in the number of errors made, but it was noted that it took the physician 46 percent more time to complete the patient's electronic chart and this led to longer patient wait times and physician dissatisfaction.

Does anyone care?

Yes. Our patients. In a study published in *JAMA*,[10] groups of at-risk patients with limited communication skills were studied to see if computer use in the office affected their satisfaction with the interactions. The results, not surprisingly, showed that visits in which the physician spent more time on the computer and had less eye contact were rated appreciably lower. Translation: Our patients feel like we care more about our computers than them.

I'm not an artist but I like to imagine a patient sitting on a bed clutching their chest while a physician struggles to get past a cartoon computer that demands time, data, and codes before it will step aside. Is this the best we can do? For thousands of years medical tools and documentation have been used to improve care and communication, and now we're supposed to invite this cartoon gremlin into our exam room and somehow make it work? Stephen H. Dart,[11] a senior director for Advanced MD, which provides EHRs for independent physician practices, said, "Legislatively directed usage will never carry the day since the physician never had his/her needs fundamentally considered in the drafting of the legislation that directly impacted their world."

But is resistance futile?

Are we able to fight back?

Many physicians in larger group practices have elected to cut back from full time to 80 percent or 50 percent in the hopes of finding a better balance of life/work. Unfortunately, they often end up using the extra time to catch up with their documentation, and ultimately this ends up hurting patient access.

Others argue with the coders and the administrators and point out the redundant tasks; they say that our current workload is unsustainable and dangerous, and they warn anyone who will listen about physician burnout. Others are well-meaning O'Briens dedicated to improving the failing system by learning all its nuances in the hopes of finding shortcuts for the rest of us. Finally, there are others who take surveys and do research to show how broken the system is and make predictions as to which poorly designed EMR will rise to the top—Betamax vs. VHS mirroring Aethena vs. Epic—with Epic seeming to be the current winner.

All of this is akin to trying to unmake a cake. As damaged as it is, the EMR is here to stay. The real question we must ask is if we can demand a different flavor of cake. Our EMR programs were built on a computer-centric model when they should have been designed to be human-centric. Isaac Asimov, one of the world's best science fiction writers, laid down the three cardinal laws of human-centric robotics in his short story "Runaround."[12]

1. A robot may not injure a human being or, through inaction, allow a human being to come to harm.

2. A robot must obey the orders given it by human beings except where such orders would conflict with the First Law.

3. A robot must protect its own existence as long as such protection does not conflict with the First or Second Laws.

Perhaps not as well known, Rob Kling writing for the National Science Foundation[13] espoused an equally important set of rules that a program needs to demonstrate to be considered a Human-Centered Information system. In the interests of clarity, I'll paraphrase these as I see them:

1. The program needs to complete a detailed study of the human tasks it is being asked to help with before it is created. (EMRs were developed for the most part by an industry with a technology bent whose federal mandate was to save money and not study what doctors do in the office and find some way to improve it.)

2. The program needs to be monitored to ensure it is benefiting the human it was designed to help. (As shown, there are a plethora of studies documenting that our current choice of EMRs are making our lives harder.)

3. The program needs to consider the skill sets a human brings to the table. (EMRs don't care how long it takes for us to fill out forms, whether the data is clinically relevant or even if anyone will ever look at it. They don't care if we arrive early, work through lunch, and go home late because there is nothing built into the system that measures the time required for a human to complete these tasks, and no bell goes off if an administrator adds one too many mandated clicks.)

4. The program needs to be able to adapt swiftly to changes in the human's needs. (Whenever a physician complains about a glitch in the EMR, it takes an act of Congress to fix it. Why? Well, it has to float up through the programming food chain until it reaches some engineering guru who will either approve or ignore the request. To add insult to injury, the concerned doctor rarely gets any feedback about the decision. A tried and true administrative technique: let them complain, agree that the problem is real, and then wait until they've forgotten about it.)

5. Having experienced first-hand the havoc a computer-centered system has on a trade; I'll suggest the fifth rule. The human operator needs to be able to say they don't want the program. (To me, this is the most important rule. By mandating conversion to EMRs, we have forced our will on the natural capitalistic ecosystem of the marketplace instead of letting products within it to evolve naturally. If the consumer can't say something stinks and wait for something better to come along, then there is no financial incentive for developers to go back to the drawing board, and the end user is left driving to work in a car with four square wheels. We can do better.)

But computers are smarter and more productive than humans. Using technology reduces human error, improves efficiency, and saves money. These are solid points. I spent a good deal of my medical school and residency poring over patient records, which had become bloated tomes. Finding the one scrap of information scribbled nearly illegibly in the margins was like unearthing gold. When you couldn't find something, you had to reorder a test or procedure that the patient swore they had already had. Technology has made it easier to identify drug interactions, set up reminders to do follow-up procedures years in the future, and share information quickly and efficiently between institutions. There is no question that patients are far better off with technology than they had been without it, but we cannot argue that computers increase productivity.

In 1987 the Solow Paradox[14] was coined when Robert Solow, a Noble Prize winner in economics, noticed that the rate of national productivity had slowed dramatically in the Internet age instead of increasing as most had anticipated it would with as more efficient computers and technology supplanted human workers. Although some have tried to refute the assertion that technology is making us less productive,[15] the Solow Paradox was supported once again by Daron Acemoglu in a paper published in 2014 for the National Bureau of Economic Research.[16] In fairness, these papers focused on the manufacturing industry. But, if you follow the breadcrumbs, you'll want to know how much growth there's been in productivity in health care. *The New England Journal of Medicine*[17] reports, "unlike virtually all other sectors of the U.S. Economy, health care has experienced no gains over the past 20 years in labor productivity ... at the same time, health care labor is becoming more expensive more quickly than other types of labor." Translation: Although technology has improved patient safety and medical documentation, it takes more time for physicians to complete these tasks.

Yet, no one is suggesting that we see fewer patients. Why not? Does the foreman in an automated car manufacturing plant stop the line because one of the workers feels like they want to get to know the individual cars better? The worker complains that they used to hand-stitch the leather seats and manually buff the car's hood before sending it out the door. The foreman checks her clipboard, shakes her head, and wonders how long it'll be before the old geezer retires. The new hires don't complain. They know this is a business.

The problem is, in my opinion, that we are a trade, not a business. We are craftsmen and women, not workers on a line. Whether or not we've clicked off all the right boxes in the patient's template shouldn't matter as much as whether we've done all we can to address the symptoms, no matter what the problem is, that led our patients to visit us. We are idealists who want to do the right thing, but who, through our inaction, ignorance, and misplaced trust, have allowed our field to become a hyperregulated monetized bureaucratic mess. We are independent problem solvers, context-free thinkers, but we don't know how to fix this problem. We just know we're in trouble.

In the last chapter, we consider what the world might look like if things went perfectly. Letting the pendulum swing in the opposite direction, let's now speculate about a darker future for the doctor-patient relationship. Bare in mind that the following is pure extrapolation and by no means represents the personal views of the author or publisher.

Censorship—Net Neutrality

The arguments for and against net neutrality have raged across the Internet. Most feel that the net represents an open source, a freedom of speech and opinion venue that should be allowed to mature and self-regulate without government intervention. Others think that businesses that pay for and maintain our access to the World Wide Web should have a say in how quickly we receive our data with those willing to pay for it getting the better and, perhaps, more accurate results. The man pushing for the change, having single-handily modified the rules under his jurisdiction as the appointed acting chief of the FCC (Federal Communication Commission) is Ajit Pai.[18] Many argue that the lobby money spent by Comcast, Verizon, and AT&T is little more than bribes to ensure their interests come out on top. As I write, a Congressional Review Act resolution is moving forward to block Mr. Pai's oligarchic move. Even if the opposition wins and stops businesses from controlling what sites we see and maintains the freedom we've taken for granted, the fact that special interests can so easily sway something, this essential hint that George Orwell's *Nineteen Eighty-Four* is closer than we thought. If corporate America doesn't succeed this time, they've proved it is possible and so will try again and again. The populous is very good at fighting a single cause for a short time but terrible fighting a complex cause over many years. Businesses know this, and they are patient.

If the FCC eventually does allow telecommunication companies to censor, limit, and slow down some sites while promoting others, you can bet drug companies and insurance companies will pay hefty sums to ensure their drugs or health-care plans are shown in the best light possible when you search. Looking up reviews of local hospitals and doctors? Guess which ones will be ranked highest? Those that pay for their results to show up.

Conversely, negative ads and poor reviews of competitors, "fake news" for the health-care industry, won't be far behind. Did you want to look up something on WebMD.com? Sorry, that site's not available now. Why don't you try BigPharmaMD.com instead? Did you want to hear about the latest research about a pill that might turn the industry on its head produced by a shoestring start-up? You won't.

Former President Obama[19] said, "Ever since the Internet was created, it's been organized around basic principles of openness, fairness, and freedom. There are no gatekeepers deciding which sites you get to access. There are no tollways on the information superhighway. This set of principles, the idea of net neutrality, has unleashed the power of the Internet and given innovators the power to thrive. Abandoning these principals would threaten to end the

Internet as we know it ... for most Americans, the Internet has become an essential part of everyday communication and everyday life. The FCC is an independent agency, and ultimately this decision is theirs alone, but ... Americans are making their voices heard and standing up for the principles that make the Internet a powerful voice for change."

But will they listen?

If we can trust what we see on the Internet even less than we do now, I predict a small fraction of the population will return to printed vetted information sources like textbooks and those few surviving newspapers that operate with high ethical standards of truth and accuracy. Unfortunately, this will leave most of us gobbling up paid advertisements that convince us to demand the newest drug or procedure from our physicians.

Freedom

In the United States, nearly everyone has a communication device that they have with them wherever they go. The tool allows them to have access to discounts, breaking news, safety alerts, and maps while simultaneously keeping us connected to our loved ones and emergency services. Unfortunately, these same helpful devices are busy collecting data about our behaviors, eating and sleeping habits, interests, and even the number of steps we've taken that day.[20] At first glance, this type of information seems harmless, and we might voluntarily elect to have our devices and Internet search engine[21] collect it. Did we want to share it? Sure. No one cares how many hours I spent in REM last night but me. Even if you elect not to put your name on it, this data is still collected. Why?

It's gold.

Imagine a future where algorisms showed that job candidates who routinely got too few hours of sleep were less productive than those who did. Imagine your prospective boss choosing a well-rested applicant over you despite your stellar curriculum vitae because they have access to your REM records. Do they need to tell you why? Nope. It was a hard decision and we had many qualified applicants. Please try again next year. Were you going to apply for life insurance so your family could stay on their feet if you were to die prematurely? Unfortunately, your rates are going to be higher than your neighbors because your GPS shows you routinely stop at the burger joint on the way home from work. Did you want auto insurance? Here again, your GPS proves to be a snitch and shows you driving ten miles above the speed limit during your commute. Did you want medical insurance? Sorry, again.

The information you uploaded to a family tree website along with a swab of your DNA to find out about your heritage suggests you've got a higher than average risk of heart disease. Cha-ching. What about your medical records? At least those are confidential. Only your doctor knows you're taking antidepressants or received treatment for an STD. Breaking news: There was a massive data breach and some entity hacked everyone's medical records. Your insurance carrier patched the hole but they don't know how much data was downloaded or from whom. We're so sorry. Next time don't share such personal things with your physician. Look at that. You've got 12 pop-up advertisements for local psychotherapists and marriage counselors. We can't imagine how they might have known.

Freedom is the power to make an informed choice and to have your options be determined by factors that you can see, change, or defend. Communication companies allow their customers to opt out of this data-harvesting bonanza, but they should be begging us to opt-in, and, dare I say it, pay us for the data we generate. Either way, we are picking up speed on a very slippery slope.

Ronald Reagan[22] said in his inaugural address as governor of the State of California that "freedom is a fragile thing and is never more than one generation away from extinction. It is not ours by inheritance; it must be fought for and defended constantly by each generation, for it comes only once to a people. Those who have known freedom and then lost it have never known it again."

Universal Health Identifier

In 1996, HIPAA[23] (Health Insurance Portability and Accountability Act) demanded that the industry assign individual health identifying numbers to every individual in hopes of better monitoring and managing patients. Congress overruled this component of the act—ironically neglecting to remove portability from the act's title—in 1998 due to concerns about patient privacy. However, with the advent of EHRs and HITECH's[24] (Health Information Technology for Economic and Clinical Health Act) requirement that medical groups show meaningful use—presumably by sharing patient information in a meaningful way with each other—the idea of an UHI (universal health identifier) is back in the spotlight.[25]

The surface concern many have about this code is that it could be used to collect and then sell unique medical information about you to unscrupulous businesses that would use it to tailor their advertising to your individual medical needs. A more profound concern is the fear that patients could elect not to share personal medical information with their doctor for fear of it falling into the hands of an outside vendor.

Thus, something that may seem harmless and convenient has the potential to strike at the heart of the confidential nature of the doctor-patient relationship and the trust that such a relationship is supposed to imbue. We need a universal code to track our mobile population of patients, and technology could do this for us as it has in Europe, yet the same technology that promises to simplify and organize our medical histories carries with it the potential to endanger our patient's privacy and our role as defenders of that right.

My Thoughts

As a child, I confronted my fifth-grade teacher with a handheld calculator and demanded to know why I needed to learn how to do math by hand if I could just punch the numbers into a machine that would give me the right answer. Calculators weren't going away, so why did I need to waste my time? She listened to me patiently, nodded curtly, and asked me to tell her how I would know if the answer the calculator suggested was wrong? The concept had never crossed my mind: Machines could get it wrong? Stunned, I returned to my desk and stared at the blackboard for several minutes before picking up my pencil and attacking my assignment with renewed gusto. There was no way I was going to trust my grade to a fallible machine.

In addition to helping me understand the nuances of math, my teacher had just saved me from automation bias. Mary Cummings describes this bias in a paper she presented at MIT[26]: "Automation bias occurs in decision-making because humans have a tendency to disregard or not search for contradictory information in light of a computer-generated solution that is accepted as correct and can be exacerbated in time-critical domains. Automated decision aids are designed to reduce human error but actually can cause new errors in the operation of a system if not designed with human cognitive limitations in mind." An example would be if I was able to use a calculator on my exam and chose to write down its answers even though they differed from my manual calculations. Paired closely with this automation land mine is the less obvious, but equally dangerous, specter of complacency. First described in an aviation manual[27] in 1976 and later revised by NASA[28] (National Aeronautics and Space Administration), automation compliance "is exhibited as a false sense of security, which the operator develops while working with a highly reliable automation; however, no machine is perfect and can fail without warning," and so can have "negative performance effects on an operator's monitoring of automated systems." An example would be the driver who, half-asleep, lets their self-driving car send them into a busy intersection despite seeing a red light, hearing horns, and seeing oncoming traffic.

While we're on them, I'll mention another common automation-induced error. Habitualization from reminders and pop-ups lead to automation fatigue. I click dozens of these a day just to make them disappear without reading them because they never say anything of value. Why are there so many? To keep liability low, a programming company will always lean toward over-warning rather than under-warning. An example is when a patient returns to the office with a new rash after completing a course of penicillin, and I inform the computer that the patient has this allergy. Immediately, a pop-up appears to tell me that the patient has recently been prescribed penicillin and is allergic to it. I know. I was the one who gave it to them, and I'm the one who marked it as an allergy a millisecond earlier. My gut response to the computer's "helpful" warning equates to "Stop telling me stuff I told you, it's redundant, annoying, time-consuming, and very much in line with 'The Boy Who Cried Wolf.'"[29]

We see all these errors and more in the newly automated world of medicine. Automation complacency was convincingly demonstrated in a breast cancer detection study where a CDSS (clinical decision support system) was used to "help" clinicians detect abnormalities in mammograms. The findings showed that doctors were twice as likely to miss a cancer on screen if an automated system made suggestions of where to look for it.[30] In this case, the radiologists believed that the system couldn't possibly miss something in the unhighlighted areas and so didn't focus on them with the rigor they devoted to the suggested areas. In his timely book *The Digital Doctor*,[31] Dr. Robert Wachter gives us another real-life example of how computer automation puts patients at risk. Pablo Garcia, a 16-year-old admitted for a colonoscopy, through a series of errors that amounted to the proverbial holes in the Swiss cheese[32] lining up, was given 38.5 tablets of Septra pills the night before. The child survived his seizure, but I can think of no rational human physician who would knowingly prescribe that many pills, nor of a pharmacist who would approve them, nor a nurse who would administer them without a mighty assist from automation bias and diagnostic momentum.

Diagnostic momentum[33] is when you accept a previously established diagnosis without sufficient skepticism, and it can be fatal. We may work with brilliant, dedicated colleagues, have caring empathetic staff, be supported by world-class technology, and have patients who trust us implicitly, but if the first step on a path feels wrong, it's up to you to force everyone to turn around and start over.

Admittedly, my calculator has yet to give me inaccurate results, and I have learned to trust it. However, I do run my calculations through it twice before I use them to treat a patient. Why? Because the results affect someone's life rather than my grade. The programs we rely on to screen for drug-drug interactions, weight-based dosing, and to warn of potential side effects are not perfect. Unfortunately, they're almost flawless, and so we can be lulled into a false sense of security or automation complacency. Perhaps, for me, this is the scariest part of how technology is changing the world of medicine. We must remember that we are the treating physician, the last line of defense, and the final human checkpoint before a therapy reaches our patients. If we let our guard down, we are letting them down as well.

Reality Check

Over the last decade, we have seen a resurgence of dystopias in literature and film. The *Hunger Games*,[34] *Ender's Game*,[35] *Snow Crash*,[36] and *Ready Player One*[37] are brilliant examples of how humans often imagine the worst so they can better avoid it. When a parent tells a child to bring an umbrella to school, the suggestion is based on experience, the weather report, and an understanding that it is better to be prepared than wet. Thirty years ago, *Star Trek* communicators and the idea we could colonize other planets were pure science fiction. Thanks to Apple and Elon Musk that future is now. Technology is a powerful tool, Pantheon's fire, and it is up to us to use it responsibly with everyone's freedom, limitations, and welfare in mind.

Chapter Three

Frontier Medicine (Old School)

Cowboy Charlie

My grandfather, Charlie Lozar, was a cowboy, a salt-of-the-earth man of action who took newspaper clippings of his rodeo days with him whenever he met a new doctor. My grandmother would censure him as much as she could, reminding him that physicians didn't have time to listen to his stories, but he was a stubborn old cuss and so plenty of young doctors learned what it was like to be thrown from a horse, ride the rails during the Depression, and drive cattle across the Wild West. I doubt every physician he met had the wherewithal to humor him, but those that did earned the old cowpoke's trust. If they told him to do something, he did it. If they told him not to worry, he believed them. This, to me, represents the purest form of the doctor-patient relationship and the element most threatened by disruptive technology. To be good advocates for our patients, we must listen to their stories, acknowledge that there is more to treating them than ordering the right medicine or procedure, and that, despite what our test scores might suggest, we don't know everything.

Indeed, if there is one constant in medicine, it is that we know far less than we think we do. Listen, observe, consolidate, germinate, postulate, and then reevaluate—these are the essential skills of a competent physician. The tools we use to heighten these six elements will change, but these principles of the medical exam must exist, or our prescribed therapy and, accordingly, our patient will suffer needlessly.

1. **Listening (Fishing)** requires that we take in everything we hear from the patient, their family members, our staff, our auscultation exam, and even what we may have heard on the radio that day. It also includes their manner of speech (respectful, fearful, defiant), their ability to communicate (senility, language barriers, youth, generational bias, and phobias—not being able to

or wishing to use technology), and their directness. Interpreting this final aspect of active listening is often the most nuanced. There are patients who will be very direct in vocalizing what they hope to achieve during your visit (a prescription, referral, or procedure). While others will wait until they realize you're wrapping things up before bringing up their real concern. Identifying a patient's mode of communication, anticipating it the next time they come in, and thus circumventing problems by proactively leading, even interrupting, a conversationalist or by taking the time to ask leading questions of a more succinct patient. Confronting a patient about their style of communication rarely, in my experience, produces any long-lasting change, so it is more prudent to adapt our approach to theirs.

2. **Observation (Fishing)** demands that we consider the patient's expressions, their body language, their clothing, their demeanor, our visual exam of their body, of test results, and their active responses to questions. It includes how they walk into the office, how they leave, what articles or medications they bring in from outside sources, and even whether they make eye contact and how often. Social nuances come into play here as knowing how to interpret a person's response to bad news (stoicism, nervous laughter, tears) encompasses how they are personally affected and how cultural norms have taught them to behave. I make a concerted effort to know as much as I can about a person's recent medical history (hospitalization records, radiologic reports, my suggestions at our last visit) before I go into the room. Invariably, the patient has concerns about one of these issues and will be reassured if you can pull a lab result or specialist's recommendation out of the air. The practice of looking at and making an effort to retain aspects of a patient's history, although time-consuming, builds a bond of trust, of shared patient-centric worldviews that lay out the canvas upon which you will soon paint your diagnosis and treatment plan. The elements of listening and observing are primarily data gathering or as if one were casting a net into the ocean. The hunter does not aim to catch a particular fish nor pretend that certain fish don't exist. They cast as wide a net as possible with no preconceived biases and pull whatever they can into the boat. Interestingly, it is these data gathering aspects of the doctor-patient relationship that are most altered by technology. We have a great deal more information at our fingertips, much of it more accurate and timelier than in the past, but we may be ignoring the dolphins in our net because our templates only ask us to count how many catfish we've caught. Not making eye contact, not letting our patients finish talking, not watching for facial cues or shifts in body language, not doing a complete exam, not connecting with our patients because we are so plugged into our computers makes us very poor fishermen and women.

3. **Consolidating (Internal)** the information we've gathered is a very inter-

nal process and not easily explained. Thus, I suspect it lies at the heart of what makes medicine an art, as it is a skill that matures with age, experience, and practice. It is the mental mechanism of sifting through all the gathered data and deciding what is pertinent and what is flotsam. For some, it can take mere seconds while others may require several minutes of serious consideration. In my estimation, it is not a deliberate action but a more profound internal activity akin to the muscle memory of a dancer or the instincts of a painter. It is the process of considering all the fish on the deck before deciding which to eat and which to jettison.

4. **Germinating (Internal)** a differential diagnosis, a list of possible causes that explain or could be hinted at by the data collected is also an internal process and closely tied to consolidation, often happening simultaneously with it in one's head. For some it comes naturally. For others it takes time to develop this skill. It can be learned through practice and lost through disuse. It can never be fully trusted, but it may act as a set of guideposts on the path to a potential answer or, sometimes just as helpfully, to rule out feared diagnoses. It can make you chase symptoms much longer in one patient than you would in another or longer than would seem prudent based on the clinical facts. Invariably, many of these "gut" feelings that I've followed during a workup have been correct and significantly altered the course of the patient's disease process. This admission is not meant to be made as a form of self-praise, as I am sure most physicians have pursued hunches that have proved fruitful, but as a concession that what occurs in a diagnostician's head is not always quantifiable nor replicable using templates.

The elements of consolidation and germination are internal processes and not visualized by the patient nor reflected in the chart or even verbally to colleagues. In many cases, these internal elements are equivocal to the artist's eye, the vital spark of the craft, and so will be the hardest for engineers to understand, mimic, and apply, as they depend on aesthetics rather than logic. These paired elements prove the most challenging for new physicians to master and to keep sharp as we age.

5. **Postulating (External)** on the possible diagnoses and the thinking process that brought you to your conclusion is not something that was done very often in the past. However, in our modern age with the advent of the Internet and Google searches, not saying the word "cancer" will not stop them from worrying about it. They've already looked it up. I routinely verbally walk my patients through my thinking process as to what we can rule in and out based on the facts, what the diagnoses could be, what seems most likely and why, and finally, what I would recommend as the next step in either treating or investigating a set of symptoms. This, in my opinion, helps them under-

stand that there is a logical thought process behind our actions, invests them in the process, and makes them more likely to be compliant with the plan and more apt to inform me if some new element has occurred that does not fit with our working diagnosis. It is not until we have moved through these steps that I turn on the computer. We then examine the labs, tests, and validate any new information that may have come up in the interview that I was not privy to earlier, and then I manually type out everything in front of them, word by word, rather than using drop-downs or smart text fill-ins. I invite them to interrupt and correct me, and I never place anything in the chart that I am not able to say to a patient's face. If they drink too much, I tell them. If they are malingering, I tell them how this may end up harming them with unnecessary and, at times, risky tests. This process gives them time to think of new questions and subsequently adds time to the interview, but I would prefer to address the concern immediately rather than with an email the next day. The advent of EMR is making it exceedingly easy for patients to look at their charts, and it is no longer possible, nor should it ever have been, to mask personal biases in scribbles or annotations. I'll acknowledge that typing the note in the office will not be efficient for hunt-and-peck typists, but if you can do it, I've found it to be invaluable.

6. **Reevaluating (External)** the other five elements, as you are applying them, adapting to new information, and actively chasing unexpected leads even if they undermine your working diagnosis, is the final part of an evaluation and possibly the most important for the long-term health of a patient. Consider a computer program that diagnoses a middle-aged man with flank pain, traces of blood in the urine, and a low-grade fever as having a kidney stone. A day later, the man develops a vesicular rash that is pathognomonic for shingles. Now, he has to start from scratch with the program diagnostician and reload his symptoms. A human physician would have suspected shingles and might have warned him to watch for a rash. At the least, they could make the intuitive leap to this new diagnosis with the patient's new symptoms. Diagnoses need to be fluid, adaptable concepts, similar to a scientist's working theory, so the practitioner doesn't fall in love with a single tree within the forest. Take a person with acid reflux, interstitial lung disease, pulmonary hypertension, and congestive heart failure. Each of these diagnoses is valid, each has a treatment plan capable of alleviating the symptoms, but if we miss the umbrella diagnoses—a unifying concept under which a group of diagnoses fits—of sleep apnea then the patient will have been underserved.

Technology seems least able to help us with these last two elements—the postulating and reevaluating of diagnoses—as the patient is and will always know their body better than anyone else. If they start with a more robust framework of understanding, it will be easier for them to communicate relevant new symptoms. A better history will allow us to better reassure a patient or take appropriate action on their complaints.

I've focused on the six essential skills of a competent physician—listening, observing, consolidating, germinating, postulating, and reevaluating—which have been tools in our arsenal since Hippocrates. They don't require technology, they are intuitive, and they will exist in some form a thousand years hence. As helpful as they are, they are only useful in allowing a practitioner to diagnose diseases and prescribe treatments for known ailments. If we didn't know a jellyfish existed, we would not know we needed to design a different net to catch and study it. As such, technology has been an undeniable boon as it has expanded our understanding of human physiology, biochemistry, pathology, and genetics, and thus our ability to treat disease processes that in the past we attributed to having been exposed to harmful air, possession by spirits, or being out of favor with our gods.

Any journey begins with a single step, but to stay on course you must occasionally look back and contemplate the path you've taken. Let's take a moment and do that now.

Tragedy Loves Ignorance

I trained in an age with antibiotics, sterile surgery, and X-rays, and so I never questioned that these might be exceptionally new advances in health care. I grew up in a time where most people who saw a doctor or went to a hospital expected to get better. Patients were treated, cured, and released. The reasons why this might not happen, excluding advanced age, fell into two simple categories: either the patient was afflicted with a particularly virulent disease or they were being treated by an inept physician or medical institution. The concept that someone would go to the hospital fully anticipating they would die there or visit a physician only to have their disease progression chronicled seems foreign to our modern ears, but these were cultural norms less than 200 years ago.

In the 1800s, the average life expectancy was nearly 35 years for men and 37 years for women, one in ten babies died in infancy, there was no anesthesia, no one suspected STDs came from bacteria (1879) or that parasites in mosquitoes caused malaria (1880), there were no X-rays (1895), and there were no antibiotics. Remember, Alexander Fleming didn't discover penicillin until 1928 nor was it used widely until 1945.[1] That's less than 100 years ago—

many of us have patients who were teenagers when all you could do for strep throat was pray you didn't get rheumatic fever or a peritonsillar abscess. Keep in mind, it wasn't until Joseph Lister presented his paper on aseptic technique to the Internal Medical Congress in the United States in 1876[2] that anyone thought to wash their hands before surgery. Still, humans are a stubborn lot. To this day, folklore dictates the application of cow manure (fecal matter teeming with bacteria) to snakebites to stave off the infection that always seems to happen if the victim survives the bite.[3]

Unfortunately, our human ignorance of the mechanics of medicine has perpetuated something of a tragic comedy of errors through the ages. Hippocrates, the founder of medicine in 460 BC, said that the brain was the organ of the mind and thought. Unfortunately, Aristotle—ironically one of the best thinkers of the time (384 BC)—argued against this theory and felt the brain was little more than a radiator to let off the heat our body generated. European physicians sold quacksalver, a salve containing the heavy metal mercury, for use on wounds and rashes and so inadvertently poisoned many of their patients. Incidentally, this is where the derogatory term "quack," denoting an unscrupulous seller of dangerous products, originated.[4] During the Middle Ages, many believed the moon's cycle had such a profound effect on humans as to turn them into werewolves, witches, or vampires. "What backward old-world superstitions," our civilized minds scoff. "We know better now." Why then do so many emergency room staff and physicians swear there is an increase in psychiatric visits during a full moon despite clear evidence that this is not the case?[5]

As recently as 1951, the brutal procedure of hammering a metal rod into a patient's head through the orbital roof and waggling it around until the recipient had trouble answering questions was considered a viable therapy for a broad spectrum of mental conditions. Eighteen thousand lobotomies were performed between 1931 and 1951 in the United States, with as many as 3,000 performed by the procedure's founder, Walter Freeman, a physician who perfected the technique on cadavers and had no surgical background.[6] The flushing out of our bowels by way of enema or colonics has been touted as a therapeutic technique since the ancient Egyptians who observed the ibis bird self-administrating saltwater enemas with its long beak as early as 1400 BC. Thinking what's good for the goose must be good for the gander, they began to mimic the bird's technique. Now, more than 3,000 years later, Hollywood elite[7] and some physicians continue to promote cleansing enemas despite there being no evidence of benefit and significant risk of developing secondary infections, burns (coffee enemas), inflammation, and even death.[8] For decades we prescribed hormone replacement to our female patients to help ameliorate the ravages of menopause, only to find out in 2002 that we were increasing their risk for heart disease, blood clots, and breast cancer.[9]

If there is any miracle to the practice of medicine, it may be that our patients still give their physicians the benefit of the doubt when we prescribe a therapy. Up until the last century, our track record has been anything but reassuring.

Hospitals Built on Bedlam

Dr. Thomas Bond established America's first hospital in 1752, but it would not have been possible without the political savvy and clout of Benjamin Franklin.[10] Now a National Historic Landmark and affiliated with the University of Pennsylvania, Pennsylvania Hospital is the site of our first surgical amphitheater and medical library. The hospital seal, approved by both Dr. Bond and Franklin, speaks to the ideals upon which the public institution was founded in referencing the Good Samaritan wherein a helpless stranger is given aid with no expectation of recompense. Indeed, most of the hospital's first physicians agreed to work without pay for a full year, and Dr. Bond didn't accept compensation for his efforts for three years. Nor was care withheld from those in need, as slaves and American Indians were treated alongside property-owning whites.

But before we pat ourselves on the back, it is important to examine the wording in the petition presented to the House of Representatives in January 1751[11]:

> That with the Numbers of People the Number of Lunaticks, or Persons distemper'd in Mind, and deprived of their rational Faculties, hath greatly encreased in this Province.
>
> That some of them going at large, are a Terror to their Neighbours, who are daily apprehensive of the Violences they may commit; and others are continually wasting their Substance, to the great Injury of themselves and Families, ill disposed Persons wickedly taking Advantage of their unhappy Condition, and drawing them into unreasonable Bargains, &c.
>
> That few or none of them are so sensible of their Condition as to submit voluntarily to the Treatment their respective Cases require, and therefore continue in the same deplorable State during their Lives; whereas it has been found, by the Experience of many Years, that above two Thirds of the mad People received into Bethlehem Hospital, and there treated properly, have been perfectly cured.

Please take note of the opening sentence wherein references are made to the mentally ill who, at the time, were creating social, ethical, and financial challenges for the general population. Reflecting on the reported success of Bethlehem Hospital in London (an institution retrospectively renowned for its abuses of the mentally ill and dubbed "Bedlam"), the state is encouraged to look at the formation of a hospital to address this public nuisance, albeit under the guise of altruism. According to the book *Bleed, Blister, Puke, and Purge: The Dirty Secrets Behind Early American Medicine* by J. Marin Younker,[12] the majority of those initially admitted to the hospital suffered from mental illness and the treatment they received bordered on barbaric. This included whippings, beatings, and, following the practice established by Bethlehem Hospital, set times of the day when the public could pay to observe the "lunaticks."

Things improved for the patients when Dr. Benjamin Rush, a close friend of Benjamin Franklin and one of the four doctors to sign the Declaration of Independence, was hired in 1783. A world traveler, open-minded observer of the medical benefits of the American Indian lifestyle, and with a medical school dropout son, John Rush, who was admitted as a psychiatric patient at Pennsylvania Hospital, Dr. Rush's leadership changed how patient's with mental health disorders were treated, his son included, and thus earned himself the title "The Father of American Psychiatry."[13] Indeed, he wrote the first published textbook on mental disease in America.[14] Notwithstanding his heroic character, he was one of only three physicians to stay behind in Philadelphia and treat 6,000 patients during the yellow fever epidemic of 1793, his son's illness must have had a profound effect on how he saw the doctor-patient relationship and inspired him to treat his charges with dignity. This then changed the culture of his hospital as well as that within new hospitals modeling their atmosphere upon his example.

Charity work and the premise that no patient should be turned away allowed hospitals to argue for tax-exempt status to recoup the losses they incurred doing pro bono work for the communities they served. As time marched on, many nonprofit hospitals lost sight of the vision of their founding fathers and began to behave as if they were for-profit institutions. Sadly, as was reported by Elisabeth Rosenthal[15] in her review of the California Nurses Association's research of 196 nonprofit hospitals receiving upward of $3.3 billion in state and federal exceptions in 2015, only $1.4 billion was spent on charity work. Again, let's do the math. That's $1.9 billion a year or $9.7 million for each hospital in unpaid taxes = profit = operating costs. Before we get too upset, maybe things have gotten better with the implementation of the Affordable Care Act. Nope. According to a report in *Modern Healthcare*[16] in 2018, "The 20 largest U.S. Health systems dedicated 1.4% of their collective operating revenue in fiscal 2016 to charity care—about the same as the previous year.... Total uncompensated care fell to a 25-year low in 2015 and held steady in 2016, according to the American Hospital Association." Okay. So, if it isn't spent on the poor, where's it going?

There's an adage in Hollywood that a genuinely successful movie never shows a profit because the accountants make sure to spend everything rather than giving it to Uncle Sam. Our health-care leaders may have been taking notes. Cigna's CEO, David M. Cordani, received $17.31 million.[17] Aetna's CEO, Mark Bertolini, received $18.7 million in compensation in 2016.[18] United-Health Group's CEO, Stephen Hemsley, made $17.8 million in the same year with a realized compensation, including stock options, of $33.4 million.[19]

So why is this important? I mean, health care is a business. We live in a capitalist society.

Let's walk through a financial scenario where an uninsured patient trips over a broken section of pavement and breaks her ankle. She presents to the emergency room with swelling, bruising, and an inability to bear weight. She receives the standard of care including X-rays, crutches, and a cast. Let's error on the low side and bill her $3,000 for this accident.[20] She can't afford the unexpected bill and so elects not to pay despite feeling guilty. Aggressive billing companies are hired but eventually give up, and the hospital writes this off as a charitable loss. Really? In my mind, a loss would be having the patient prove that she can't pay and then the hospital volunteering to write her debt off as a charitable community service—end of the story. Having tax payers absorb the cost, sending predatory collectors after the patient, having her credit score destroyed, and making her think twice before seeking help the next time she's injured isn't a fair trade-off when a paper-pusher is making $20 million a year.

Remember that the physicians who worked in America's first hospital did so without pay.

I guess history doesn't always repeat itself.

A Doctor's Doctor

"A good physician treats the disease: the great physician treats the patient who has the disease."[21] This statement is attributed to William Osler, the father of modern medicine, which every graduating medical student would do well to tattoo on the back of their hand. As related in *Bleed, Blister and Purge: The History of Medicine on the American Frontier*, physicians in America during the 19th century could become doctors by (1) apprenticeship or (2) attending medical school or by simply purchasing a diploma.[22] That's right. If you had the money, you could pay off a licensing mill and walk away with a degree to practice medicine. It wasn't until around 1853 that the states started demanding that physicians demonstrate credentials to practice medicine. So naturally came the institutionalization of the medical training program of which Dr. Osler, one of the four founding professors of John's Hopkins Medical School, was a well-respected constituent. Having written the landmark textbook *The Principles and Practices of Medicine* in 1892, he is also accredited with forming the first post-graduate residency program for specialty training. If you've ever been on rounds, this is the man who is credited as the first to take medical students to the bedside of the patients afflicted with the diseases being studied in class.[23] His dedication to hands-on training is exemplified in another quote attributed to him: "He who studies medicine without books sails an uncharted sea, but he who studies medicine without patients does not go to sea at all."[24]

Although it had a laudable start with an inspiring teacher and a training program that focused on a trade-like apprenticeship, Dr. Osler's residency program has been much abused and changed over the years. As related in Elisabeth Rosenthal's book *An American Sickness*,[25] in 2014 hospitals received about $15 billion annually in government subsidies to underwrite losses attributable to running residency programs. This works out to be about $100,000 per resident while researchers found that each resident performed about $332,726 worth of work for the hospital per year. Yes. Staying up all night doing scut work makes a difference. Senior staff bill insurance companies for the patients they admit to teaching hospitals so do not always need to be paid but instead are happy to have residents hold down the fort while they see patients in the clinic and get a good night's rest.

So let's do the math: $332,726 (the annual value of each resident), minus $0 payments to the teaching attending, minus a resident's average yearly salary of $55,000 in 2015,[26] and a residency training program can expect to make $277,726 in profit for each of its students. Since there are about 28,000 residency slots offered per year and most programs are at least three years long, we have approximately 80,000[27] residents a year. Eighty thousand residents multiplied by $277,726 is $22 billion of pure profit being racked in by training programs annually. Not a bad business model for the hospital, but it begs two big questions. (1) Why is the federal government subsidizing highly profitable programs with tax payer money? (2) Why are newly minted doctors graduating with an average of $166,750 in debt[28] being paid so little for their hard work? Sadly, I have to wonder if Dr. Osler wouldn't have come up with another quote similar to "a good residency program produces doctors who can heal the sick: a great program produces doctors with the financial freedom to walk away from the craft but who choose to stay."

Why not pay back the residents' medical school loans as they go through training? Pay them $80,000 a year *and* pay off their loan at $50,000 for every year of residency they complete. At the end of residency, they'll either be able to become fantastic physicians or have the option to walk away and do something else. Too many physicians are trapped in jobs they are ill-suited for because they have no other way to pay back their debt. Patients deserve doctors who want to be there, and doctors have earned the right to leave a job they no longer love.

Don't feel too bad for the programs; they'll still be making $202,726 a year on each resident they train and could write off the $50,000 as a business expense.

Sawbones

Having completed a preliminary surgical year in downtown Chicago after two stints of trauma surgery at Cook County, I have a special place in my heart for the sawbones. I turned down an offer to follow that path but cherish the experience and lessons I learned before pursuing family practice. The sleep-deprivation, stress, responsibility, the nearly immediate feedback on choices, and, above all, the daunting awareness that, at times, you're the only one in the room that knows what to do next, was as terrifying as it was life changing. If I called my chief resident in the middle of the night and said I had admitted a child with what I thought was appendicitis, he would ask why I hadn't done labs. The next child I admitted with appendicitis I made sure to get labs before calling but was then asked why I hadn't called in the OR staff and prepped the patient for surgery. When I called about the next child with appendicitis, having accomplished all the above, I was asked why I hadn't already done the surgery. The take-home lesson: "If you know what to do next, stop asking permission and do it. You're a doctor."

Charles Darwin (1809–1882) aspired to be a surgeon in his youth, but at the time there was no anesthesia and patients were often tied down or restrained as the doctor performed the procedure. Having watched two such bloody operations, the future progenitor of the concept of survival of the fittest decided to take a different path.[29] It wasn't until the advent of nitrous oxide and then ether (surprisingly discovered before nitrous but not used for sedation until 60 years later) that surgeons were able to demonstrate the full scope of their skills. No longer hindered by patients who fought back or died from the sheer pain of surgery, procedures were done more often, and fewer deaths occurred. That's not to say mistakes evaporated. Floating kidneys that were said to meander around the abdomen like ghosts were surgically tied in place, unnecessary tonsillectomies were performed, and to this day we may be performing elective C-sections far more often than is medically indicated.

John Hunter (1728–1793), arguably the "father of surgery," attained many cadavers for dissection from grave robbers, and young medical students in the colonies mirrored this practice with less public acceptance. The New York "Doctor's Riot" of 1788 shone a spotlight on the problems caused by the need for fresh bodies for physicians in training to practice on while learning anatomy. Richard Bayley, a surgeon who had trained under John Hunter, hoped to pass on some of his knowledge but needed bodies.[30] It was not uncommon, nor was a great deal of fuss put up, when the potter's field was plundered for bodies, but when a white woman's hand was reportedly waved out of a window at a peeping boy who was told it was the arm of his mother things got complicated.[31] The boy ran home and told his father who dug up the grave of his recently deceased wife and found it empty whereupon he recruited friends and workers and proceeded to form a mob that descended on Columbia College's anatomy lab. The mayor and sheriff intervened and place some of the doctors in prison to protect them. Their efforts were in vain as the mob grew to 5,000 angry citizens the next day, a mass far too large for the town's police force to hold back. In all, 20 died in this single event. Over the next 90 years, there were 17 more violent riots across the states.

The people wanted their dead to be left in peace.

Riots led to the earliest medical licensing systems in the colonies. No longer could you buy a medical degree. Now, physicians had to apprentice under an established and respected doctor, pass a rigorous exam, and have attended at least two years of medical school. So, we have grave robbers and an overzealous anatomy class to thank for today's accreditation process.

Apothecaries

For the early colonists, an apothecary shop must have felt a bit like a hardware store for what ailed you. Apothecaries listened to your complaint and then either mixed something up or pulled down a prefilled bottle of syrup. As most physicians of the time universally recommended bleeding for everything, this was an alternative approach to addressing illness and may have had better results in some cases. Notwithstanding the risks of poisoning or consuming a placebo, many of these pharmacies stored ingredients that the American Indians had been using for thousands of years. Some of these would even go on to become well-known therapies in our modern age: aspirin (willow bark), irregular heartbeats (foxglove), and treatment/prevention for malaria (quinine).[32]

As always, medications have risks as well as benefits. Heroin, in different forms, was used to treat a variety of illnesses such as a cough, alcohol addiction, and hangovers. In liquid form, which amounted to mixing it with alcohol, it was called laudanum or tincture of opium and was used for toothaches. Mixed with camphor, it was renamed paregoric and was used to sooth teething babies, calm asthma, and slow down loose bowels. As its use was so endemic, those who prescribed it were often thought to practice heroic (a play on the word heroine) medicine.[33] Notwithstanding the explicit issue of addiction, overdoses and deaths were not uncommon.

Cocaine was manufactured from the coca plant grown in Peru and used to treat aches and pains, as a local anesthetic, and as a way to treat hemorrhoids. Colonel John Pemberton developed Coca-Cola as a patented medicine to address practically anything from anxiety to bowel disorders. The fact that this mixture of alcohol and cocaine was addictive didn't hurt business, and it wasn't until 1905 that the company removed the cocaine.[34]

Why?

The Wiley Act went into effect in 1906. It was designed to help protect consumers from dangerous chemicals that might be mixed into drugs or elixirs and marketed to the public. Interestingly, the law didn't require that the drugs work, as many of them didn't, but made it illegal to put things in them that might harm a patient. Despite its well-intentioned creation, the law did little to test or regulate what was being sold as the assumption was that companies wouldn't sell bad products as they would lose business.

That was unless the potential benefits seemed too good to pass up in the publics' eyes. DNP (Dinitrophenol) was used in World War I in the manufacturing of munitions and later as an herbicide and chemical for the development of photographs. Looking for other uses, a study done at Stanford University in 1933 showed that this chemical could induce rapid weight loss in humans by increasing a person's metabolic rate. Although it did cause rapid weight loss, this chemical was responsible for many deaths and cataract associated blindness. The FDA knew of these side effects but could do little more than warn consumers with flyers as it had no power to stop products from being sold to the public.[35]

It wasn't until the Elixir Sulfanilamide incident in 1937 that politicians rethought their assumption that a capital-driven marketplace would only produce safe products. At the time, Sulfanilamide, in powder form, was a useful drug against streptococcal infections, but a salesman suggested that there was a demand for the drug to come in liquid form. S.E. Massengill Co.

responded by having their chemist mix the medicine with diethylene glycol, which produced a raspberry flavored elixir. Neglecting to test the concoction for toxicity, they immediately shipped 633 bottles and killed 100 people in 15 states.[36] Diethylene glycol, you'll remember, is antifreeze and thus a deadly poison. This single event convinced Congress that it needed to exert tighter control over the pharmaceutical companies. The Food and Drug Administration (FDA) now prohibited false therapeutic claims and demanded that the manufacturers prove the drugs they sold were safe.[37]

Fast forward to a real American hero, Dr. Frances Oldham Kelsey, who refused to approve thalidomide for use in the United States despite its use in many other countries as she was not convinced of its safety. Despite being a new hire at the FDA and under intense pressure from the drug company, she stuck to her guns and stopped the disastrous birth defects seen throughout the world from taking place here. For her fortitude, she was awarded the President's Award for Distinguished Federal Service in 1962 and will forever stand as an example of why physicians must value integrity over profit.[38]

The Nightingale's Song

Without a doubt, the most underappreciated people in health care are our nurses and medical assistants. In 1854, Florence Nightingale dropped the mortality rate in the British military hospital where she worked from 40 percent to 2 percent by isolating infected patients, physically cleaning the rooms they were housed in, and washing the linens of the injured soldiers. The American version of Florence Nightingale was Mary Ann Bickerdyke, aka "Mother Bickerdyke," who helped set up and manage 300 field hospitals under General Ulysses S. Grant as he fought the Confederate army.[39] Of note, the infamous Harriet Tubman worked as a nurse and a spy during the civil war.[40] In 1916, Margaret Sanger, a trained nurse, opened America's first birth control clinic and was promptly shut down. She fought the system, published sex and health education geared toward a female audience, and finally opened the first legal birth control clinic in 1921.[41] The founder of the American Red Cross in 1881, Clara Barton was a nurse in the Civil War and used her experience to help organize this global institution. Mary Eliza Mahoney was the first African American professional nurse and a founding member of the American Nurses Association. As an author, my personal favorite is Walt Whitman. He is well known as a poet, and few remember that he served as a volunteer nurse during the Civil War, which influenced his later work.[42]

An entire book is required to do justice to the sacrifices, tragedies, and heroic measures nurses and medical assistants have made for their calling. I will only say that I have had the privilege to work with these unrecognized, undercompensated, and inspiring individuals throughout my career, and they represent the backbone of what it means to care for another human being. They listen to their patients, gently guide new physicians away from making tragic mistakes, bear the brunt of patient tirades meant for their doctors, and interpret the often alien scrawls and vague messages of their physicians. They stock, document, clean, and manage every part of our medical practice so that the doctor-patient encounter can proceed as smoothly as possible, and they have been just as dramatically affected by technology as the rest of us. When we complain there is too much to do, too many mandates or procedural templates to complete, these mundane tasks are delegated to our nurses and assistants. When patients can't get their medications refilled, or sign on to their websites, or get their records transferred, or remember their immunization history, these are the calm, meticulous, professionals that fix it. When equipment fails, codes are called, someone needs to be triaged, or the world is ending these are the men and woman we call.

With or without technology, the doctor-patient relationship would suffer immeasurably without these unsung heroes.

My Thoughts

For centuries there has been a robust esoteric battle between vitalism and mechanism, with the mechanist running victory laps for the last two decades. However, now with computer scientists postulating a day when we will be able to create a digital representation of our minds to upload into another body or copy it dozens of times and use it as a base for artificial intelligence, we need to reexamine the virtues of vitalism and reboot the concept to meet our modern needs.

Vitalism may have started with Aristotle's argument for a soul but his ideology didn't coalesce into a school of thought until Georg Ernst Stahl (1660–1734) argued that although the body was dependent on the laws of physics, it was animated by an unseen force, a vital element that opposed the tendency to die. This vital spark or driving power kept our various organs working in harmony, helped us to fight off disease, was inseparable (this being the key point) from the body, and was the thing that was extinguished when our bodies died.[43]

René Descartes (1596–1650) took the mechanistic view that our bodies were merely well designed parts, like gears or pistons, that worked of their own volition when healthy, and that our souls were separate from this corporeal form much as one might add or remove a hard drive from a computer's shell. Without the hard drive, the computer's fan and screen might work, but the machine would not be able to "think" or behave as if it were alive.

One of the more powerful arguments against vitalism was the observation that specific body parts continued to act as if they were alive after death as exemplified by peristalsis in the bowels. If the vital spark were extinguished upon death, as vitalists asserted, then the gears should immediately stop moving, whereas if, as the mechanists proposed, the body were the framework that held the soul, then the engine could continue to run, as seen in the growth of nails in the deceased, even if the hard drive were broken.

So here we stand at the dawn of a biotech revolution having discarded vitalism in favor of the idea that if a soul exists it much be independent of the machine we call our bodies. But if a human body is a machine then we should be able to reverse engineer it so flawlessly that the manufactured machine body would be indistinguishable from the original. Having done this, we would then need to decide if what we'd created was "alive" or merely a convincing facsimile of life. For instance, if a well-crafted decoy can fool a flock of ducks, how do we know that this mechanical human is anything more an expensive craft project? To complicate matters, let's say we made an exact duplicate of the neuromatrix, the nervous connections in our human brains that make us think the way we do, and downloaded this pattern into our machine body. In doing so, would we have duplicated a person's soul or simply made a more convincing decoy duck? Thus, the mechanistic view sticks us with the AI equivalent of Schrödinger's cat: If we were able to perfectly replicate our minds and bodies, how would we explain where that manufactured creature's soul, the hard drive running the machine, came from other than to say that "life" was never anything more than a series of mechanical switches firing in the right sequence. This then would disprove the existence of a soul and in so doing undermine the mechanistic edict that the soul left or became separated from the body when someone died.

If, however, we reject mechanism in favor of vitalism, we can avoid this embarrassing paradox. In the vitalist's view, there is something individual and unique about each body, something vital to its singular existence, and this vital spark cannot be duplicated, removed, or transferred into another vessel. Indeed, each perfectly manufactured body described above would be a new person with autonomous thoughts, desires, and rights to self-preservation. Vitalism saves us from having to worry if a duplicated neuromatrix that carries the same value as the original and leaves us only wondering what kind of kindling is needed to create a vital spark.

Bringing Us Up to Date

From sawbones to sanatoriums, the evolution of our profession has been an adventure. Admittedly, things like bloodletting, mercury poisoning, and tinctures of opium made it a bumpy ride, and yet patients, for the most part, trusted their doctors and respected those who earned it. Frontier doctors had to be self-reliant, confident in their craft, and willing to take some measure of responsibility if something went amiss—which it inevitably did. Medical knowledge, or the absence of it, may have cost the early colonists more lives than any of the physical hardships, but the intention of the treating physicians was never in question. They did the best they could with what they had, and their patients expected little more.

Things have changed.

If technology has done nothing else, it has expanded the pool of knowledge the general population has access to explore. In so doing, it has undermined and called into question the physician as a medical authority. We no longer have the final word on any topic. Patients routinely check Google for second opinions (sometimes while we're talking to them), question side effects, and are less forgiving of human error. Worse, the future promises more of the same. How long will it be before the standard of care includes automated computer templates, complete with Siri-like questioners to triage patients or even provide prescription medications? How long before artificial intelligence protocols get the diagnosis right more often than the family physician? When that day comes, where do we fit into the New World Order? Are we going to be the data entry clerks, the fall guys for the lawyers, the tour guides on the therapeutic digital highway, or decorative tchotchkes, holdovers from a bygone era?

I don't know what we will be.

But I can tell you that we won't be in charge.

The future of medicine will be one in which physicians and patients strive to work together as equal partners to develop individual treatment plans built on open communication, shared but realistic health goals, and the patient (being fully informed of the risks) accepting full responsibility, but not admonishment, for the life choices they make. If we hope to make this partnership work, we will need to develop a meaningful frontier-style relationship with our patients, one in which we can listen to their cowboy stories and remember that they are our brothers and sisters rather than ICD codes. Conversely, our patients will need to believe that we are doing the best we can for them with what we have and, perhaps, that will be enough.

Personally, I don't think we can recapture the simple trust of the doctor-patient relationship so long as there is money to be made from people being sick.

Chapter Four

Beam Me Up, Scotty (Telemedicine)

Unexpected Consequences

When we fail to see the difference between good marketing and good medicine, good people die. In our modern world, the line between flashy advertising and verifiable therapeutic outcomes has blurred to nothing. They tell us the future is here. We can email our physicians directly, participate in video consultations on our phones, have our phones monitor our heart rates and alert us if we develop dangerous arrhythmias, and we can book appointments with our physician online without going through a triage process. Being on the cusp of this wave is so essential that many medical groups spend more time advertising their technology to the public than the skills or medical pedigrees of their physicians. Why? The patient as a consumer of health care has become convinced that medical technology is safe and possibly more accurate. According to a 2015 survey of more than 2,000 doctors and consumers, twice as many patients preferred to use technology (smartphones, genetic testing, being able to view the doctor's note online, and EMRs) to come to a diagnosis than did physicians.[1] Not that we don't have reasons for concern. Take Dr. Frankenstein's fictional attempts to defeat death with electricity and the subsequent unexpected consequences he suffered. We stand at the dawn of a new era, uncharted waters in which we may find limitless bounty balanced against unimagined risk.

Putting my Luddite tendencies aside, there are real patient safety concerns associated with the wiring of medical care. Will patients make life plans based on mail-in genetic sequencing test results? Will their data be sold to or stolen by companies who could then alter the life insurance policy choices offered to a patient based on their DNA? How reliable and useful will data gathered by a patient's wearable device be in directing care? If a home monitor shows consistently elevated blood pressures or pulses, should a doctor act on those results or the contradictory reassuring results they see in the patient's office visit records? Will the wireless connectivity of home morphine pumps, pacemakers, and diabetic insulin infusions put those patients at risk for network failures or malicious viruses? What would happen to us if a massive electromagnetic pulse caused by the purposeful explosion of a nuclear device in our atmosphere turned all our gadgets off? A scary thought, but one that may no longer be science fiction. What if our whole network crashed due to a cyberattack? What if all the tests, procedures, medical notes, and allergy histories we've diligently logged into a patient's EMR vanished overnight? What if a trade war made manufacturing these tools cost prohibitive? Are we missing something when we use telemedicine to evaluate patients who live two blocks away, and if we do and the patient dies or receives substandard care, whose fault is it? Was the patient offered the option of a phone, tele-visit, or office visit and chose the technology or were they told that they would have to wait for an office visit but could have video visit the same day? Did the physician approve the telemedicine appointment or was it booked because the group mandates a certain number of these tele-visits each day?

Despite convenience, speed, and consumer confidence, medical innovations have dramatically changed the benefits and risks our patients are exposed to when they seek treatment. An FDA study published in 2013 found that surgical robots were directly involved in 144 deaths and 1,391 injuries.[2] Of these errors, 14.7 percent included broken/burnt pieces of instrument falling into the patient, electrical arching 10.5 percent, and 8.6 percent were due to the robot making unintended movements. More than 10 percent of the time the robotic procedure needed to be restarted, converted to a manual procedure, or rescheduled. This is that awkward part of medicine where the hype meets the health of the patient. A robot doing our surgery sounds cool. Being sent home with parts of that machine having accidentally dropped into the surgical site—not so much. FDA safety concerns around external infusion pumps used to deliver pain medications, fluids, and other medications found that there were 56,000 adverse events during a four-year period that led to injuries and deaths.[3] The government recalled 87 infusion pump models during this time with 14 of them falling into a Class 1 level of concern wherein there is a reasonable probability that the use of the device will cause a severe health consequence. In 2017, implantable cardiac devices made by St. Jude Medical were recalled due to cybersecurity vulnerability concerns which, if exploited, could allow an unauthorized user to remotely access the device and either turn it off or deliver unneeded and life-threatening shocks.[4] No documentation of this happening has occurred, but these patients were told they needed to have surgery to replace their devices because someone could potentially kill them with a few keystrokes. Welcome to modern medicine.

Even if we haven't seen it happen yet, the very real possibility that medical devices implanted into our bodies could be hijacked led Dr. Suzanne Schwartz, the director for the Office of Strategic Partnerships &Technology Innovation at the FDA, to issue this warning in 2016. "All medical devices that use software and are connected to the hospital and healthcare organizations' networks have vulnerabilities ... [which] require vigilant monitoring and timely remediation.... Today's draft guidance will ... safeguard patients from cyber threats by recommending medical device manufacturers continue to monitor and address cybersecurity issues while their product is on the market."[5] In a sense, she was putting the software developers on notice. It was no longer enough for them to create a functional program and walk away. They were also responsible for protecting those programs, and the patients they were designed to help, from nefarious influences as long as they were in business.

Prior to his death, Professor Stephen Hawking said in a BBC interview that "efforts to create thinking machines pose a threat to our very existence ... [and] could spell the end of the human race.... It would take off on its own, and re-design itself at an ever increasing rate. Humans, who are limited by slow biological evolution, couldn't compete, and would be superseded." Technology entrepreneur Elon Musk, the man spearheading the dream of colonizing Mars, mirrored our times greatest theoretical physicist's concerns in calling AI "our biggest existential threat."[6] Musk went on to say, "I'm increasingly inclined to think that there should be some regulatory oversight, maybe at the national and international level, just to make sure that we don't do something foolish."[7] In the statements of these two inspiring thinkers, we see real fear. These are not cultural bystanders nor backwoods extremists. These are people who have proven that we should listen when they talk, and they are saying "tread lightly."

This is not to say that we should unplug our computers and lives. I've had several patients follow-up with me after an emergency room visit where vague symptoms of indigestion and fatigue were found to be atrial fibrillation. The ER physician was then able to use the patient's Fitbit to isolate when the arrhythmia started and so decide if the individual was a candidate for cardioversion. I've received digital pictures of moles from patients which led to earlier diagnoses of cancer. I've reviewed thousands of downloaded home blood sugar results, assessed the resulting graphs, and used these charts to modify my patients' diets or change their medications. EEG (electroencephalography) machines tell us if a patient is at risk for seizures. EMG (electromyograph) machines show us which peripheral nerves are being compressed and how severely. Digital CT scans and MRIs allow us to find and treat pathology tens of times faster than in the past. PET (positron emission tomography) scans will enable us to monitor the body's metabolism and thus screen for metastasis. Gama Knife surgery allows for the noninvasive treatment of previously untreatable brain cancers. Deep brain stimulators offer real promise to Parkinson's patients, and genetic testing, with trained guidance, may indeed allow patients to make better-informed decisions about the risks they may pass on to their offspring. Organ transplants, regenerative medicine, gene therapy, and genetic engineering are pushing the envelope of what we can do, and our nature is one where we will continue to test our limits.

But, as both Professor Hawking and Mr. Musk espouse, we may need limits, brakes to keep us from gliding over the singularity cliff to stand midair, humanity's Wile E. Coyote moment, before noticing we've gone too far.

Luddites

In the late 18th century, a mythical character called Ned Ludd, a skilled textile artisan, is claimed to have smashed a textile machine when requests for government aid to protect the artists' livelihoods were ignored. In 1811 in Nottingham, British weavers and textile workers revolted against the modern factories that were taking their jobs. These were trained artisans who had learned their craft at their parent's knee, but now found themselves out of work because the industry had designed automated looms that could produce the same product despite being operated by unskilled labor. The weavers begged the government for help and were ignored. Taking matters into their own hands, they broke into factories with sledgehammers and took out their frustration on the machines that were robbing them of a livelihood. As one of the most memorable rebellions against the Industrial Revolution, they left manifestoes and threats under the name of Ludd although no evidence exists that their leader ever existed. You see, much like Robin Hood, "General Ludd" lived in Sherwood Forest and so was never captured. Not that the same could be said of the Luddites, as many ended up being shot or hung by company guards and soldiers. Indeed, the British government passed laws that made machine-breaking punishable by death, and the worker's uprising against the machine age died under the iron heel of the bureaucracy.[8]

The first weaver-type jobs to fall victim to our hunger for more medical technology are the radiologists and dermatologists. As described at length in *The Digital Doctor*,[9] and in *An American Sickness*,[10] radiologists were the first to embrace technology. They saw it as a way to more accurately view the patient's internal pathology, to work remotely, and to compare new and old films. Indeed, as first adopters, or the first weavers trained to use the equivalent of a pre-industrial loom, they reaped a short hiatus from the disruptive consequences of this new tool. Now, we are beginning to use pattern recognition programs like the facial recognition ones used by Facebook, to find cancers and identify radiologic anomalies. It's only a matter of time before the machine algorithms surpass the experience the human radiologists accumulated after years of training. To survive, they will now need to hone their skills in interventional radiology or become analysts who review and modify requests for particular tests. The fact that dermatologists interact with patients, do procedures, and see children, will cushion the effect that the same software protocols could be used to identify skin cancer using a photograph of a mole. This is happening as we speak. A computer scientist at Stanford created an artificially intelligent diagnosis algorithm for skin cancer that does just as well as its human counterpart as published in Nature in 2017.[11] A similar breakthrough in 2017 in radiology showed that algorithms could now diagnose pneumonia better than radiologists.[12]

There is intrinsic value in what technology is doing for radiology and dermatology. Programs that can identify cancer faster and more efficiently than the human eye will not be less accurate at the end of the day. High-resolution smartphone pictures taken by patients of nevi they wouldn't have bothered making an appointment for will be found to be malignant and lives will be saved.[13] These are good things, admirable benefits of the innovations we're making in the field, and perhaps that's why these professions have not created a "Doctor Ludd" to follow.

However, if they do, I would recommend they recall the story of the sledgehammer-wielding weavers who were sentenced to death and hung for breaking machines.

Humans love their technology.

Taylorism

Frederick Winslow Taylor was the first to use scientific management to improve a workforces' efficiency. In 1890, he began working for the Manufacturing Investment Company where he instituted production planning, real-time analysis of daily output and costs, and a modern accounting system. As a consultant for many firms, he went around with a stopwatch and clipboard and started watching how different employees did their jobs. At the time, workers took great pride in their work, and many learned their trade from their fathers or from having spent time as an apprentice under a senior steelworker. Thus, they each had unique ways of completing their tasks, and this was reflected in their work. Taylor felt this was inefficient and therefore analyzed how long it took each employee to do their job, found the most effective way to do that procedure, and standardized those movements so that everyone had to follow a set protocol. His efforts significantly improved the factory's productivity and created a management revolution that swept across the United States and into Europe in the early 1900s.[14]

Indeed, Taylor's theories and results caught the attention of Henry Ford in 1908 who was looking for ways to build his Model T faster and at a lower cost. At the time, it took a team of workers an entire day to manufacture a single car that sold to the public for $825.[15] After hiring Taylor in 1908 to observe his employees (there is some debate about this as some claim Taylor would get hired as an employee at different factories, work among the men, write a report, and then demand payment for his unsolicited observations[16]), Mr. Ford began to implement Taylor's scientific management theory and discovered that a great deal of time was wasted bringing parts to the car. His solution was to have workers drag the vehicle past stationary employees who only had to do one repetitive task. In 1913, he moved to a power-driven system that would carry a car down the assembly line allowing a single car to be built in 93 minutes. That vehicle sold for $575 and allowed Ford to capture 48 percent of the automobile market.[17] From an economic perspective, this was a staggering success. From a laborer's perspective, this was an unmitigated disaster. Taylorism and the assembly line led to the de-skilling of the American factory worker whereby a person who had been able to build an entire car from scratch now only knew how to attach a headlight.

As highlighted in Matthew Stewart's book *The Management Myth: Debunking Modern Business Philosophy*,[18] Frederick Taylor fudged more than a little of his data allowing his results to support his theories. As so much of what we consider standard practice rests on the premise that if we all do something the same way, the product will be better. The labor union rebelled against what they felt was "stopwatch" management, and the entire workforce walked off the job at the United States Watertown Arsenal in 1911. This led to congressional hearings that banned the practices promoted by Taylor in government facilities.[19] However, this mandate did not extend to the private sector and so elements of the scientific management style can be found in nearly all our daily work lives. There's a protocol for everything, a manual of standard best practices, a procedure you must follow when you wish to complain about a new procedure, and in most cases the voices of the people doing the job never get heard.

In medical practice, the dialogue goes something like this: Going home late again? Why don't you do things like Jimmy? Alice completed the most health-care goals for her patients last month. Why haven't your scores been as good? Although you have no control in booking appointments, we've noted your patient access has been poor. Can you do better? Although you've counseled your patients to stop smoking, many of them haven't quit. You've received poor patient feedback for not giving a drug addict their pain medications. You've given too many antibiotics this month. You didn't click off enough boxes to get full reimbursement for your last patient visit. Please do an addendum. Apparently, you are not motivated to accomplish the goals the administration feels are best for most patients. Why don't we link your paycheck to our mandates and see if that helps? What? You think patients are individuals and not numbers? You believe some patients take longer to treat than others? You think it's more important for the living patient to be healthy than for the one living on the computer screen to appear healthy?

Sorry, wrong answers. Please try again.

Physicians don't have unions to defend the interests of the doctor-patient relationship. Indeed, due to fears that such a group might collude to price fix medical care, it is illegal for doctors to form unions (we'll talk more about this in Chapter Nine). Amazon, Facebook, and Google are just fine. Really?

Despite what they might like us to think, the AMA and all the other specialty group associations are not unions. They do lobby for physician and patient rights, but they do not speak for most doctors, and their boards have, in my opinion, far too many fingers in other people's pies to stand on a soapbox and say they are working solely in the best interest of their members.

So we've lost the game. Taylorism wins. We are well-paid cogs in the wheel. How much longer before physicians devolve into de-skilled data entry clerks that scan our patient's implanted digital health adviser into the mainframe and tell them what pills they've won from Big Pharma.

I hope not.

The unique difference between physicians and autoworkers is that the product of our labor is a living, breathing human who can say for themselves if they want to be on an assembly line.

I'm betting they don't.

Dumb and Dumber

In the book *World Without Mind: The Existential Threat of Big Tech*, Franklin Foer talks about how technology has dramatically altered the landscape of journalism and the intrinsic value of the written word. One of his most telling examples was in describing how Amazon's Jeff Bezos introduced the e-book. "By unilaterally setting the price of the e-book at $9.99, far lower than paper, Bezos falsely implied that the cost of producing a book resided in printing and shipping, not in the intellectual capital, creativity, and the years of effort."[20] Amazon, Google, and Facebook don't care what an individual book or blog costs. They care about digging in as social axis points, places we go to buy anything, get information about the world, and talk to friends. As gatekeepers, they are positioned to be keen observers of our buying habits, searches, and social networks and can use this information to build personality profiles.

Invisible online algorithms are working behind the scenes to make product suggestions, tweak our results, and decide which of our friend's posts we are likely to see. Although this is done under the auspice of improving our online experience, it is ripe for abuse as was demonstrated in the Facebook and Cambridge Analytica fiasco where 87 million individuals had their data stolen, sold, and used to manipulate them and their friends.[21] They did this by using a personality app "thisismydigitallife," which created a loophole in Facebook's privacy firewalls. Surprisingly, Facebook knew about the breach in 2015 but abstained from acknowledging it until 2018. The billionaire Robert Mercer, a Trump supporter, gave $15 million to Cambridge Analytica where Steve Bannon, President Trump's chief strategist, sat as a board member at the time. Aleksandr Kogan designed the malicious personality app through a company called Global Science Research. Of note, Mr. Kogan received grants from the Russian government to research Facebook user's emotional states.[22]

To continue with another excerpt from Mr. Foer's book, "That's why the present moment feels so profoundly uncomfortable. Our faith in technology is no longer fully consistent with our belief in liberty.... The proliferation of falsehood and conspiracy through social media, the dissipation of our common basis for fact, is creating conditions ripe for authoritarianism. Over time, the long merger of man and machine has worked out well for man. But we're pulling into a new era when the merger threatens the individual."[23] If algorithms can be designed that understand our personalities well enough that they can manipulate our actions in the real world, how many of our future decisions will be our own? If "fake news" is already influencing our political choices and global policies, how hard will it have to push to get us to believe a newly patented drug or procedure is going to change our lives. How long before we stop questioning if this is true or checking the source material? How long before that source material is as fake as the advertisement?

Pride, respect, and responsibility are the three pillars upon which every craftsperson relies. We are proud of our skills, the sacrifices we've made to attain them, and how our hard-earned abilities make us uniquely suited to do things that positively affect the world around us. We respect those in our profession that have made similar choices, the products of their labor, and the craft itself. We acknowledge the responsibility we have to stand as role models, as bastions of good faith, and as the last immutable barrier to chaos. Unfortunately, it is these very pillars that technology has destabilized. How can we have pride in a job that a machine can do better? How can we respect those who have sold or devalued their skills to make the machine better? How can we be asked to accept responsibility for results we only played a small part in producing?

Professor Stephen Hawking said, "The automation of factories has already decimated jobs in traditional manufacturing, and the rise of artificial intelligence is likely to extend this job destruction deep into the middle classes, with only the most caring, creative or supervisory roles remaining.... The internet and the platforms that it makes possible allow very small groups of individuals to make enormous profits while employing very few people. This is inevitable, it is progress, but it is also socially destructive."[24]

The sadist part: we are doing this to ourselves.

My Thoughts

In writing this book, I spent countless hours researching the available literature in the field of medical technology and innovation. As a whole, I was impressed with the majority of the writers I found, but Dr. Eric Topal's book *The Patient Will See You Now* was not one of them. If it's not clear from the title of his book, he suggests physicians will not be needed in the future. Indeed, he spends a fair part of his time arguing that once we train patients to collect their vital statistics, they will be able to use algorithms to treat themselves. He talks about the paternal nature of medicine—the old boy's network—and how in the future we won't even need hospitals. Why? Because hospitals are dangerous places where 440,000 people die each year due to preventable medical complications.[25] He references an author who notes this is like having four jumbo jets crashing a week, and then he presumes to imply that the medical community is sweeping these deaths under the table.[26] I cannot say that there may not be an element of truth to his assumptions, but I have to point out that the people on jumbo jets are healthy and those admitted to hospitals are not. It's like he's saying we should blame lifeguards because the studies show that people who go swimming seem to be at much higher risk for drowning than those that stay on land.

Sadly, he spends much of his time promoting technology for situations that he has no experience performing. For one, he suggests that voice recognition programs could document the verbiage of an office visit and thus free nearly half our time to do other things.[27] This lets him say it's not a big deal for us to ask our patients to bring in reams of home collected data and have us sift through it. Okay, so where's that voice application? It's not in my office. Please, don't hand out work to physicians who see three to four times more patients in a day than those in your specialty. I know cardiologists struggle to get through the day, but I don't presume to tell them that it's okay if they feel overworked because it'll be all better when everyone starts doing stents at home with their cell phones. Stay in your lane.

What irks me most is that I keep thinking about England's Luddite rebellion and how it destroyed the lives of countless craftsmen and woman. You see. Someone had to tell the automatic loom manufacturers how to weave cloth; they had to sell out their profession in the name of innovation and then skip on home with their seven bits of silver. I'm not saying that change isn't inevitable or that we shouldn't have manufactured clothing, but I do think some of the blame of the hardships we experience because of technology lies at the feet of those that promote it, regardless of the unexpected consequences it has on the people it affects. Not all physicians are paternal, not all hospital deaths are due to errors, not all manufactured clothes are as good as the hand-sewn ones made by professional tradespersons.

Dr. Topol is fond of suggesting that there's an app for just about everything. Really? Is there an app that tells you you've developed terminal cancer but that it will be with you the whole way? Is there an app that explains to you that you've contracted HIV but that we have medications that can help you live a normal life and that it's taken care of plenty of patients who have done just that? Is there an app that calls your loved ones after you've died and tells them its sorry for their loss, that you were an inspiring person, and that it will be happy to help in any way it can with the grieving process? Is there an app that doesn't believe you when you say you don't drink or do drugs, that asks you again, and then gets you the treatment you need? Is there an app that tells you that having worked with you for 20 years, it thinks you're depressed and would benefit from counseling even though you think you're coping fine with your wife's death and the loss of your job? Is there an app that cares?

Topol references the RAND study of 2005[28] as one of the reasons we need to push forward with technology, but we've already seen how flawed that study was and how the companies that funded it were the same that profited from it. He seems to think primary care physicians have nothing better to do than use email and Skype to manage all their patient's needs without physically examining them. On average, I manage 30 urgent messages, more than 100 lab and radiology results, 50 medication refill requests, five cc notes from specialists, three cc notes from colleagues, have two or more scheduled phone interviews, and see 20 patients in my office each day. I arrive at 7:30 a.m. and leave at 6:30 p.m. (on a good day). The patients I see are not simple social visits. They consistently have at least five "acute" complaints and seven chronic issues I have to address. I enjoy my job, but I wonder where exactly I'm going to find time to FaceTime with patients that don't have a clinical reason to see me in the office. He suggests that in the future we won't need hospitals because we'll all have high tech homes that will monitor our vitals and send the data to our physicians. Really? Did the United States win the galactic Powerball? Where is this money coming from and how can our patients get it? All those Tony Stark high-tech gadgets sound incredible, but clinics in our at-risk communities struggle to keep their lights on and doors open. Indeed, many would be overjoyed to have enough of the stethoscopes Dr. Topal thinks are so antiquated.

Perhaps I'm unfair, but Dr. Topol has maneuvered himself into the public eye as a spokesperson for medical technology, and as such he can expect some constructive criticism. Unfortunately, those of us in the trenches have been too busy cleaning up the mess technology has made of our field to give Little Boy Blue the feedback he needs to hear. Open sourcing medical information and patient collected data might work for the twenty-somethings, but most of my practice consists of low-tech baby boomers and patients who grew up reading the newspapers and pulps. My resistance to his suggestions has little to do with wanting to be reimbursed (he said as much in a 2018 interview with the *Wall Street Journal*[29]) and more to do with not believing that my 90-year-old will open her emails. Additionally, I worry about my patient's privacy and fail to see how we can say the health benefits he thinks data-mining patients will provide can outweigh the real risk their medical information will be stolen and used against them as we saw with Cambridge Analytica.

I've made and will make predictions about the fantastic benefits technology may bring to the office encounter, but I don't pretend to think that these things are practical solutions now. I know the difference between science and science fiction.

We've all seen the videos of people who are so invested in their cell phones that they've walked into fountains, heard of deaths caused by drivers texting, and know someone who can't last a full minute without checking their messages. Dr. Topol suffers from this same dissociation from the real world when it comes to his high-tech toys, and I fear that those who follow him too closely may lead their patients into the open ocean.

Not to worry.

If anyone drowns, we can always blame the lifeguards.

Prescribing Caution

This chapter has been about the unexpected consequences of change. Our job is to do no harm, to reduce our patient's suffering, and to act as a guide for them as they move from one end of life's path to the other. For centuries, we've done this, to the best of our abilities, by relying on experience, trust, and communication. Although we live in the age of communication, it feels like we do anything but talk to each other face-to-face. We are more secluded, more distrusting of our neighbors, and more fearful than at any other period in recorded history. The pendulum swings for all things, but we must be cautious when it carries us too far.

Information overload, poorly researched online articles written by inexperienced authors, fake news, and the expectation of a painless cure has led to unrealistic demands on a health-care system that was doomed to fail when we monetized our health. Because we value money more than care, office visits are short and overloaded with data entry. Patient education is done through online learning classes or group meetings rather than through individualized physician counseling. Fear of legal repercussions and the ease of practicing defensive medicine with a click of a button leads to higher bills and validates unfounded patient fears. Why would my doctor order that test or give me antibiotics if they weren't worried I had something? Answer: It takes less time, you wouldn't believe them if they said you were fine, and if they didn't do it, you might give me a bad review on Yelp.

We've all played the game where you link two cups together with a thin piece of string and talk over a long distance. It's fun, educational, and unreliable (as something frequently gets lost in translation). That might be fine for a kid's game, or even one of Dr. Topol's adult communication toys, but when a patient's life is at stake, nothing can replace a face-to-face office exam done by an experienced human physician.

Chapter Five

The Healing Touch (Origin Story)

Lifting the Hood

Have ever you gone to an office visit, sat across from your physician on the mandatory crinkly exam room table, your clothes folded neatly on the chair, the awkward gown of too many ties draped inexpertly around your shoulders, and describe, while you shivered in the frigid room of antiseptic smells, your symptoms? Did your physician listen carefully, recount the possible diagnoses, order the appropriate tests and therapy, print out some informational pamphlets, arrange a follow-up, and leave—without examining you? How long did it take for you to realize the missing element? Did you feel like maybe you should say something but then realized that the doctor had ordered a chest X-ray or CT scan or even a full panel of labs and so decided this was as good as having them listen to your lungs or press on your belly. This is not the norm, but it happens far more often than it should. The physical exam is being replaced by tools that should validate and clarify findings found through the physician's skill rather than supplant them. As our profession abandons the art of the exam, it orphans skills that took 300 years to evolve in favor of practices favored at the time of Hippocrates where diagnosis and therapies didn't rely on the physician touching their patients. It was during this time that disease was thought to arise from an excess of one of the four humors (cholera: yellow bile; phlegma: phlegm; sanguis: blood; and melancholia: black bile[1]).

Hippocrates believed that all diseases originated in these humors, and it was the physician's intellectual job to figure out which one was out of balance with the rest. Imagine if your mechanic said they could fix your car by guessing if it had too much gas, motor oil, windshield washer fluid, or brake fluid. Although these things are important, they pale when compared to the diagnostic power of lifting the hood or crawling under the chassis. Being a competent human mechanic means physicians must get their hands dirty. It means we must have the right training, skills, and the appropriate tools for our job. We wouldn't expect even the most experienced motorhead to change a tire without a socket wrench, so diagnostic tools and techniques best augment our evaluation of the human machine.

The son of an innkeeper changed all this when he introduced one of the most essential exam tools we have, the technique of percussion (learned from his father's habit of tapping on wine barrels to find out how full they were), to the world in 1761. Leopold Auenbrugger described his technique for tapping on the body to understand the densities of the underlying organs in his treatise *Inventum Novum*, but it was not received well until Jean-Nicolas Corvisart, Napoleon's physician, showed how it could be used in practice in 1808. Thus, the idea that actions taken on the outside of the body could provide clues as to our internal functioning took hold and may have influenced René Laennec, one of Corvisart's students, in his inspiration to place a rolled up cone of paper over a patient's heart and initiate the creation of the stethoscope. Publishing his findings and techniques in 1819 in the journal *On Mediate Auscultation*, Laennec termed words we appreciate even today such as "rales" and "egophony."[2]

Extending the concept that the individual health of internal organs could affect how patients felt, Johannes Müller wrote the groundbreaking book *Handbook of Human Physiology* and taught Hermann von Helmholtz who would go on to invent the first ophthalmoscope in 1850. In 1871, Carl August Wunderlich noted in his article "Medical Thermometry and Human Temperature" that the temperature of sick people was markedly different from that of healthy individuals and so should be considered one of the vital signs essential to monitoring human illness.[3] Twenty-five years later, Scipione Riva-Rocci invented an easy-to-use sphygmomanometer that measured blood pressure, demonstrating how pivotal a patient's blood pressure could be in treatment.

The discovery that we could not only hear but see into the body as described by Whilhelm Conrad Röntgen in his article "On a New Kind of Rays" in 1895 marked a shift away from a proximity-dependent evaluation process. Now we could use X-rays to capture pictures of the inner organs and evaluate them well away from the ill individual. The visual representation of the human body evolved[4]:

- 1903: The electrocardiogram (ECG)—Dr. Willem Einthoven
- 1924: Electroencephalogram (EEG)—Dr. Hans Berger
- 1942: Ultrasound (U.S.)—Dr. Karl Theodore Dussik
- 1955: Mammography—Jacob Gershon Cohen used it for cancer screening in healthy women
- 1971: Computed tomography (CT or CAT)—Dr. Godfrey Hounsfield

- 1974: Positron emission tomography (PET)—Michael E. Phelps, Edward Hoffman, and Michel M. Ter-Pogossian[5]
- 1978: Magnetic resonance imaging (MRI)—Dr. Raymond V. Damadian
- 1992: Automatic DNA Sequencing—Dr. Leroy E. Hood
- 2008: Fusion of PET/CT scans for molecular imaging

Each of these tools has expanded our understanding of the human body and disease processes, but they have also allowed us to gently push our patients further away. At the beginning of the 21st century, we can see how telemedicine is the natural evolution of this process. Consider this scenario: "No, Mrs. Jones, we don't need you to come to the office. I can see the blood-streaked sputum you've coughed up on screen, I have the vitals, blood sugars, oxygen saturation, and peak flow you've collected at home, and I'm concerned you may have cancer given your smoking history and recent weight loss. I've ordered a STAT CT of your lungs, pulmonary function tests, and arranged a follow-up with a pulmonologist to review your findings. I will email you all the appointment times and locations. If you have acute changes, please go to the emergency room and do try to stop smoking. Have a wonderful tele-day."

Many would argue the above is well within the parameters of our modern standard of care. The patient is stable, has symptoms that are not life-threatening, and I've ordered investigative tests to determine and document how ill she is, warned her to seek additional help if her symptoms changed, while also advising her to stop the likely trigger of her symptoms. To me, it feels wrong. It seems like I'm being told that since I know how to fly an aircraft, I'm suddenly somehow qualified to be an air traffic controller. Really? You see, despite what the technology gurus would have us think, most patients don't want to fly their own planes any more than they want to change the transmission in their cars. Some might call my attitude paternalist, but I think it's simpler than that. If your vehicle broke down on the side of the road, would you send your mechanic a picture of the smoke, an audio recording of its engine, and measurements of its tire pressure and fuel gauges and wait for them to tell you how to fix it? No. You would tow it into the shop because your mechanic loves to fix cars, they've been trained to do it well, and that's all they do all day long. Why would we treat our bodies with less respect?

The Power of Proximity

When I enter a patient's room, I do my best to be entirely present during the encounter. This means that I block everything on the other side of the office door from my mind. I'm not thinking about other patients, labs, home, finances, or anything but the individual sitting in front of me and their history, concerns, risk factors, and our communication dynamic. This is not easy to do, and it took me years of training to live in the absolute moment of that visit, but the benefit of achieving this singular presence is enormous. It lets me use the tools we presented in Chapter Three—listen, observe, consolidate, germinate, postulate, and then reevaluate—to the best of my abilities, and it earns me my patient's trust. There is something about working with someone face-to-face, that is wholly different, more real, than when we communicate over the Internet or phone. It's likely an instinct built on the pretense that if I'm close enough to touch someone, then I've got skin in the game. Face-to-face dialogue counts as a pact, an agreement between equals who want the same thing: the patient's good health.

The other benefit of having an office visit is the nonverbal cues that both I and the patient exchange. If I'm leading them in the wrong direction, I may notice changes in their body language or expressions that would be easy to miss over the phone or even via a teleconference. These clues tell me a great deal about how to present information, how much to provide, and whether the patient is receptive to the path I'm suggesting. In reverse, they can read my posture, eye contact, and facial expressions and know if they're giving me information that will help narrow our differential or not. UCLA professor emeritus Albert Mehrabian's 1970 study became widely quoted for showing that 93 percent of effective communication was nonverbal.[6] Detractors pointed out that the study's results applied to discussions involving strong emotions and were not meant to be a universal rule. This is demonstrated in our ability to successfully book a haircut or order a pizza over the phone. But in situations involving plans for the end of life, cancer prevention, and even the risks of hormone replacement therapy, emotions can run high, and so nonverbal cues are critical to achieving a good outcome.

Telehealth does have a place in appropriate circumstances such as when seeing a patient in the office would cause them undue hardship. Parkinson's, multiple sclerosis, quadriplegia, next day follow-ups after surgery or an office exam seem like reasonable targets. Patients who are ambulatory, live three blocks away, and just "don't have the time" to have their lungs listened to when they have a high fever, wheeze, and underlying asthma do not. When I was in training, our attending physicians would have frowned and had a stern talk with any resident who ordered antibiotics over the phone just because a patient "wanted them." This is becoming the norm.[7] Worse, health-care groups are integrating tele-visits into their scheduling templates and so forcing physicians to evaluate patients who might be better suited for an office visit. Patients booked in this manner are given the misleading impression that their complaints can be managed over the phone and so can become upset when this does not prove to be the case. Such practices create high-risk appointments that needlessly put the doctor's license and the patient's health in jeopardy. Tight screening parameters that rule high-risk patients out of phone visits even if they demand them seems like the safest solution for all involved.

The Death of the Physical Exam

In 2012, a Cochran study reviewed 182,880 participants from 14 randomized controlled trials over the median of nine years of data and found no benefit from routine general health checkups.[8] This caused a stir both within and outside the medical community. If the annual exam was useless, why were insurers paying for it? If it did nothing to reduce an individual's risk of death, why were patients going for them? If it did nothing to reduce the risk of cardiovascular disease or cancer, why were physicians asking their patients to come in once a year? Were we all wasting our time?

The problem with this study lies with there being no way to create a valid control, a twin who does the opposite of what the physician recommends. Because of this, our mention that the patient is gaining weight and should consider joining a gym or convincing them to take a baby aspirin once a day or counseling them on how to deal with their teenager without blowing up isn't reflected in the outcome. As physicians, we rarely do a simple physical, pat our patients on the back, and ask them to come back next year. We ask them questions about their lives, about their fears, and make suggestions on lifestyle or attitude that never make it into the chart. We talk to them about anxiety, depression, sleep disorders, and life plans. We build a rapport, a level of trust, and so can act as a bellwether of stability upon which they can weigh outside life stressors. The value of any office exam lays hidden in the things that don't happen, the paths steered clear of, and so will prove as elusive as a snipe to the number crunchers.

I believe M. C. Hammer's colloquial term for this was "you can't touch this," with the Latin equivalent being *non ut metiretur*.[9]

Case Studies

Mr. Carlton

Years ago, as I was starting to develop my panel of patients, I had an older man walk into my office complaining of a swollen forearm. He had no fever or chills, no cuts on his body to indicate an entrance wound, but his arm was erythematous, warm to the touch, and mildly tender. He had a steady pulse, both his arms had the same blood pressure, there was no fluctuance (induration suggestive of pus) to the soft tissue, and neither appeared swollen or indicative of a blood clot. His arm pain had been going on for more than a week, he had recently returned from a trip to Costa Rica, and he had been having trouble sleeping because his arm felt like it was alive. As the swelling under the paper-thin skin of his forearm had begun to break down, I placed a strip of Xeroform (a petroleum-based occlusive dressing) over it, started him on an oral antibiotic for a presumed cellulitis, drew labs, and asked him to see me back in the office in two days.

I received a message the next day that he had been up all night because his arm kept moving by itself and couldn't he have some sleeping medications. Concerned that his age and infection may have pushed him into delirium, I checked his labs and found them to be within normal range. I called him up and found out he felt fine, was completely lucid, but felt like his arm was angry with him. Rather than changing antibiotics, providing a sleep aid, or waiting another day, I had him come in to see me in the office. Pulling back the bandage, I found the glistening brown heads of five larvae sticking out of Mr. Carlton's arm. They were very active and happy to have air as the Xeroform dressing I'd placed the day before had been suffocating them.

Using forceps, I drew them each out and put them in a specimen container. They were large, white, healthy grubs, and the holes they'd left in my patient looked clean with no pus or underlying infection. Mr. Carlton had been right to complain that it felt like his arm was alive and that it was angry, it had been, and I hadn't given him enough credit for his choice of words. His trip to Costa Rica and the botfly population it harbors was the part of the history I had not had enough clinical experience to recognize as the key to the puzzle. Botflys capture mosquitoes and lay their eggs on the bloodsuckers before releasing them. The mosquitoes drink blood from their victims and inadvertently lay the botfly's eggs in the host's skin. The half-life for their maturation varies, but Mr. Carlton's trip was about three weeks before his presentation. The locals treat early infections with camphor and later ones by tying raw meat over the affected area, so the larva will dig their way up through it to get to the surface and breathe. My application of Xeroform had a similar effect but with no egress and so had made Mr. Carlton's stowaways more than a little upset. Pinching the larva out with your fingers is not recommended as their bodies burst and so can induce anaphylaxis in susceptible individuals.

* * *

Five. The Healing Touch (Origin Story)

Learning point: Just like when we go to the movies and suspend disbelief when we watch someone fly or demonstrate magical powers, we must do the same for our patients and always take them at their word.

Mrs. O'Neil

Mrs. O'Neil had mild senile dementia for several years. It wasn't bad, and she could drive and accomplish all her daily chores with little help from her family who she never wanted to burden. She took her medications, followed up for her annual exams, did her labs, and overall was a cheerful and pleasant person who cared a great deal about her grandchildren. Her husband had passed several years ago due to Alzheimer's disease, and so she had moved to my town to be closer to her family.

So it was sadly ironic when she appeared for an appointment with her family after a hospital stay during which she had a complete workup for a rapid progression of her dementia. Her CT and MRI/MRA revealed age-appropriate white matter disease with only mild carotid stenosis, her ECG was stable with no arrhythmias, her chest X-ray was negative, and her urine was mildly positive, so she was discharged into the care of her family with Bactrim for a presumed urinary tract infection. During our interview, her mini-mental exam (MMSE) had fallen from 25/30 to 17/30, and she was quick to confabulate about why she been walking down the street in her pajamas in the middle of the night. Her family was worried but reassured that she seemed to be making some improvement. They would sleep at her house and let me know if anything changed. I reviewed all the hospital tests, ordered a few more, arranged home health, and booked a follow-up appointment.

Two weeks later, Mrs. O'Neil had an MMSE of 19 but was confused about the year and claimed that she had driven herself to the appointment when her family had brought her. Her urine culture from the hospital had been positive, and a urine dip in the office was negative. She had no fever, motor loss, or loss of appetite. She was glad her family was spending more time with her but couldn't remember her daughter's birthday. It bothered me that her mental status change had been so rapid and had persisted even though her UTI had cleared. I stopped all nonessential medications, despite her having been on many of them for years, and ordered additional labs including an RPR for syphilis.

Mrs. O'Neil turned out to have tertiary syphilis, and she made a miraculous mental recovery after a series of high dose penicillin G injections. Her VDRL dilutions improved along with her memory and functional status. In retrospect, it seems likely that her late husband's progression into dementia was from the self-same tertiary syphilis that had been eating Mrs. O'Neil's brain.

* * *

Learning point: Listen to your gut. Keep looking for causes if something doesn't feel right. Sometimes the right answer isn't simple or likely. Tertiary syphilis does happen in the elderly: check for it.

Ms. Ferguson

Ms. Ferguson presented with her parents after finding a mass in her axilla that increased in size over the course of three days. She had a low-grade temperature, felt tired, and had been losing weight for the last two weeks. An MRI done in the ER revealed a 3 cm mass in her axilla with surrounding lymph nodes. Her WBC was mildly elevated with a small left shift. She had been told that there was a chance of lymphoma and referred to interventional radiology for a biopsy. She was distraught and wanted the biopsy as soon as possible as well as a referral to oncology.

We discussed lymphoma, the diagnostic process, and what was involved in doing a biopsy as well as how long it might take to get results back from pathology. I did a full exam, and the mass was mobile, mildly tender, non-fluctuant, and her arm had begun to swell from venous congestion. An ultrasound done in the ER had ruled out a DVT, and she had strong distal pulses and no apparent signs of cellulitis. On the plus side, her nodes would be easily accessible by radiology. On the negative side, lymphoma did seem like a possibility. What bothered me was the localization of the mass on the right side with no lymph nodes or findings anywhere else. I reexamined her arm and found two small scratches on the wrist. They didn't have pets, but Ms. Ferguson remembered that she had been at a friend's house a week earlier. Her friend's kitten had scratched her when they were playing a game with yarn. She hadn't given it another thought until now.

I started her on azithromycin and consulted infectious disease who felt we should proceed with the biopsy.

Her bartonella henselae immunofluorescence assay test came back positive, and the biopsy confirmed the diagnosis of cat scratch fever. A vet evaluated and treated the kitten, and after several months of close observation, Ms. Ferguson made a full recovery.

* * *

Learning point: It's okay to reexamine a patient, to look at the same area you've already screened for something you might have missed. Treating the right problem is more important than your pride.

Author's Note

I don't describe the above cases to promote my diagnostic prowess (I've missed far more odd diagnoses over the years than I've caught) but to provide the reader with practical examples of how an exam contributes to the diagnostic process. Human pathology is complex, intriguing, and challenging, but it is also mercifully finite. There are only so many diseases, and only so many things that can go wrong. Our job is to think of every possibility, so the one thing that doesn't fit rises to the surface. Medicine is a messy, imperfect science that relies on luck, intuition, and the active suppression of assumptions, but it is also one of the most intellectually and emotionally rewarding professions in the world.

Appearance Is More Than Skin Deep

We've talked some about body language and nonverbal cues to establish how critical it can be for a patient to have an office visit. One of the nonverbal aspects of any encounter is appearance. Is your doctor older or younger than you, are they well-groomed, overweight, what's their ethnicity, do they look tired, male or female, do they have a language barrier, and are they dressed appropriately? Although it takes time, many patients begin to ask personal questions of their doctor so that things like political views, religion, and ethics can start to influence the relationship. Some physicians try to keep things professional and quickly steer patients onto other paths, others recognize that part of a healthy relationship involves sharing.

As physicians, we mistakenly think we are the only ones making critical judgments during an interview. A patient's anxiety, trust, comfort level in asking questions, and ultimately compliance, can be influenced by what they think of the person giving them advice. Only share as much as you feel comfortable. Never overshare (this is the patient's visit) but understand that opening up about yourself can demonstrate that you are a fellow human with struggles that are similar to their own. If they know that you were bullied as a child, changed a flat tire, or dreamed of winning the lotto, they may feel these shared experiences make you a more reliable partner in their health care.

Along those lines, I'll share here that I once created a company called Beyond the Light Bulb. It was to promote an invention I'd filed a patent for called the Disposa-Tie. I'd noticed that fewer and fewer male physicians wore ties. I understood the rationale as recent studies had found that the clinician's tie was one of the dirtiest things in the office. It rarely gets cleaned, is touched daily, and follows the doctor around like a dirty rag from one sick patient to the next. I mourned the passing of the tie, however, as, in my opinion, it contributed an element of professionalism to the interview. My solution was a disposable paper tie that could be pulled out of a box much like a pair of gloves and disposed of at the end of the day. I developed several beautiful prototypes that felt and looked the same as their silk ancestors, pitched the idea to venture capitalists, but ultimately couldn't get the traction I needed to develop the product. The pushback from investors: Why does a doctor need to wear a tie? If it's dirty, they should go without it. Financially, this was good advice as the golden rule is that you must show that there is a demand for something. I no longer wear a tie, but I do miss them and wonder if my patients might see me wearing a Disposa-Tie around my neck as a nonverbal cue of my professional attitude.

You Can't Arrest Me

At 15, I volunteered in an emergency room. The bustling chaos of what was undoubtedly the daily grind for the staff felt to me like I was in the middle of a war zone. I did my best to keep up, to help where I could, and to observe.

One of the patients who stuck with me was a middle-aged man screaming profanities at the doctors and nurses and accompanied by a police escort. Mr. Phillips threatened their lives and families and swore he would sue everyone in sight. Strapped to the stretcher as he was, I took solace in his inability to write any of our names down. My physician mentor, Dr. Llampa, discovered from the officers that Mr. Phillips had washed down a hundred sleeping pills with a bottle of wine in a suicide attempt. We started IVs, a nasal gastric tube, and administered activated charcoal. Concerned that we might save his life, Mr. Phillips became even more violent and produced a new string of colorful insults. Then, abruptly, his heart stopped.

Dr. Llampa called a code, ordered meds, performed CPR, but the patient's heart remained stubbornly inert. He charged the crash cart paddles, yelled the mandatory "Clear!" and shocked Mr. Phillips. Instantly, our patient's belligerent heart restarted, and the monitors above his head stopped whining. Opening his eyes, Mr. Phillips continued his furious rant as if nothing had happened.

Five. The Healing Touch (Origin Story)

As gently as he could, Dr. Llampa told his patient to calm down as he had just suffered a cardiac arrest. To this, Mr. Phillips said, "No one's going to arrest me. I know my rights. You can't arrest me for this."

Doctors and patients sit on opposite sides of a knowledge divide, a chasm, really, that can at times interfere with productive communication. As the above example illustrates, words mean different things to us than they do to our patients. Nonverbal cues, unquantifiable variables, and being fully present in an encounter are ways to bridge the gap between our medical training and the real-world expectations of our patients. Providing the opportunity to build this connection and the common ground it fosters is what makes office exams such valuable tools, and why I hope it never goes the way of our ties.

Chapter Six

Go Gently into That Good Night (Death)

Waiting for Godot/Death

As we enter the 21st century, our patients expect miracles. They think science and technology will soon help us live forever, cure cancer, reverse the aging process, and, at the very least, provide patients with lab-grown replacement organs. Worse yet, many believe doctors should want to help create this future because our job is to fight death. Really? As a thought experiment, please take a moment and do an Internet search for pictures depicting physicians doing battle with the specter of death. Your imagination says there must be a slew of marble sculptures, images, and oil paintings showing this epic battle. What you'll find is that there isn't much out there aside from the 1959 metalwork *Keeping Away Death* by Julian Hoke Harris, found on the side of Fulton County Department of Health and Wellness building.[1] Most of the art before the 19th century shows death as an unstoppable, fearsome, and often angelic force of nature whose duty it is to usher the dying into the next world. Except for Ponce de Leon's search for the Fountain of Youth, death was no more the enemy to this pretech population than the setting sun. It was natural, inevitable, and often thought of as an escape from the torments of life. "We are not Gods," said Gilgamesh in the epic poem of his deeds written circa 1400 BC. "We cannot ascend to heaven. No. We are mortal men. Only the Gods live forever. Our days are few in number and whatever we achieve is but a puff of wind. Why be afraid then since sooner or later death must come?"[2] Thousands of years later, Michelangelo said, "death and love are the two wings that bear a good man to heaven."[3] Finally, the great bard Shakespeare wrote, "if I must die, I will encounter darkness as a bride, and hug it in mine arms."[4] Contrast this with the futurist Ray Kurzweil's paraphrased statement in *WIRED* magazine that "the first AI's will be created as add-ons to human intelligence, modeled on our actual brains and used to extend our human reach. AIs will help us see and hear better. They will give us better memories and help us fight disease. Eventually, AI's will allow us to conquer death itself. The singularity won't destroy us. Instead, it will immortalize us."[5] Bear in mind, Mr. Kurzweil works for Google and so has a vested interest in keeping our hopes up. But he did predict wireless cell phones, laptops, the integrated World Wide Web, and wearable tech, and so his views on life extension may represent the expectation of a growing number of our patients.[6]

Most patients' beliefs about death lie somewhere between Gilgamesh and Kurzweil and finding out where they stand on the acceptance/resistance slid-rule is part of our job as their physicians. In opening this discussion, it is important not to pass judgment or allow our beliefs to influence our patients, but to position ourselves as experienced facilitators capable of helping them see where the boxes they check off will lead. This is critical as someone may start out with strong convictions about their code status only to reverse course when they better understand what their choices mean. These are not easy or comfortable conversations, but they are dialogues that need to be undertaken. Despite what the transhumanists, biohackers, and immortalists proclaim about the coming of the singularity, it hasn't happened yet whereas death has a long track record of happening much sooner than anyone of us would like.

So, until the computers take over, it makes sense to prepare for the end.

How we might do this with some level of dignity and control is addressed in Dr. Samuel Harrington's book *At Peace: Choosing a Good Death After a Long Life*.[7] In it, he explores the six most common chronic diseases that lead to death in the United States (congestive heart failure, cancer, chronic obstructive pulmonary disease, stroke, dementia, and diabetes), how to recognize when one of these illnesses is nearing its natural conclusion, and what options a patient might have other than the aggressive care measures medicine offers. He talks about both his professional experience managing death as a gastroenterologist as well as the personal growth he experienced in helping his parents face end-of-life choices. In her book *With the End in Mind: Dying, Death & Wisdom in an Age of Denial*, Dr. Kathryn Mannix uses patient stories from her 30 years as a palliative care physician to demonstrate how accepting the end can lead to a more dignified and less disturbing death.[8]

Our expectations of the end of life are built on our understanding of the world we live in and the choices it promises. In the past, death was an absolute and so could not be postponed except in fantasy and science fiction. Today, we are told that technology will soon free us from our mortal bonds. "Tell me more," demands our monkey brain. "There's a way to avoid pain and suffering? Who knows these secrets? What must I do to learn them?" This interest is natural given our inherent drive for self-preservation. What we might not have predicted is how the growing belief that there is a way to escape the cycle of life would heighten our anxiety and fear about death. Raise a puppy inside a five-by-five-foot wooden cage, and it will be content. Let it watch another puppy escape to run unleashed in the fields, and our puppy will whine and paw at its prison walls for the rest of its life. We are content because we don't believe there is a way out, but if even one person achieves immortality through science, mankind may destroy itself trying to replicate the process.

Accepting Death

Why do we fear death?

Perhaps it is death that should fear the coming of man, for no other creature is more conflicted about having been alive. We have questions, demands, grievances, and concerns about those we've left behind: What did it all mean? Did I do it right? Am I to be punished or rewarded? Will someone else be made to pay for my death? Is there justice in the universe? Is there an afterlife or is there nothing but the absence of self-awareness? Am I supposed to do it again? Is there a heaven? Is there a hell? Were all my actions predestined and, if so, how can I be judged as I had no power to alter the course of my fate? How does it all end? Is there a god? Whose? Why do we have to die? Was life an accident? Is there life on other planets? How long do they live?

Many expect to be debriefed, but few are confident that they have accomplished the goals of their life's mission and so are rightly anxious about "judgment day." Helping our patients come to terms with the end of life requires that we step back from the religious and moral framework and consider what death represents to the human mind. For many, it means the end of something they hold dear, the loss of control and authority, and the raising of a wall between them and the people they know and love. If an entity, especially an unknown, threatened to do all this, why wouldn't we resist it?

Indeed, the human mantra has always been to oppose that which limits us, to soldier on, to be discontent with the status quo, and to sacrifice everything for a glimpse beyond the ridge. The myth of the indomitable human spirit is canonized in our oral history, literature, and film. A perfect example of this is found in the film *Monty Python and the Holy Grail* in which one knight is hacked to bits by another while suggesting that his missing limbs and the fountains of blood spewing from his forced amputations are mere "flesh wounds."[9]

Six. Go Gently into That Good Night (Death)

The not so subliminal message: We enter this world resisting the inevitable, bloody and helpless, why should we not exit it in the same manner? Even if you are nothing but a bloody torso, you should fight to your very last breath or, as the poet Dylan Thomas presumably begged his father, "Do not go gentle into that good night, ... Rage, rage against the dying of the light."[10]

In this, we see the denial stage of the model Elisabeth Kübler-Ross laid out for us in her 1969 book *On Death and Dying*, in which she outlines what she felt were the five emotional states a person travels through to achieve acceptance.[11] As she later clarifies, we do not move through these stages sequentially, nor are all required, but anger, denial, bargaining, depression, and acceptance do seem to be recurrent themes.

Imagine you're playing a four-person board game, and it is clear you will lose. Are you angry? Do you retrace your moves and look for where things went wrong? Do you blame the other players or the game? Do you overturn the board and scatter the pieces? A patient's anger at being given a terminal illness is justified and rational. They may blame the physician, the system, or even family members for something that no one could have predicted nor avoided. Indeed, in many cases, the etiology of a disease can be traced back to the individual's personal choices such as smoking or poor diet. The patient may perceive that a delay in diagnosis or treatment by a few days carries the same causal responsibility as the damage they've done to themselves over a lifetime. Expecting and absorbing this misdirected anger rather than resisting it requires that we understand how this stage plays into the Kübler-Ross model.

For depression, imagine a movie in which the main character sacrifices her life so that her family might escape some terrible fate. Would the audience be satisfied if the film ended abruptly when the heroine died? They should. What happens to the supporting characters is immaterial to the main character's story. Yet, if the film stopped the minute she took her last breath, the critics would demand their money back and label the rendition as "pointless." Consider how much better the story might be received if the director showed how the mother's choice helped save her children and thereby altered the course of human history. Suddenly, we feel her life had meaning, and her death was justified. Why? Would her life have been more or less significant if her children died despite her choice? Was her death more or less justified because it became a big-budget movie? This is a hard perspective for the living to grasp as we will forever be the audience and so take up the position of the critic. For the soon-to-be-deceased, it feels like they are being sent home early from a packed movie theater. Anyone would want to know how it ends.

Returning to our board game, acceptance of death allows players to shift gears and use their resources to help one of the other players still in the game. This evolution of action, from selfish to altruistic, mirrors the perspective change we experience as we age and watch our children grow into adults. We begin to want to leave something behind, some wisdom or financial legacy, which will mark our existence and, in some way, contribute to our progeny's success. From an evolutionary standpoint, this makes perfect sense as it lends a selective advantage to that individual's line of DNA.

Technology has inserted itself into the denial and bargaining stages and so has become an almost insurmountable speed bump on the road to acceptance. The mind understands that if it can disprove the primary theorem, it is dying, it will not need to travel through the other stages, and so it is willing to expend a great deal of energy in denying reality. Promises of immortality, life extension, cryopreservation, and even biodome duplication make patients think there may be a way out, and so can delay, distract, and prevent them from enjoying the final stage of the Kübler-Ross model. As physicians, we need to be well informed about the stories our patients are being told so we can provide a scientifically-grounded argument against these distractions. As noted by a consensus article written by 51 of the world's leading aging researchers in *Scientific America*, "No currently marketed intervention—none—has yet been proved to slow, stop or reverse human aging, and some can be downright dangerous."[12]

Ask yourself this question: Is it better for a millionaire to spend her entire fortune prolonging her life by five years or to use the money to ensure her five grandchildren get a quality education and can lead productive lives?

Much of death is about perspective.

Immortality

Immortality means different things to different people. Christians believe that their soul is immortal. Buddhists believe their essence will be reborn repeatedly until it achieves enlightenment. Evolutionary biologists think our bodies are the machines that allow our immortal genes to propagate. Artists feel that their work will make them immortal. Martyrs trust their actions will earn them immortality. The unifying common denominator to all these concepts is that none try to convince followers that the physical body they currently possess will become immortal. Thus, the promise of immortality becomes a thought game in which the player must believe that there is more to them than flesh and blood. In his book *Immortality*, Stephen Cave breaks the narrative quest for immortality down into four key groups[13]:

I. **Staying Alive:** The idea that something like an elixir (the Fountain of Youth), science, a curse (vampirism), or some entity more significant than ourselves will allow us to continue on in our current bodies indefinitely.

II. **Resurrection:** The idea that despite having to experience death we will at some later point be brought back to life in another, the same, or a facsimile of our bodies.

III. **Soul:** The idea that there is something immaterial that exists outside ourselves that cannot die but continues in this ethereal state after our mortal death.

IV. **Legacy:** The concept of indirectly leaving behind some lasting afterimage of our lives in the form of familial reputation, art, literature, heroic deeds, or infamy.

As mentioned in the last section, we are influenced most by technology in the bargaining and denial phases of the acceptance process. As the narrative of staying alive meshes best with these, we see a great deal of patient interest in ways to prolong life by slowing down the aging process. In his book *Heavens on Earth*, Michael Shermer does a superb job of addressing the antiaging theories.[14] Additionally, he provides rational arguments as to why humans cling to these theories despite the discouraging evidence:

A. **The free-radical/mitochondrial theory of aging:** The idea that cellular respiration causes the buildup of oxidative free radicals that damage an organism's DNA by leaving it with an unpaired electron. The therapy being antioxidant supplements.

B. **Gene-regulation of aging:** The idea that cells age due to changes in the way genes are expressed later in life, either by having aging turned on or by repair mechanisms turned off, and so could be modified using genetic engineering or stem cell manipulation.

C. **The telomere theory of aging:** A theory that is based on the idea of the number of times a cell can successfully divide depends on the length of its telomere, which is foreshortened with cellular turnover and whose wearing out is slowed by the enzyme telomerase. Thus, lifestyles (plant-based and exercise rich) that promote telomerase may extend life.

D. **Engineered Negligible Senescence (SENS):** A research approach supported by Aubrey de Grey that focuses efforts on the seven aspects of our biology that lead to aging. As these seem to be a list of the bad things that cause aging rather than solutions, I'm not sure it stands on its own as an antiaging theory.

If we accept that stopping the body's aging process is far more challenging then we thought, perhaps we should focus on the most essential part of the body—the brain. In early 2018, Yale researchers announced that they had kept a decapitated pig brain alive for 36 hours.[15] The breakthrough was announced at the brain science ethics meeting at the NIH (National Institute of Health) in a bid for funding and ignited a firestorm of debate including if the technique could be used on humans. If it could, wouldn't the individual quickly develop a psychosis from the complete sensory deprivation? If the brain were kept sedated to counteract this, would people elect to have their brains preserved for implantation in new bodies down the road instead of their current practice of cryopreservation? Keeping in mind that there is no evidence we will be able to transplant a human brain anytime soon, Professor Sestan has used his technique on hundreds of pigs and sees no reason it couldn't be successful on larger animals such as primates. Predictably and rightly, Dr. Sestan and others are now seeking ethical guidelines under which to continue their work.[16]

Death Is Not Our Enemy

Death is not our enemy or that of our patients. Death is as much a part of the cycle of life as birth and if more of us addressed it this way it might be better managed. Pregnant women are given due dates, asked to develop birth plans, and attend Lamaze classes with their partners to prepare for the delivery date. They talk to other pregnant women, share their anxieties and concerns openly, and understand that even when one adjusts for every contingency not everything will go according to plan. There are smooth births, and there are ones that require medical personnel and interventions to avoid complications. Why don't more of us treat death the same way? To be sure, we've improved. Many patients have durable powers of attorney, have documented their code status, and know that both hospice and palliative care services are available. Our society may not yet be ready for classes titled "What to Expect When You're Dying" or having an estimated death date stamped on our charts, but thanks to technology, these things may not be that far off.

Imagine a death-day app that monitored your vitals, knew your medical conditions, medications, diet, family history, recent labs, exercise routine, geographic area, stress levels, sleep patterns, marital status, alcohol intake, smoking history, gender, race, and telomere length based on a mouth swab you sent into the company. With this information, such an app could make a relatively accurate prediction as to the year, month, and day of your death. Lifestyle modifications such as taking up running might push the estimated date into the future. A broken hip might accelerate the countdown. Putting aside the storm of legal issues such a tool would incite (people who committed

Six. Go Gently into That Good Night (Death)

suicide rather than reaching their end date or gave away all their possessions but didn't die), this type of feedback might entice people to lead healthier lives. It would also act as a reminder that none of us lives forever and discussions about death should not be as awkward as they are now.

There would need to be laws in place to make it illegal for businesses and insurance companies to discriminate against people based on the app's estimated death date, but we wouldn't be able to regulate inevitable social interactions. Would you date someone who might die 20 years before you? Would there be more gold-digger marriages where the spouse knew they would get a payout in a matter of months rather than years? Would we elect an official who might not be able to finish their term? Would people try to make their EDD (estimated death date) come sooner on purpose to see how close they could come to death before changing their behavior? Could someone hack your app and make you think you were going to die sooner than the unmolested algorithm estimated?

What if this same app were found to be accurate and someone decided they didn't want to go through all the pain and suffering usually associated with the end of life? Currently, five states and Washington, D.C., have death with dignity statues.[17] In California,[18] a patient may medically end their life when they have a terminal illness that will end their life in six months. How would an approaching EDD be any different? Do our patients have the right to die?

Dr. Philip Nitschke thinks we do and has built a "death machine" to help us.[19] In a recent article, he said that "if we are talking about a good death," referred to by the Greeks as "euthanasia," then why isn't this the goal for all of us? Why do you have to be terminally ill (i.e., almost dead) to die with dignity? The Sarco is a self-contained capsule that asphyxiates its occupant using liquid nitrogen to bring down the oxygen levels after a series of failsafe buttons are voluntarily pressed. The process is proposed to take about a minute, and Dr. Nitschke wants to make it available to anyone over 50 via his nonprofit organization Exit International.

Thus, do we take one step closer to the euthanasia practices portrayed in the dystopian film *Soylent Green*?[20]

Since the time of writing this, I've discovered that something similar to the death app I describe above has been developed: It's called Deadline.[21]

My Thoughts

I think philosophers disguise themselves as fiction writers so they can create worlds for the concepts they wish to explore with their readers. Baring this in mind, I'll share an excerpt from the science fiction novel I'm writing called *The Juncture*. In this scene, Turtle Beowulf, a police officer in a society in which humans have achieved immortality by transferring their minds into new bodies (fluxing), reflects on the teachings of his Graydu—a Nar Van Master—who wants his students to reject this process.

> Consider, suggested the Graydu, how much fun it had been to play tag as children. It was one individual against impossible odds, against everyone else, and yet the game felt right, perfect. It didn't matter who was "it" at any one time. It was the game that counted, and everyone had a role to play. Now, imagine what would happen if the child who was "it" decided they were too special to continue playing the game. They wanted to be "it" forever because they were better than everyone else. The conflict was gone, and the game died.
>
> This same sense of self-importance was what made humans think they should live forever. Fluxing wasn't a way to fight death. It was a way for individual humans to say they were too special to play the game of life.
>
> Whereas, Nar Van students understood that it was the game that counted and not the individuals who played it.
>
> Having been raised to want to extend his own life, to think this was the path to fulfillment, Turtle had struggled with his new mortality. Graydu Quiko sensed his distress and pulled him out of class. Together, they sat on the roof of building five and watched the stars twinkle through the cone. "You are upset."
>
> "Yes," agreed Turtle.
>
> "Do you know why people die, Van Beowulf?"
>
> "If everyone lived forever, we would run out of resources. Once a species reaches a certain population density, disease and violence kick in and knock off the weakest members of the group. Dying is nature's way of rotating the crop."
>
> The Graydu nodded, considering the answer. "Death keeps us humble. Knowing that life ends forces us to appreciate it, to respect it in all things. Without death, humans begin to think of themselves as gods. They become too important, too powerful, for the world ever to lose. Thus, any action they take to prolong their existence is justified. A coward's pride makes them run from death. A warrior opposes death by making every breath count."
>
> "I am not a coward."
>
> "I know," agreed the Graydu somberly. "You understand that life is conflict. To be alive, truly alive, we must oppose death instead of running from it. The fluxing process is designed to extend life indefinitely in the same way the child who is 'it' plans to make the game of tag last forever by not playing. But refusing to play defeats the purpose. We are meant to die because it is in opposing death that we learn to live."
>
> "So, we should fear death?"
>
> "Death is an alien place for the living for it is the absence of all opposition. It is absolute stillness and complete harmony. The dead have no pain, no suffering, no conflict because they are not alive. We should not fear that which we resist, but we must respect its power."
>
> "Our nature is defined by what we oppose."
>
> "Nar Van warriors see death as the ultimate opponent, the finest chisel with which to carve away the vanity, the sense of entitlement, and the pride that we all carry with us. What is left behind, the universal humility of life, is the essence of Nar Van."

Turtle nodded. This was the talk he needed, the scaffolding on which to hang his scattered misgivings. "I understand."

"You understand only the petal," said the Graydu with a gentle shake of his head. Reaching inside his robe, he withdrew a small black book and offered it to Turtle. The title read in deep gold letters: *The Art of Nar Van*. "But one day you will see the stem and know that all things have roots."

A Good Death

A good death will mean something different to every person, but we all want one. It should be painless, under our control, at a time of our choosing, and after we feel we have made a difference. Most would like to die in our home, surrounded by familiar people, smells, sounds, and material things. We want as much dignity as the process will allow. Helping our patients achieve these moving targets is a skill that takes time, empathy, and a widened perspective on what death means to each of our charges. As every birth is unique and unpredictable so, too, is the process of dying, but the experience can be a rich and fulfilling one if family and friends are willing to help.

Physicians are no longer found at the bedside of our patients at the moment of their deaths but instead receive a notice from hospice, the coroner, or from a loved one. Even if the patient's death is expected, smooth, and without incident, I would encourage every physician to call and speak to someone who was there, to express your condolences, and to answer any questions they might have about your patient's passing. As many patients as we have, as busy as our practice or day might be, as little contact as we might have had, we must remember this person and the family they have left behind have experienced one of the most monumental events of the cycle of life. It can be tragic, inspiring, humbling, and terrifying for those who observe it and providing them a venue outside of the immediate family to share their thoughts can be as informative for you as it is therapeutic for them.

I believe it is telling that the deathbed is the one place in medicine that you are least likely to find technology. Dying is a personal, intimate, and uniquely human activity. Ask any technology guru, Google executive, transhumanist, or Silicon Valley devotee this simple question, and you will see what I mean: Would you, on having taken your last breath, be more likely to reach for your cell phone or a loved one's hand?

When it comes right down to it, no computer will ever understand what it means to step onto Charon's boat.

Chapter Seven

Lawyers, Doctors and Lobbyists, Oh My (*Mala Praxis*)

Mala Praxis

The term "malpractice" sprung from the Latin term *Mala Praxis*, which was coined by Sir William Blackstone in 1768 and translates to "bad practice." Ironically, the word "practice" in laymen's terms suggests that one is not yet skilled at something and so is likely to make mistakes in gaining experience; ergo, it allows that the one acquiring this skill is not yet proficient in the art. However, in use, practice means the day-to-day application of the ability the physician has attained up to that point in their career and suggests that they should be behaving in a way that is like that of most of the people in their profession. Imagine if you went to a cobbler and paid for shoes only to be sent home with a pair of gloves. Would you go back to that professional? Most malpractice centers on the concepts of duty and negligence or the idea that a person in the profession has a responsibility to act in a socially appropriate way, and when they don't, they are negligent of their duties. Take a firefighter who kicks his feet up and watches the house across the street burn because he doesn't feel like putting the fire out.

With modernization, there was a cultural decline in religious fatalism. Gradually, the belief that all misfortunes were acts of God and predestined or retribution for a person's moral transgressions was replaced with the thought that the concept of determinism, in which human actions, either by the individual or those around them, caused outcomes. This then opened the door to the acting human to be accountable for their actions or, in the case of medicine, the doctor rather than God was to be held responsible for the poor outcome of surgery or therapy. The number of malpractice lawsuits rose accordingly with this shift in thinking, and so began a search for guidelines by which cases could be tried.[1]

The landmark English case that set up the framework for most of our litigation was the 1957 John Bolam incident in which a depressed patient was given electroconvulsive therapy without muscle relaxers, and the procedure left him with two broken hips.[2] The patient argued that he had not been informed of the risks or the option to have relaxers. The court ruled against Mr. Bolam as it said the burden of proof to show that something is not the standard of care lies with the claimants. About this, Kim Price reported in *The Lancet*[3] that "since Bolam, modern medical negligence law can be whittled down to three fundamental factors: one, confirming the patient was 'owed a legal duty of care' by the health practitioner who is the 'defendant' in cases of medical negligence; two, establishing that the defendant was in 'breach' of that duty of care in failing to reach the standard of care required by law; three, proving that this breach of duty caused or contributed to the damage or injury to the patient." The take-home point, although often forgotten, at the time was that if a physician broke a compact with a patient, but there was no or negligible injury to the patient, then there may not be a case for malpractice even if the patient is unhappy or the actions of the doctor appear grossly inappropriate. This was an important point to remember when negotiating treatment plans with patients as our refusal to provide something that was inappropriate but which the patient demanded because they believe they should have it may not have been considered malpractice. However, many believed that this case put too much power in the hands of the physician as the medical profession determined the standard of care. Recently, the Bolitho decision, again in England, showed a change in perspective as it allowed the jury or judge to decide if a physician's actions, or lack thereof, put the patient at unnecessary medical risk. Thus, the jury could decide in favor of the defendant if they felt the physician's actions were not reasonable or logical even if the doctor did what most in the profession would have done.

There has been a 56 percent decline in the number of paid malpractice lawsuits between 1992 and 2014, but the payout for each has increased by 23 percent, from $287,000 to $353,000.[4] Many think this change is due to tort reform that effectively capped the amount a claimant could win and so made malpractice suits less financially rewarding for lawyers. As discussed in a CBS News article, the most common claims, up to 63 percent of them, were due to missed diagnoses, cancer, and heart attacks which led to death.[5] In this same piece, Dr. Richard Anderson (CEO of the physician-run medical malpractice insurer The Doctor's Company) addresses the mixed message most physicians face: "You can't afford to be wrong and if you're only wrong once every 10 years or once in your career, we'll take you to court. But the second message is medical care is too expensive; we're ordering too many tests."

Indeed, as I'll mention in later sections, defensive medicine is one of the key reasons many doctors order superfluous tests. These tests can lead to complications, false-positive results, and the accruement of extraordinarily high medical costs to prove that there was nothing wrong in the first place. Additionally, tests ordered to pacify a patient or physician's anxiety rather than to evaluate a clinical concern can lead to symptom validation. This is where a patient assumes they were justified in presenting with a trivial complaint as the doctor responded to it by ordering an expensive test. Notwithstanding the reassuring results, the patient observes that the physician ordered a CT or MRI to rule out a brain tumor for the patient's complaint of a minor headache and so will feel justified in demanding similar definitive tests in the future.

So the question remains: Should the firefighter who hoses down a house because the occupant smelled smoke be held liable for the resulting water damage or should they choose to wait to see the smoke themselves and be held negligent for not acting soon enough to stop the fire from doing damage?

In either case, the firefighter's livelihood is at risk for a fire they didn't start, in a home they don't own, and for actions taken based on unverifiable complaints.

Welcome to modern medicine.

Sharks in the Water

Often forgotten or overshadowed by his impressive political contributions, Abraham Lincoln was a malpractice attorney. His most well-remembered case occurred in 1855 when he defended a doctor who had splinted rather than set the legs of a man who had a building fall on him as the physician did not think the man would live. When the disabled patient survived, he sued the physician for not adequately treating his fractures. The doctor lost the case in a lower court, but Lincoln thought he could win it on appeal. He didn't. One could argue that this was because Lincoln was spread too thin: He was running for the senate, debating Stephen A. Douglas, and defending two murder cases. But it is equally likely that no one could have won this case. The growing popularity of determinism in which people rather than fate was at fault for human suffering made defending malpractice cases that much harder.[6]

Indeed, as discussed in a well-written *JAMA* article by Dr. James Mohr titled "American Medical Malpractice Litigation in Historical Perspective," there had been an explosion in malpractice suits.[7] Although the direction of malpractice law in England was monitored, it wasn't until around 1840, with the relaxing of rules surrounding filing civil tort proceedings, that we saw an explosion of medical malpractice suits by American lawyers. Between 1840 and 1860, the cases heard by the state appellate courts rose by 950 percent. Initially, professionally-trained physicians saw malpractice litigation as a good thing as they thought it would discourage charlatans and quacks. This opinion quickly changed when they found that lawyers were predisposed to file cases against defendants, professional doctors, who had money to pay their clients.

Ironically, it was the physicians' own formalized training that put them at risk. The herbalists and holistic practitioners made no promises, had no standardization of practice, and generally sold a product (tea or a poultice) instead of a cure. Physicians' textbooks were used against them in court as were visible deformities, a foreshortened limb from a poorly healed fracture, which tended to sway juries and judges. Bear in mind that such injuries had led to amputations in the past and the disability was only evident because doctors had been trying to do more to save the limb. Dr. Mohr goes on to point out that many physicians found it easier to forgive patients' medical bills or settle out of court than to risk their professional reputation and security in a legal battle. This spilled blood, money, in the water and promoted even more predatory litigation in which doctors were sued for refusing cases or for procedures that were done decades earlier.

At the height of the malpractice lawsuits in 1847, a group of elite doctors founded the American Medical Association. This organization worked tirelessly to regulate, standardize, and license physicians to create a unified base of practice and a united front to defend its members against frivolous lawsuits. But how best to protect doctors against something that is hard to prevent, predict, or recover from once it occurred? Answer: Medical malpractice insurance entered the stage promising to pay for lost lawsuits and to protect individual doctors from going bankrupt if they lost.[8] Problem: Physicians had forgotten that money was the reason lawyers had gone after them, instead of the quacks, in the first place. Malpractice insurance created an ocean of cash and, not surprisingly, the sharks thrived.

Bad Medicine

Recently, Dr. Harold Bornstein admitted that the letter he released to the public in 2015 stating that "if elected, Mr. Trump, I can state unequivocally, will be the healthiest individual ever elected to the presidency" was dictated by the then-presidential candidate. Aside from the clear question of fraud, by both parties, the fact that we, the public, would believe a physician would say "his physical strength and stamina are extraordinary" of anyone is an indictment of the times.[9] Dr. Bornstein said he felt "raped, frightened, and sad" when Mr. Trump sent his henchman to forcibly retrieve documents from his office. These were Mr. Trump's medical records, but the way they were taken made the physician feel abused. Still, before we rush to his defense, Dr. Bornstein's admission to the press that Mr. Trump used Propecia for hair loss several days earlier was a breach of patient confidentiality and so a fair reason to end the relationship.[10] As one of the more visible examples of how far the pendulum has swung, we see that the doctor felt compelled to break his code of ethics in writing a misleading letter but was held accountable and fired the minute he tried to gain notoriety by providing the media with confidential information. Physicians are no longer running the show, and we haven't been for some time. Afraid of what our patients will say on Yelp, on surveys sent to their homes, to potential clientele they meet, and on social media sites to friends and family, some thin-skinned personalities would sooner cave than say no. Abusive patients know this and will go doctor shopping to find someone they can bully or coerce into giving them pain medications, work notes, and legal documents.

This abuse happens from the other side of the table as well. Recently, the idea of "paying for performance" has gained popularity in the reimbursement venue. In this model, doctors are encouraged to get their patient's cholesterol or blood pressure under control and so may be enticed to prescribe medications to produce these results even if they know that promoting diet, exercise, and weight loss would be the best option. In this, we can see the hand of technology and data points. There is no easy way to bill for the 15 minutes a physician spends talking about low-fat diets, but starting medication and seeing a patient's cholesterol levels drop on the next test is something we can plug into our pie chart. A physician risks her bonus at the end of the year or having her salary docked if her patients' scores don't meet the arbitrary guidelines her employer sets.[11]

It's important to remember that doctors are people. Most physicians want to help our patients lead healthy, successful lives, but many also want our patients to like us, and we all have bills to pay. It is not uncommon for a physician to find themselves at the middle of a three-way tug-of-war between what their patients want, what the statisticians demand, and what they feel is the best clinical approach. If this weren't enough, there are those who add in the element of personal gain, and in these cases the stage is set for them to be drawn and quartered.

Sadly, there are bad people out there, and some of them are doctors.

In this, I am grateful that we have a legal system and lawyers dedicated to getting rid of these criminals.

The USA Gymnastics doctor, Larry Nassar, sexually abused hundreds of young girls and was sentenced to 40–175 years in prison.[12] Dr. Sundiata El-Amin was convicted of running a "pill mill" where he wrote hundreds of thousands of prescriptions for oxycodone, often without ever examining his patients.[13] Salomon Melgen, the highest billing doctor (2008–2013), was recently sentenced to 17 years for Medicare fraud and ordered to pay back $42.5 million to the government.[14] Harold Shipman is suspected to have killed more than 200 patients over 27 years using diamorphine to earn the title of Britain's worst serial killer, or "Doctor Death," before he hung himself while in prison in 2004.[15] Unfortunately, this list goes on and on. In the United States, a fair comparison would be Dr. H. H. Holmes who built his Chicago home with secret passageways, fake walls, and trap doors.[16] There was a hidden lab in the basement where he did dissections on the young women he gassed with pipes that led to the rooms he rented out. He sold many skeletons to local medical schools, and the remains of more than 200 victims were discovered on his property. Erik Larson paints a haunting description of Dr. Holmes's life and crimes in the *Devil in the White City*.[17]

Although these are exceptional examples of abuses of the doctor-patient relationship, they serve to remind us why the adage "Trust no one" still exists.

Money Talks, Doctors Walk

In a telling Medscape report for 2017, 89 percent of 4,000 responding doctors who had recently been sued felt the suit was unwarranted. Forty percent took more than three years to close, 30 percent were settled before the trial, and nearly 60 percent of physicians were encouraged or required to settle regardless of their feeling that the case was unjustified. Sixty-three percent of plaintiffs received more than $500,000 in compensation with 28 percent receiving more than $1 million. The result was that 32 percent of these physicians either chose to leave medicine (6 percent) or said they no longer trusted their patients[18] (28 percent). If we examine these numbers more closely, there seems to be a disconnect between a sense of wrong-doing on the part of the physician and what the courts and malpractice carriers were willing to pay out. Indeed, nearly 40 percent of the doctors would have done nothing different and yet were actively discouraged from having their day in court.

Why?

Money.

The medical malpractice litigation system is not so interested in justly assigning blame as it is in making sure the wheels, and palms of those involved, are well greased with money, from the lawyers who cherry-pick cases to the malpractice insurance companies who find it cheaper and easier to settle, as it also ensures their clients, the doctors, will see how important it is to have malpractice coverage in the first place. The system is broken. It's a bizarre feedback loop, a financial worm hole that survives and grows by swallowing its tail.

Lawyers promise their clients justice, compensation, and that the system will change.

It won't.

Why not?

Because no one is admitting fault. At the end of arbitration money is paid and the case is closed. This is despite nearly 90 percent of the doctors in the survey feeling their lawsuit was unjustified. In this report, one-third of the cases were settled before trial with 40 percent of the physicians unable to think of anything they would have done differently. The truth is that bad things happen, and our culture demands that the injured party receive some form of compensation. After all, we can't blame a higher power, and no one wants to point out that the plaintiff's smoking, genetics, obesity, and drinking contributed to the diagnosis the doctor was slow to catch, so let's sue; their malpractice insurance will cover the damages. Please note, I'm not saying that most of these cases don't have merit or shouldn't be prosecuted. I'm suggesting that the institutionalization of a litigious process where the primary focus is to produce money instead of retribution is unlikely to change behavior. The insurer writes a check, the lawyer takes their percentage, the doctor goes back to work, the patient remains injured, and the system keeps on chugging away.

Nothing changes.

Wait. I'm wrong. There is one change.

The malpractice insurance rates go up.

Defending the Castle

As disturbing as the structure of malpractice insurance is in the United States, a more significant problem is the defensive style of medical practice it induces. In a large-scale survey done by Jackson Healthcare in 2010, between 73 and 92 percent of physicians self-reported ordering tests and procedures, which may not have been clinically necessary, to protect themselves from lawsuits.[19] This equated to upward of $850 billion or up to 34 percent of our annual health-care costs in the United States. Simply put, one out of every four dollars spent in 2009 or $2.5 trillion in health-care cost was defensive. The practice of ordering tests to "rule out" something that they thought was unlikely was widely acknowledged as a way to quell the fear that they might miss something and be sued. Some might argue that it was profitable for physicians to order or perform these tests, but only 6 percent of the physician's income was found to come from the tests they ordered. Compared to private sector physicians, those working for the federal government practiced significantly less defensive medicine, as they felt protected by the Federal Tort Claims Act. "Under the Act, health centers are considered Federal employees and are immune from lawsuits, with the Federal government acting as their primary insurer."[20] Further evidence for how risk aversion induces defensive practices can be found by noting that physicians practicing in New Zealand, Canada, Sweden, and the United Kingdom are not subject to personal liability suits. According to the Jackson study, these physicians said they never ordered tests just to prevent a lawsuit.

If you're a physician, take a moment and consider a world in which you didn't feel compelled to order an ankle X-ray for a sprain, a CT scan for a minor headache, or rib films to prove there's a fracture when the lungs are clear and the therapy won't change. Imagine a system that didn't make you feel like you should order labs annually in a healthy person just because you might find something. Wouldn't it be nice not to feel like some lawyer is whispering sweet nothings into your ear as you evaluate an overweight smoker with diabetes, hypertension, and sleep apnea who wants a testosterone level? What about the smoker who has no symptoms but wants a chest X-ray to make sure they haven't developed cancer—yet? What about the middle-aged patient who wants a lumbar X-ray for four days of back pain with no radicular symptoms?

Thirty-nine percent of the physicians in the previously cited 2017 Medscape survey said that the fear of a lawsuit made them order tests that they might not need. Why? Don't we have systems in place, organizations like the American Medical Association that claim to lobby for physician rights? Yep, but only 7 percent of those surveyed felt that these groups were doing enough to reduce frivolous malpractice lawsuits.[21] If they didn't see it coming then how else can we protect ourselves but by practicing defensively?

There is another way to fight back.

Doctors have sued and won cases against lawyers who filed unjustified lawsuits. In an informative article published in the *Aesthetic Surgery Journal*,[22] a doctor must prove that:

1. The underlying malpractice lawsuit was filed not only without justification but maliciously.
2. The doctor won the case.

The author goes on to explain that "justification—in legal terms, *probable cause*—is based entirely on what the lawyer knew when the lawsuit was filed, not on what was later discovered. Malice is inferred from the absence of probable cause, and whether the doctor won—in legal terms, a *favorable termination*—depends wholly on the outcome of the case." What this means to me, keeping in mind that I'm not dispensing legal advice, is that if a lawyer files a claim without probable cause but only because they want to stir the pot and see what floats to the surface (even if they find something of interest) but then lose the case in court (not settled in arbitration), they may be liable for acting in malice against the physician or group and so guilty of false claims and responsible for the damages, both financially and emotionally, that these allegations caused the physician.

One of several examples given in the article describes how the lawyer of a patient who had a heart attack and fell and broke their shoulder, sued the hospital for having caused the break even though records showed that the patient arrived unconscious with the shoulder already broken. Another case involved a lawyer who lied about having spoken to a doctor knowledgeable about the case before filing the lawsuit.

Maybe if more lawyers found themselves defending their actions, proving that they had a real probable cause, they would think twice about frivolous litigation. More importantly, if physicians knew they could sue the plaintiff's attorney, they might be more prone to demand their day in court rather than settling cases they felt were unjustified. Could we take this a step further? What if we got rid of settling altogether? If every lawsuit had to be either dropped or tried, there would always be a winner or a loser. Lawyers who brought cases that were good enough to settle but not likely to win would run the risk of being sued if they lost and so would be more selective in picking cases. Physicians who lost lawsuits would have defended themselves on the stand and so might then try to be better doctors if they were shown to be wrong.

In such a world I suspect there would be fewer malpractice cases and so physicians would be less prone to order unnecessary tests "just in case." If we want to see the rising tide of our nation's health-care costs recede, we should start thinking of ways to reduce the need to practice defensive medicine.

Politics Is a Shell Game

If you've ever had the urge to understand how politics works, Steven Brill does an excellent job of walking his readers through the intricate steps involved in passing the Affordable Care Act in his book *America's Bitter Pill*.[23] I will warn you that some of the material is dry, factual, and mundane, while other parts involve juicy, underhanded, last-minute deals that will make your head swim. This is real reporting as it gives the reader the facts as they occurred, the cause-and-effect of concessions made to special interest groups, and, above all, a feel for how many greedy fingers are stuck in American's health-care pie.

A successful politician is like a magician in that they distract their audiences with one hand while magically making our money vanish with the other. Despite the incessant political rhetoric, Americans are not so gullible as to think elected officials are altruists. These are humans who know how to read people and manipulate systems so that they get what they or someone they work for wants. Humans can be duped, bribed, blinded by religious and moral platitudes, and threatened with public disclosure of previous indiscretions. They worry about losing their jobs, their power, and their social status. Such people are for sale.

Who buys, collects, and pulls strings in Washington? The lobbyists.

Were you ever curious about how much gets spent each year in Washington, by whom, and for what? Check out OpenSecrets.org.[24] In 2017, lobbyists spent $561 million "educating" our elected officials about how they should vote on health-care related topics. We live in a democracy where one citizen gets one vote, one chance to pick the person they feel best represents their views, while Washington lives in a democracy where campaign contributions and fancy lunches buy the buyer far more than a single vote. All this money must be influencing someone to do something for someone. Why else would special interest groups, physician and hospital factions included, funnel all that cash through these high-priced deal-makers? What about my vote or that of my patient? Do you think any politician would choose to sit down with me for lunch and a $25 donation when they could have a feast at a five-star restaurant and accept several hundred thousand dollars from a professional lobbyist?

American democracy is supposed to be one citizen, one vote? Good luck with that.

My Thoughts

It may feel like this chapter took a bit of a detour, but I believe that the law so strongly influences the actions of both the patient and physician that the excursion was valid. Laws were initially designed to address situations where there was malicious intent by one individual to harm another. Yet today, we find the offspring of these tools being used to punish well-intentioned individuals for circumstances over which they have had only limited influence. You could argue that a physician who is slow to diagnose a smoker with lung cancer failed in their duty, and so the patient suffered and died sooner than they might have if they had seen another provider. Currently, our law says that this doctor's delay in identifying the problem qualifies as negligence, and so the family of the deceased should be compensated and the physician punished with the loss of their license or probation. But this fails to acknowledge the causal nature of smoking. Each time the patient bought a pack of cigarettes, lit up, and inhaled, they were choosing to put themselves, and nearby family members, at risk by releasing known carcinogens into the air and into their bodies. Each time they chose not to stop the habit, they were accruing responsibility for the potential outcome—lung cancer—for which, when it eventually occurred, society says their physician should bear both financial and professional liability. Why wait for cancer? Why not sue the doctor the minute they fail to take the pack of cigarette or e-cigarettes away from the teenager who just started experimenting?

Humans like taking risks. We don't like taking responsibility for the consequences.

But smoking is addictive, it's hard to quit, and so it's not entirely up to the individual once they start. Nicotine receptors in their brains are being turned on, triggering deeply engrained neuropathways that are almost impossible to rewire.

Do you think the FDA would let me sell 1% milk produced by cows I'd genetically engineer to produce nicotine enriched milk? No. Why not? Milk is better than smoking. It contains calcium and vitamin D, so it helps prevent bone loss and subsequent hip fractures. The public's addiction to my 1% milk fat product would draw 2 % and whole milk drinkers away from the fattier alternative and so reduce obesity. The outcome would be "all natural" just like the genetically enhanced tobacco the smoking industry uses to double the nicotine in their plants as reported by *The New York Times*.[25]

I'm afraid it wouldn't fly.

Why not?

Seven. Lawyers, Doctors and Lobbyists, Oh My (Mala Praxis)   93

I don't have millions of dollars to spend on lobbyists and to throw at pliable candidates as campaign contributions. Granted, the amount spent lobbying on "old school" tobacco has declined from $72 million in 1998 to $6 million in 2019[26] due to the 1998 Tobacco Master Settlement Agreement.[27] But, this has been more than made up for by the $3.4 billion growth we've seen in e-cigarettes after Lorillard merged with Reynolds to make it the largest tobacco manufacturer in the United States and the leading seller of e-cigarettes.[28] Altria and Reynolds spent a combined $23.6 million lobbying between 2014 and 2015 with measures like that attached to the FDA funding bill at the last instant by senators like Tom Cole from Oklahoma, which exempt all e-cigarette products on the market from having to determine their effect on our public health. What about the laws against advertising cigarettes to adolescents? Sorry, they don't apply to e-cigarettes.[29] With two million American middle and high school students using addictive e-cigarettes in 2016 despite age restrictive laws, it's hard to see how this won't blossom into our next health-care crisis.[30]

Don't think I won't mention the silent monster "chillin'" in the closet—marijuana. Few people realize that one joint a day is equal to from five[31] to a pack[32] of cigarettes a day in lung cancer risk[33]—yet we've said this is okay in nine states and Washington, D.C.[34]—and there is a push for legislation to make it legal in all 50 states. The National Organization for the Reform of Marijuana Laws has donated more than $100,000 to our candidates to normalize its recreational use.[35] How is this even vaguely okay? Marijuana is an addictive, federally illegal drug, which has been shown to cause COPD, lung cancer, and actively rewire our children's brains[36] while destroying their ambition, and somehow, it's fine for our candidates to take money to make it legal.[37] What if there was an organization pushing for the legalization of methamphetamine? If we know that these inhalants cause cancer, that addictive substances started in adolescence are hard to quit, and that these things lead to emphysema and cancer later in life, why is this okay? We complain about high health-care costs caused by defensive medicine, spend billions of dollars screening for, treating, and researching ways to stop metastasis, but we refuse to look at the cause—money, profit, greed—and a political system that tolerates lobbyists who throw special interest money at our elected officials so they'll look the other way as our children "experiment" with increasingly accessible products that we know as adults destroy their chances at a healthy life.

At heart, I don't think our politicians are evil, stupid, or misguided. I think most of them make concessions, telling themselves white lies, so they can stay in office and push laws they feel will improve the overall quality of life for their citizens. They need money to do this, and the lobbyists are happy to provide. The politician who refuses contributions from groups they feel are morally corrupt will soon find themselves campaigning against well-funded opponents who did not share their qualms.

If we got rid of the lobbyists and kicked special interest groups out of Washington, if we (the public) paid attention to what our politicians said and held them accountable for delivering on their campaign promises, and if we voted, I think we could, as a nation, cut our health-care costs in half and improve our country's health within one election term.

Case Closed

In the 1800s, physicians thought malpractice lawyers might make the world a better place by chasing away the quacks. Instead, the lawyers went after the professional physicians' deeper pockets. Malpractice insurance succeeded by promising to reduce the risk that a physician would lose their home during a lawsuit. Instead, this led to a larger pool of money for the lawyers to salivate over. Lawyers began suggesting settlements through arbitration to avoid protracted court cases and the risk of damaging a physician's reputation. Instead, malpractice insurance went up, more people sued, and physicians began to practice defensive medicine. Health-care costs skyrocketed. Perplexed by the nuances of the health-care system, politicians turned to lobbyists to help educate them. Instead, special interests funneled money through these conduits to influence the laws in their favor. The 2005 RAND study we mentioned in Chapter One serves as an example of how far off track the promise of financial gain can lead us.[38] The study said that national adoption of the EMR would save us $81 billion annually. Instead, we now face a predicted $5.7 trillion health-care expenditure in 2026[39] as this overpriced billing machine transformed our doctors into an army of data entry clerks.

Trying not to cry over spilled milk, we acknowledge that technology isn't going away.

How can we use it to improve care and drive down costs?

As long as a physician follows what their network shows to be the algorithmic standard of care, mistakes will be less likely to happen. Physicians will not order tests they don't need because the computer will not suggest them and actions that deviate from the accepted algorithm would, by definition, not be the standard of care. Patients that want a test or procedure because they feel they need it could pay for it out of pocket, but a physician who refuses to order something would not be liable. Integrating Bolam and

Bolitho rules into every algorithm could thereby nullify malpractice lawsuits before they began.

Ergo, if we fully integrate algorithmic medicine into our system there would be no defensive medical expenditures and malpractice suits. If we apply the supposition that one out of every four dollars spent in health care is unnecessary, such a system will save us $1.43 trillion annually by 2026.

That's a lot of pocket change. We rush to mandate best practice algorithmic medicine to save lives and reduce costs.

As a result, we destroy the practice of medicine.

Why would a physician play a hunch, try an unproven medicine in a hopeless case, or even bother to think outside the box? Any attempt to deviate from an algorithm would put the physician and the organization they work for at risk. Predictably, the question will arise: If the physicians of the future will do little more than what the computer says, why will we need them?

We won't.

Thus, this book.

Chapter Eight

Medicine Is Dirty (Don't Bring It Home)

The Training Gauntlet

I was abused, and I still turned out to be a good doctor. To teach them how to cope with stress, we need to make student doctors' lives as miserable as possible. If we torture them enough in medical school and residency, only the ones who are smart and tough enough to handle the real world will graduate. It's for their own good. They need to be willing to put their family life aside during training because medicine should come before all-else. To mold them into doctors, we need to break them. Even a small mistake could kill someone. So, when they make a tiny mistake, we should make them feel like they did kill someone, so it never happens again. Training is hard, but this is the way it's done. Suck it up or quit.

This is just a small taste of what the culture of medical training was when I was going through it. As we will see, things are changing for the better, but we have a long way to go. In 1978 Samuel Shem (Dr. Stephen Bergman[1]) wrote *The House of God* to provide the public with a rare, if somewhat shocking, glimpse of what life was like for a doctor-in-training.[2] He went on to write the sequel *Mount Misery* about his time as a psychiatric resident.[3] Some of it is clearly fictionalized for public consumption, but we cannot ignore the nuggets of truth and the underlying cry for help.

I vividly remember doing morning rounds and being grilled relentlessly about every nuance of a patient's labs, symptoms, life outside the hospital, diagnosis, and treatment. It took me a while to figure out that the questions didn't stop until you didn't know the answer. You might have all the clinical information down pat, but if you weren't able to quote the journal article that supported your response, hadn't committed the textbook pathophysiology of the disease being treated to memory, or if you had neglected to write down the patient's aunt's second cousin's dog's name, you

Eight. Medicine Is Dirty (Don't Bring It Home)

were worse than pond scum. Why did you need to know this? Because your patient's life depended on it. Really? Most residents learned that no matter how hard they worked they would never know all the answers. Indeed, this malignant "pimping" is designed to publicly humiliate straight-A students in much the same way a marine drill sergeant might destroy their recruits' wills in boot camp before rebuilding them into Marines. On rounds, we're great at tearing down a student's dignity and confidence. What we tend to forget is the rebuilding part. Based on the Socratic method, this abusive style of teaching is far from what the great educator would have recommended.[4]

But, when intellectual bullying doesn't do the trick, we can rely on sleep deprivation to weed out the unworthy.

During my surgical residency, I was on call every third day or Q3. This meant I arrived at the hospital at 5 a.m. to pre-round, rounded with the chief, did surgery all day, did post-op checks, did ER admissions, ran to every code, put in central lines all night and assisted in emergency surgery all night, got maybe an hour of sleep, did pre-rounds and surgery all day with post-op checks before going home around 7 p.m. the next day after a 38-hour shift. I spent 10 hours at home, went back for a regular 14-hour day, had 10 hours at home, and then was on call again for another 38-hour shift. This meant I lived at the hospital, working 128 hours of the 168 hours in a week, was paid minimum wage, and diagnosed, operated on, and treated patients while extremely sleep deprived. Did this affect my competency? I remember holding a retractor during an open cholecystectomy and hallucinating due to lack of sleep that the gallbladder we were removing was a dehydrated apple with the face of an elderly woman who was smiling at me as we detached it. Happily, the surgery went well.

Did I say anything? Nope.

Changing to a family practice residency the next year, I was on call every fourth night, which was significantly better, but weekend calls, with me as the only professional in the clinic in the backwoods of Barre, Massachusetts, went from Friday morning until Monday night or 64 hours straight. Despite this, I will say that family practice was a more intellectually stimulating experience. Whereas surgical residents did an enormous amount of physical and procedural work, family practice demanded a better understanding of the "why" of things and this suited my personality better.

I will add that I loved both training experiences, learned more than I had at any earlier period in my educational life, and felt both programs prepared me well for my current practice. "Wait a minute," you'll say, "didn't you just finish telling us how terrible it was?" Yes, and yet it gave me the skills I still rely on to this day. This is why it has taken so long for the culture of physician training to change. Institutionalized abuse produces self-confident, well-educated doctors with thick skins who work well in emergency situations. In some, it also leads to physician burnout, suicide, being abusive toward others, and professionals who are continually looking for an escape hatch—a way to retire early or transition into an administrative position. Much like organized religion, members of our social construct are expected to regulate, treat, and reprimand its own members because no one on the outside world would understand what it is to be a physician. As we've seen time and again, this closed and secretive ideology lends itself to abuse and manipulation.

While I was in medical school I inadvertently became an intellectual threat to another student's ego. I don't remember the specifics, but she saw me as competition and so had the resident in charge of medical rounds, who I suspected she was sleeping with at the time, lie about my capabilities and recommend I repeat the class. This hurt not only my resume but also my confidence, social standing, and most certainly my educational trajectory. Within two weeks of the new session, my new chief resident and attending physicians voiced their dismay, as they found no defect in my knowledge base or ability. I could have gone to the dean and complained that I believed my fellow student's inappropriate relationship with my superior had influenced his judgment of my skills. Unfortunately, the cultural backlash of such an accusation would have been enormous. You didn't accuse anyone of letting their personal relationships influence their medical opinions, especially someone higher up the food chain. I would have been labeled a "whistleblower," and this would have damaged my chances of graduating further than retaking a class. A medical student's social and intellectual standing among their peers, the "rumor mill," was the first impression most evaluators had of you on rounds. If you were the social "runt" of the litter, it didn't matter how smart you were or how hard you worked to redeem your status; you were the punching bag, the target, and the weakest link. Welcome to our professional version of *Lord of the Flies*.

Not that I'm innocent of following in the footsteps of my predecessors. As a surgical resident, I grilled medical students until they cried. As a chief resident in family practice, I handed out impossible tasks to the interns and berated them when they couldn't finish in time. I subjectively evaluated and treated students based on what I'd heard from the "rumor mill." Abuse begets abuse but that doesn't make it right, and I am sorry and do apologize to anyone who felt I was unfair or too harsh.

I was wrong.

In 1998, the Libby Zion law was passed in New York State in response to the death of an 18-year-old while under the care of what the family believed to be an extremely overworked resident physician.[5] This groundbreaking law limited the number of hours a resident or intern could work in the hospital to no more than 80. In July 2003, the Accreditation Council for Graduate Medical Education (ACGME[6]) passed regulations that similarly limited the work hours of all physicians in training throughout the United States.[7] I commend ACGME for their work and recommend anyone reading this book to visit their website as they are strong advocates of physician rights and patient safety with protocols in place to report and have abuses corrected. However, not everyone follows their mandates as is exemplified in their follow-up assessment of the Libby Zion hour restriction. In surveying training programs in 2016, they found many had not fully implemented their restrictions and even more had excuses as to why doing so would harm both the physician's education and the patient's safety.[8]

Rules only help if they are enforced, and it is nearly impossible to change a system that produces a profit (see Chapter Nine).

Thus, we need more people who are willing to point out injustices.

This is our profession, our calling, and we will only fix it when enough people agree that we are living in an abusive home with damaged parents and younger siblings who don't need to suffer the "training" we endured to be fantastic doctors.

Dividing Up the Family

Hippocrates felt all diseases originated in five basic groups, and it was the physician's job to figure out which ones. How different is this from our modern predilection to send patients to different specialists: joint aches go to rheumatology; cardiovascular issues go to cardiology; strokes go to neurology; anxiety goes to psychiatry. By compartmentalizing medicine we have developed experts who are infallibly well trained to take care of one part of our patients but often neglect to see or feel ill trained to take care of something outside their scope of training. Should a dermatologist prescribe blood pressure medications? Should a cardiologist perform a prostate exam? Should an oncologist deliver a baby? Would you like your radiologist to treat your child's sore throat?

Why not?

All these physicians went to medical school. They are doctors and by rights could do these things. In fact, they can legally do all of them as long as nothing goes wrong. However, if there is a poor outcome, we hit them with malpractice lawsuits and rebuke them for stepping outside the lines we've drawn in the sand. How dare they take care of or address a problem that isn't in their "field."

Rather than suggesting that our gynecologist begin doing brain surgery, I'm pointing out that the most effective thing abusers can do is isolate their victims. They are told they are different, "special," in some way and so they deserve accolades but must, in turn, be willing to make sacrifices. When they point to someone else and complain that they have it easier or harder, they are told that it isn't a fair comparison because they're different.

We are all physicians. We all want our patients to receive the best care possible.

Yet we have a different medical association for each subspecialty. They lobby against one another to gain funding, beneficial laws, and social standing in much the same way children might fight to win their parents' favor rather than realizing that they should be working together to escape an unhealthy environment. Every dictator knows that the easiest way to stay in power is to encourage your citizens to fight each other while you go about your business unnoticed.

In this, technology may provide us with an advantage as it allows for open and uncensored dialogue on the Internet and within group practices. More and more physician bloggers are standing up and calling foul. Today, some of the most dissident voices are: KevinMD.com,[9] Dr. Wes,[10] and Rebel.MD.[11]

Testing the Monkey

So, you want to be a doctor?

You love helping people. You're intelligent, relatable, compassionate, and dedicated to the craft. Your interpersonal skills are solid and you don't mind long hours as long as you're doing something meaningful. You can think on your feet and tend to be the calmest one in the room during an emergency. You have excellent pattern recognition and can spot a funny looking skin cancer across the room. You need no more than four hours of sleep to perform well. You're good with your hands and have no problem with blood, cutting, or giving bad news in the most empathetic way possible.

Terrific. I'm so happy for you.

Now, here's the crucial question: How good a test-taker are you?

Planning for Medical School

Undergraduate degree: 4 years
Average total cost: $25,000–$50,000[12]

- Biology, chemistry, physics with some medical schools also requiring calculus, English, biochemistry, and psychiatry. Having a 4.0 GPA in these classes keeps you in the running, but it is not enough.
- MCAT—on average taking more than 300 extra-curricular hours to prepare for and with the need to score at least 500 out of 528 to be competitive. How important is your score? If you have a perfect GPA and a 500 you will have 74 percent acceptance rate. If you get a 490, it will drop to 9 percent.[13]
- Demonstration of health-related field work: volunteering, shadowing doctors, and research projects.
- A personal statement describing why you want to be a physician.
- Apply to the American Medical College Application Service (AMCAS[14]).
- Get stellar letters of recommendation.
- Nail the interview.
- Have a willingness to take on enormous debt—according to the American Medical Student Association 86 percent of graduates finish with debt ranging between $150,000 and $350,000, which is 4.5 times higher than was reported in 2003.[15]
- Be emotionally stable with 50 percent of students experiencing burnout and 10 percent having suicidal ideations.[16]

Planning for Residency

Medical School: 4 years
Average total cost: $150,000–$350,000
Average total 4-year income if not attending medical school: $230,000[17]

- Pass the three steps of the United States Medical Licensing Examination.[18] Scoring well means the difference between matching and not matching at all. More than at any other part of your career, this is a numbers game.[19]

   Step 1: tests basic concepts and principles of science and takes a full day or 8 hours.

   Step 2 CK: tests the student's ability to apply medical knowledge to clinical problems: takes a full day.

   Step 2 CS: tests the student's clinical skills on standardized patients in the office setting.

   Step 3: is a two-day test designed to assess both clinical knowledge and judgment through written and patient case simulation evaluations

and you may not sit for it until you've received a medical degree from your school.
- Registration with the National Resident Matching Program which matches applicants with hospital residency programs.
- Gather letters of recommendation, do research in your field of interest, write a personal statement, revise your curriculum vitae, and achieve a solid Medical Student Performance Evaluation[20] that is written by your dean of student affairs in collaboration with faculty members.
- Decide what type of medicine you want to practice for the rest of your life.
- Go to interviews at the different programs you're interested in to ensure both the people and location match your personality.
- Ensure eligibility for the Supplemental Offer and Acceptance Program so that you can scramble for a position if you are unmatched.[21]
- Apply for a Medical License and DEA approval for the state within which you'll be practicing.

Planning for Employment

Residency Program: 3–7 years
Average annual income: $52,000[22]

- Complete an accredited residency program.
- Decide if you want to enter the workforce or do a fellowship. Start the fellowship application early.
- Network with friends, family, and faculty to find a position.
- Have an active or pending application for a medical license in the state you want to practice.
- Have no lawsuits against you.
- Be proficient with your local EMR.
- Make sure you have malpractice tail coverage for when you transition to your new position.
- Have letters of recommendation from the faculty at your program.
- Have an idea of where you want to establish yourself long term: You've likely been jumping around the states for the last 12 years. Where you land this time might be permanent so don't sign the first job offer that comes your way. You've put in your time. You finally have the power to negotiate. Don't sell yourself short. Consider getting help looking over the contract that comes with the offer.
- Study for and pass your boards. This is not a given. The pass rate has dropped from 90 percent in 2009 to 78 percent in 2013.[23]

Planning for Retirement

Average Time in Active Practice: 36 years[24]
Average annual income: $217,000–$316,000[25]

- Join the ranks of the more than one million doctors (active and retired) in the United States.[26]
- If you didn't pass your boards, pass them soon or your program may not offer you a permanent position.
- Expect to perform 3,500 office encounters a year if you are primary care and 2,700 annually as a specialist with visits ranging between 13 and 16 minutes.
- Forty percent of active physicians work evening and weekend hours.
- Learn the local EMR.
- Make it through the first three to five years of probation designated in most practices before you're offered a full partnership.
- Try not to overspend. It's hard to resist the temptation to buy the car, house, clothes, and lifestyle all your friends have accumulated while you've been in school. They don't have your debt. You make a lot and you owe a lot. Trust me and live below your means and you will have far more control of your life in the future.
- Pay back your student loans as quickly as you can.
- Stay current with your CME.
- Protest the corrupt Maintenance of Certification tests—see Chapter Nine.[27]
- Find something outside patient care and your family life that validates your personal identity. I write. Your reading keeps me sane.
- Save and invest for retirement. Average retirement age is about 65 years.[28]
- Buy a home, put the kids through college, pay medical insurance, try not to get sued, save lives, and get used to hypocrisy.

Cannon Fodder

So, it's not so easy to become a doctor.

But at least once you've got your degree, state license, and DEA number, you'll have the respect of your patients and colleagues.

Nope. You've got to earn that.

New physicians entering the workforce are generally placed on probation and monitored closely by patients, peers, and administrators. Despite all the challenges up until this point, the rigor of study and practice, they remain the new kid on the block. Make one mistake and your knowledge base will be questioned. Make a recommendation to an established physician's patient that contradicts their practice style and you've made a potential enemy for life. Fail to see patients fast enough, document things well enough, meet practice guideline mandates, or keep your patients happy and you're on notice.

What's the easiest way to keep patients happy? Give them what they want. Why do we want satisfied patients? Medicine is a business, and the consumer is always right.

Wait.

I thought medicine was an art, a calling, and don't we have an ethical mandate to do the right thing?

Yep. Good luck with that.

It's hard to do the right thing, to say no, to upset the people around you by pointing out problems. It's even more difficult when you're the new kid on the block, which is sad as your fresh outside perspective could be transformative for a clinic stuck in its ways.

So, you've decided to put your foot down and refused to prescribe chronic pain medications to a drug-seeking patient with a positive drug screen for methamphetamines. He writes a scathing critique of your medical skills and sends it to your member service department, threatens to sue, and starts following you on social media. You begin seeing him hanging around your car at the clinic. He won't leave your panel even though you've made it clear he needs to be in drug treatment before you'll consider refilling his medications.

You complain to your superiors and are told everyone has patients like him. It's the job.

He suggests he knows where you live. Your heart races anytime you get a message from him or see him on your schedule. He glares at you during office visits. He says he hopes at some point in your life you feel pain like his so you'll know what it's like to suffer.

You make sure security is around nearly every time he visits the clinic.

You don't want to escalate things. It'll make it look like you don't know how to handle your patients.

New doctors are targets for drug seekers, psychiatrically demanding, and high-maintenance patients. These individuals know how to manipulate the system, how to bully physicians, and what to say to get what they want. They know how vulnerable you are, and they will use this against you.

The best advice I can give you: Don't give in to them. Word gets out very quickly within this community as to who is an easy target. If you bend the rules for one, you'll suddenly have 20 of them. Defend your practice style, the things you will and will not do, and in five years your panel will have self-

Eight. Medicine Is Dirty (Don't Bring It Home)

adjusted to carry patients who know how you work. Give in and you'll forever have the patients no one else wants.

"But," your compassionate mind will say, "someone needs to take care of them. They have real issues."

This is true, but they also need to have limits set and understand that there are basic rules and behaviors that will not be accepted in a professional setting—by anyone. If they find someone who gives them what they want when they act up, they will never change.

Keep in mind that this problem is not unique to new physicians. Take the recent case in Indiana where Dr. Todd Graham refused to give inappropriate pain medications to a woman only to have her husband return two hours later with a semiautomatic weapon and murder him in the parking lot.[29]

The dark secret few physicians admit to in public is how patients abuse us.

A 2017 survey of more than 800 U.S. physicians found that 59 percent had heard offensive remarks about their character in the last five years. These remarks were directed at their youthfulness, gender, race, religion, weight, and ethnicity. Nearly half of the patients who made these comments changed doctors because of their biases. Perhaps more concerning is that 51 percent stayed and may allow their prejudice to taint the advice their physician provides in the future.[30] Physicians have unconscious biases toward their patients, but it goes both ways.

As reported in the *New England Journal of Medicine*, between 2011 and 2013 there were annually 24,000 reported workplace assaults with 75 percent of them occurring in the health-care setting.[31] These altercations, directed against both physicians and nurses, included violent crimes such as assault, stalking, rape, and homicide, with the most common complaint being verbal abuse. Yet the medical culture remains one where we are expected to turn the other cheek. Our patients are at their lowest point. They are afraid, angry, grief-stricken, and poorly informed. We must forgive them for acting out. Besides, abuse is a part of the job, and the law will always side with the patient.

Not true.

These are excuses. The author of an article in *NEJM*, Dr. James Philips of Harvard Medical School, told Reuters Health that "our Industry is, statistically, the most violent non-law-enforcement industry in the United States." He goes on to write, "One reason health-care providers are reluctant to report these is that we have compassion for our patients, and we don't want to treat patients like criminals or the enemy. So we make excuses when we shouldn't, and we overlook patients who are intoxicated or on drugs, and other patients who have altered mental status because of chronic dementia or acute delirium.[32]"

Despite the documented escalation of violence, little is being done to protect health-care providers. Indeed, there are no federal rules explicitly protecting workers from violence. Recently, state laws, many pushed by the American Nurses Association, have been passed in California, New York, Illinois, and New Jersey that requires employers to take prevention measures.[33] While helpful, what may be more useful are laws such as Bill 1219, which unanimously passed in the Pennsylvania House of Representatives and makes assaulting a health-care worker a felony instead of a misdemeanor.[34]

That's one state out of 50.

Abuse is abuse; there is no excuse.

We need to do more.

We need federal rules designed to protect the people who have devoted their lives to helping others.

Quitting Life

There are approximately 400 physician suicides a year. In men, this is twice as many as the general population. In women, it's almost three times more than the average.[35] The methods used are typically drug overdose, hanging, and firearms. The incidence of suicide among family members left behind is increased, and every year nearly one million patients are left without a doctor due to suicide.[36]

Most patients will never know why they've been assigned to a new physician.

In her thoughtful and timely book *Physician Suicide Letters—Answered*, Pamela Wible, MD, reviews the hazing, bullying, and abuses young and senior physicians experience in training and practice. Recognized for her work by the American Medical Student Association and colleagues, she has forced open the can of worms no one has wanted to acknowledge until now.[37]

According to a 2018 investigative report conducted by Medscape, physicians now have the highest suicide rate of any profession with 4 out of every 10,000 doctors ending their life by their own hand. This is double the national average and even higher than the military.[38]

Many point to depression, substance abuse, unrecognized mental illnesses, and a fear that by asking for help physicians and students will identify themselves as unworthy, weak, or unhirable. It is doubtful that our medical student selection process is so twisted that we are inadvertently choosing candidates who have a predilection for suicide. Indeed, just the opposite is often the case. Medical student inductees are well-adjusted, high-functioning, intelligent, empathetic, goal-oriented, diligent youngsters who know their profession demands they make sacrifices for the good of others. They know the path will be hard, that some lose hope and commit suicide, but they never think it will be them. They are stronger, smarter, and more well-rounded than those who have come before them. They will do better.

Every single doctor who killed themselves must have thought the same way. Why else would they have signed up?

Medicine changes you.

The training, sleep deprivation, abuse, sense of powerlessness, responsibility, and the secret knowledge that they are fallible, transform some of our enthusiastic young recruits into depressed alcoholics with active suicide plans.

In initiating therapy, technology may come to the rescue as recent studies have shown that mobile health apps were effective for serious mental illness.[39] As many medical students and professionals are worried that their depression or mood issues will affect their career path, the autonomy of this approach holds a great deal of appeal. With time, they might then be comfortable enough to ask for more substantial help with a trained human therapist.[40]

The National Suicide Prevention Lifeline number is 1-800-273-8255. Please call right now (not later—put down this book and call) if you need help or visit their website www.suicidepreventionlifeline.org.

Before taking off, flight attendants will explain that should the cabin lose air pressure the adult passengers should put the oxygen masks on themselves prior to helping their children.

A two-year-old will not know how to help their unconscious mother.

We must help ourselves first if we hope to help others.

You don't need to feel this bad.

Call: 1-800-273-8255.

The Sterile Glass Ceiling

Even though females make up nearly half of all the medical students in the United States, those entering the workforce, irrespective of the field, may face an approximately $17,000 pay gap when compared to their male counterparts. According to a 2011 article in *Health Affairs*, this gap is more massive than it was in 1999 when the gender divide was only $3,600.[41] In the past, this gap was said to be due to women choosing jobs in traditionally lower paying fields like primary care in hopes of having a more flexible lifestyle. Newer studies show a shift in this trend with just 30 percent of women entering primary care in 2008 compared to 50 percent in 1999.[42] Yet the gap seems to have widened.

In 2018, Doximity surveyed 65,000 U.S. physicians from more than 40 different specialties and found that female doctors earned $105,000 less annually than their male equivalents with female physicians earning nearly 30 percent less than male physicians across all specialties.[43] What about academic medicine? Teaching institutions that run courses designed to help young female doctors negotiate for better pay, where lectures are given supporting gender equality, must have better numbers than those in the general workforce. Sorry. A 2016 article published in *JAMA* showed staggering evidence that even after accounting for specialty, rank, research publications, and clinical revenue, women were paid substantially less.[44]

There's more to it than the money. Only 13 percent of department leaders at the top 50 NIH funded medical schools in the United States were women in 2015.[45] There is a pattern of women being passed over for academic awards[46] both here and abroad where *The Lancet* reports only one in ten awards are given to women.[47] Only 34 percent of research papers published in high impact medical journals (*BMJ, JAMA, The Lancet, NEJM*, etc.) listed a woman as the first author.[48]

As disappointing as these findings are to see, technology makes it easier to track down and illuminate the problem. Groups like the American Medical Women's Association are leading the way, and I recommend everyone review and join their fight for equality.[49]

Mamas, Don't Let Your Babies Grow Up to Be Doctors

Current projections show that there will be between 42,600 and 121,300 shortfalls in overall physicians by the year 2030 with 14,800–49,300 of those being in primary care.[50] This is due in part to the aging population with growth in this demographic to reach 50 percent by the study's endpoint. If we expect most active primary care physicians to have panels of about 2,300, somewhere in the range of 34 and 113 million patients in the United States will not be able to find a doctor—because there won't be one.

Current physician burnout is at an all-time high jumping from 45 percent in 2011 to 55 percent in 2016 according to a Medscape survey of nearly 16,000 doctors.[51] A 2017 survey by Ipsos Public Affairs, found that 83 percent of physicians feel they don't have enough time to spend with their patients and end up writing scripts or placing referrals so that they can move on to the next person (54 percent).[52] These same physicians admit that 87 percent can't keep up with all the medical advances and research and 76 percent don't get enough sleep because of time constraints and stress.[53]

Is it any wonder that surveys consistently reveal physicians would not recommend a career in health care and would not do it over again themselves?[54]

What about the money?

I suggest you run the numbers. It can take more than two decades to pay off our medical school loans and even then many of us are still writing checks.

We'll talk more about this in the next chapter.

My Thoughts

A Doctors' Bill of Rights

On November 10, 1999, the first Doctors' Bill of Rights Act HR3300 was introduced to Congress, but it was never enacted.[55] A second attempt was made in 2012 by Dr. Elson Hass but failed. It has been nearly 50 years since the Patients' Bill of Rights was introduced in 1973. Why don't we have a compendium of our own? We are mistreated by our mentors and the institutions where we train. We are second only to the police in our exposure to violence and experience the highest suicide rate of any profession.[56] Physical and verbal abuse directed at us by belligerent patients only qualifies as misdemeanors in 49 states. Those of us that are female or minority are underpaid, poorly represented in leadership positions, and rarely acknowledged. We are on the verge of having decades of hard-earned skill and knowledge transformed into computer algorithms designed to increase corporate profit and efficiency.

It's not right, and I'm not alone in saying we need to fight for our rights. Dr. Elson Hass,[57] Dr. Michele C. Parker,[58] Dr. Erika L. Adler,[59] Dr. Elliot Abemayor,[60] Dean Sittig, PhD,[61] and many more have written versions of what they feel constitutes reasonable demands. I reviewed these and many others, studied the concepts and concerns, and drafted what I think maybe a concise, fair, and inclusive list to act as a starting point for negotiations.

THE DOCTORS' BILL OF RIGHTS

All physicians should be guaranteed the following freedoms:

1. To form a union (see Chapter Nine).
2. To enact laws and policies that limit the number of safe hours a physician can be expected to work with financial penalties levied for noncompliance on teaching, private, and institutions providing health care.
3. To receive rightful and prompt reimbursement for services rendered.
4. To utilize human-centric EMRs designed to improve real-life clinical

workflow rather than data-centric ones geared toward optimizing billing or administrative data collection.

5. To modify schedules to reflect the nearly 40 percent increase in time required for data entry, telemedicine patient management (emails, texts, digital consultations), and coding.

6. To sue lawyers or law firms for false or unfounded litigation filed against them.

7. To be informed prior to any digital recordings being made of the physician and have the right to refuse such a record being made, used, or posted on social or other public media sites.

8. To earn equal pay for equal work irrespective of gender, race, or educational pedigree with income transparency.

9. To be treated with respect and as a professional by patients, colleagues, and administrators.

10. To work and train in an environment that does not tolerate abuse, physical or emotional, and takes steps to separate the parties and reeducate perpetrators with no recrimination against those who bring charges.

11. To be judged on clinical abilities rather than on patient surveys.

12. To end a relationship with a patient who is abusive, manipulative, or deceitful or whose willful lack of compliance is likely to result in legal or material action against the physician by the patient's surviving family or representative.

13. To treat a patient in what they feel are the best interests of the patient rather than the demands of the physician's employer, the patient, or a third party.

14. To only be required to perform professional maintenance tasks or take recertification exams that have been statistically proven to benefit patient care and that are administered by non-profit organizations that behave as non-profits.

15. To work as a solo or small-group practitioner in a community where larger group practices or institutions are not allowed to use economic pressure, negative advertising, or selectively restrict access to care or services to undermine the provider's ability to maintain a sustainable medical practice.

16. To write off medical school loan repayment (both interest and principal) as a work expense on taxes irrespective of income.

17. To have access to all medical literature and research without fees or membership requirements.

18. To be protected from predatory loan companies.

19. To be guaranteed a residency position if the doctor graduates from an accredited medical school.

20. To have medical malpractice insurance from a single comprehensive carrier who offers competitive and transparent set rates, rules, and choices

that do not differ across state lines nor by gender, race, years of practice, or educational pedigree.

The American Hospital Association introduced a Patients' Bill of Rights in the early 1970s. It was edited and improved in 1992, but no single version was established as each state was expected to refine the basic tenets to fit their patient population.[62] As guideposts, the Health Insurance Portability and Accountability Act established a consumer bill of rights,[63] and the Association of American Physicians and Surgeons published their recommendations.[64] Then, on June 22, 2010, President Barack Obama introduced regulations associated with the Affordable Care Act that helped refine the rights of patients when dealing with insurance companies. Specifically, it prevented insurance companies from denying coverage to those with preexisting conditions and assured that most patients would get preventative health screening without extra fees.[65]

As a patient myself, I applaud the Patients' Bill of Rights.

As a physician, I am appalled that we have not been allocated similar protections from abuse.

The Not-So-Perfect Match

As you may have gathered from number 19 of the Bill of Doctors' Rights, there are not enough residency positions for the number of graduating medical school students. How could this be when we need more doctors in the field? The Balanced Budget Act of 1997 put a cap on the number of the residency positions the federal government would fund through Graduate Medical Education.[66] This left residency programs to pick up the slack or, out of the goodness of their hearts, to create more slots for the increasing number of medical students entering training. As we will see in Chapter Nine, this doesn't make much fiscal sense and so is unlikely to happen to the extent it needs to without incentives or laws (carrots and sticks).

According to the 2018 National Residency Matching Program, there were 37,103 U.S. and international medical and graduate students applying for 33,167 positions.[67] Sadly, 213 graduating medical students didn't have a match even after the Supplemental Offer and Acceptance Program. These individuals may have had knowledge or personality deficiencies, but many will have been perfectly well-adjusted professionals. Having these dedicated young doctors walk away from the match, their wings clipped, with a diploma and $270,000 of debt but no easy way to pay it back (they cannot practice medicine without a residency) is inexcusable.

The fact that it happens every year is abusive.

We are taking steps to improve things with the Training Tomorrow's Doctors Today Act, the Resident Physician Shortage Reduction Act of 2015, and the Affordable Care Act's push to train primary care physicians in non-hospital settings, but we need to do more. If a student graduates from an accredited medical school, it means that the school feels they are competent to practice medicine. If the graduate student is unable to find a match, the system has failed the student, and their debt should be forgiven.

P.S. The match page[68] is an excellent source of data and statistics, but they make it surprisingly tricky to decipher how many U.S. medical students don't match annually even though this seems like it should be front and center on their website—I challenge them to make this number available next year and in perpetuity. We can't fix something we don't look at because we are afraid or ashamed to admit it.

Technology May Clean Up Medicine

In this chapter we focused on the training process as it was, as it is now, and what we need to do to improve it so that we produce qualified physicians to meet our society's growing demand. I discussed the abuses my generation experienced before the laws changed but then revealed that little is being done to regulate the new mandates. We talked about the division of the specialties, the steps needed to complete training, and the abuse physicians can expect to experience. Suicide, gender inequality, and workplace violence set the stage for a profession many would not choose to do again. Physicians deal with tragedy, social injustice, abuse, addiction, and death daily. They are trained to empathize, treat, and move onto the next patient while understanding that theirs is not a nine-to-five job and working off the clock is expected. They know that patients can be terrified, stressed, and angry and that some level of stress and abuse is unavoidable.

But that doesn't mean that there shouldn't be limits.

Using technology to promote, educate, and regulate the 20 elements of the Doctors' Bill of Rights may allow us to reclaim our profession and so be better caregivers for our patients.

I want to be able to tell a newly minted medical student that they're doing the right thing, that they have a fantastic and rewarding career ahead of them.

Currently, I have a hard time meeting their eyes.

Chapter Nine

It's the Money, Stupid (Terminal Economics)

How Much Is Your Life Worth?

When we talk about the "C" word in medicine, many immediately think of cancer when corruption may be the real *"gros mot."*[1] Confronting an uncomfortable topic is the first step in treating it, and this chapter will address what happens when we link human illness to profit in a capitalist society. Herein, technology is a double-edged sword. Self-serving entrepreneurs find computers have made it easier for them to hide their unethical behavior but unwittingly leave a trail of digital breadcrumbs for determined investigators to follow back to the rat hole in the wall. Medical compensation has always influenced the doctor-patient relationship, but the 21st-century remuneration has depended on the patient's ability to pay. After the brutal medical ethics travesties committed during World War II, the World Medical Association (WMA) updated the tenants of the Hippocratic oath to better reflect the evolving moral framework of the times. In 1948, the Declaration of Geneva was adopted and set a code for international medical ethics that said, "A Doctor must always maintain the highest standards of professional conduct ... (and) practice his profession uninfluenced by motives of profit." It was deemed unethical for doctors to participate in "any self advertisement ... collaborate in any form of medical services in which the Doctor does not have professional independence ... receive any money in connection with services rendered to a patient other than a proper professional fee, even with the knowledge of the patient."[2] In 1957,[3] the American Medical Association (AMA) adopted codes of conduct that seemed to agree with the WMA and included in their principles of Medical Ethics the provision, "In the practice of medicine a physician should limit the source of his professional income to medical services actually rendered by him, or under his supervision, to his patients. His fee should be commensurate with the services rendered and the patient's ability to pay. He should neither pay nor receive a commission for referral of patients. Drugs, remedies or appliances may be dispensed or supplied by the physician provided it is in the best interests of the patient."[4] However, this clear and financially restrictive clause was removed from the AMA's 2016 Code of Conduct. Of note, no link or easily accessible record to the old mandates are found on the AMA's website; that doesn't seem that ethical.[5]

Why did they feel their codes needed to be updated?

Things have changed.

The Health Maintenance Organization Act passed by Congress in 1973 is a federal law that legitimized the ability of outside groups to influence the outcome of a doctor-patient interaction under the auspice of reducing health-care costs.[6] From that point, the reins of health-care policy, price, and delivery were given to the bean counters. Statisticians, rather than physicians, decided what to charge for a diagnosis, what medications were in our formularies, and how many hospital days each person should be allotted. Suddenly, health care was the ugly duckling turned swan, and entrepreneurs rushed to lay claim to one of her golden eggs. Since then, the dominoes haven't stopped falling. The Balanced Budget Act of 1997 put a cap on the number of residency positions the federal government subsidized, and thus how many practicing physicians enter the United States workforce each year.[7] Under the 2010 Affordable Care Act, Medicare began rewarding providers who formed groups that accepted "bundled" payments. This reimbursement framework paid organizations to provide care to a large number of patients, regardless of their diagnosis, and so gambled that businesses would work to keep their panels healthy to avoid spending money later on preventable illnesses.[8] A worthy idea built on a glaring loophole: ours is not a closed system, and so patients are free to move from one carrier to another annually. If a CEO wants to save money for their group, they can subtly raise the annual fees or co-pays of a high-risk subpopulation and so encourage high utilizers to migrate to a different group. If profit instead of health is the goal, humans will find a way to manipulate the system for personal advantage.

Our Founding Fathers relied heavily upon the writings and philosophies of John Locke in constructing the framework of our modern democracy. Locke believed that primitive humans were fundamentally good at heart and could live happily off the land without the interference of human laws. In this ungoverned state, we had natural laws, unalienable rights, which any just system we adopted to regulate ourselves should not take from us. A modern government that discredits or abuses these rights is therefore broken and the people have a duty to revolt against its oppression. In his groundbreaking work *Second Treatise of Civil Government*, he wrote "that being all equal and independent, no one ought to harm another in his life, health, liberty, or possessions."[9] These words were used, nearly verbatim, in the July 4, 1776, *Declaration of Independence of the United States*,[10] with the clause "pursuit of happiness" used to encompass things like property and health. The system we've adopted over the last century to regulate our health care does not follow John Locke's principals nor the intentions of those who founded our great nation. Should the CEOs of our hospitals and medical organizations be paid millions of dollars each year while uninsured or indigent patients are forced into bankruptcy by aggressive collection agencies?[11] Should lobbyists for marijuana, alcohol, and tobacco be better positioned to influence our nation's laws than the patients suffering from the apathy, lung cancer, and addiction they cause?[12] Should pharmaceutical executives be able to hide behind teams of high-priced lawyers after having promoted the off-label use of a drug known to cause birth defects in newborns to pregnant women and their doctors without fully disclosing the risks?[13] The health-care laws of our country have been corrupted, undermined, and misused so that they best serve the interests of the few rather than the many, the greedy instead of the needy, so we, the people, must voice our discontent and demand change.

The public Medicare claims database released by the Obama administration can be used to determine how much individual doctors billed and were paid using taxpayer money through Medicare.[14] The Associated Press looked at this data and found that 344 out of 825,000 physicians were extremely high utilizers, together receiving $1.5 billion in 2014 or more than $3 million each.[15] Most notable of the abuses was Dr. Salomon Melgen, convicted for having defrauded Medicare out of $73 million, and his questionable relationship with New Jersey Democrat Bob Menendez.[16] Menendez, who received more than $1 million in undisclosed gifts from Dr. Melgen, often went to bat for his friend's billing practices. In 2018, the congressman was cleared of corruption charges but doesn't feel he needs to follow the ethics committee's recommendation that he pay back the "gifts" he received and is now running for reelection.[17] Like cancer, corruption has metastasized to nearly every corner of our system. Think education is safe? Think again. Lois Margaret Nora made nearly $700,000 in compensation as president of the American Board of Medical Specialties, a nonprofit organization that spent more than half its annual revenue paying its board members while administrating tests that contributed nothing to the practice of medicine nor to the health of our patients.[18]

If we hope to fix health care, to rebuild the trust our patients once had in us, we must force those who abuse the system into the light so that they can be publicly shamed and vilified.

To do this, technology may be our greatest ally.

The Maintenance of Certification (MOC) Scam

Having dyslexia, test taking has never been easy. It takes me more time to process certain words, to confirm both my answer and the question being asked, and to make sure I don't skim over important details. I'm sure these same issues arise for all test takers, but those of us with dyslexia have tricky minds which, at times, like to replace words and numbers with ones that aren't there. Luckily, I've trained myself to diligently and systematically run through a myriad of mental fail-safes before moving on to the next question. I apply this same internal system of self-correction when reviewing my patients' labs and test results. It takes time, but I've found that knowing I have a learning disability and taking steps to compensate for it has helped me to catch far more normal human errors than I might have otherwise. Still, timed test-taking remains a struggle. I understand the need to test to confirm that knowledge or skill has been learned and retained. Additionally, I concede that testing helps a student consolidate what they've learned and identify deficits that need to be patched up with additional reading. I also agree with the need for graduates, especially in medicine, to continue learning so they can provide the best possible care to their patients.

What I find abhorrent is the mandated testing of trained professionals to create income for a self-appointed group of individuals who care more about profit than principles. What makes my stomach churn is how easily they used fear and ignorance to convince lawmakers and the public to institutionalize this Maintenance of Certification (MOC) testing process despite there being no evidence that it was needed nor proof that it would make things better. What makes my eyes turn into my skull is the knowledge that they are listed as a nonprofit when nothing could be further from the truth. The American Board of Medical Specialties (ABMS) has wasted our time and money and has created the real possibility that a licensed physician could lose their livelihood just because they didn't fill in the right sequence of spots on a computer screen as opposed to if they can do their job in the real world.

Shame on you, ABMS!

Shame on us for not stopping you sooner!

Consider a report published in the *Journal of the American Medical Association* in 2017 showing the revenues and expenditures for the 24 U.S. boards in the fiscal year 2013 wherein they reported $263 million in revenue ($230 million coming from test fees) and $239 million in expenses with only $51 million being spent on administering the test while twice that amount, more than $100 million, spent on officer and employee compensation. Add to this the ridiculous assertion that this group is a nonprofit when the net balance of assets held by the board rose from $237 million in 2003 to $635 million in 2013.[19] Yet despite their apparent windfall, they saw a need to increase the fees charged to physicians. Why? As was revealed by Kurt Eichenwald in a *Newsweek* opinion article, they cooked the books by counting unpaid but expected payments from physicians in the future as deferred revenue. Charles P. Kroll, a certified public accountant specializing in health care, did an investigational audit and found that the ABMS used this technique to show a $39.8 million loss on the books over the five years before 2013 while paying $125.7 million to senior officers and staff.[20] Rightly upset, many physicians have banded together in grassroots movements on social media to introduce legislation in nearly 20 states to curb the ABMS's power and antitrust behavior. In 2016, Oklahoma was the first state to prevent hospitals and insurers from requiring MOC certification for physicians to practice with Georgia; Maryland, Missouri, North Carolina, Tennessee, Washington State, and Texas was soon to follow.[21]

We're making progress, but corruption is as tenacious as any cancer and it never dies without a fight.[22]

In 2015, ABMS spent $450,000 it had collected from physicians under the auspice of certifying us on a public relations firm to help it improve its image and so continue to exist.[23] Just one of the results of this was the "certification matters" campaign they launched so the public can look up their doctor's name and find out if they are complying with MOC. Why? There is little evidence that passing their tests improves a physician's ability to care for their patients.[24] It is merely a social media scare tactic and PR stunt to validate the ABMS's existence.

So as not to leave you with the impression that my disillusionment with ABMS is motivated by a personal vendetta, I am fully licensed and credentialed. I play the game, pay their fees, and participate in their banal recertification process because the system has been rigged to punish those who fight back. But what if you refuse? In the past, board certification was a voluntary process, and a physician's medical license or ability to practice medicine was not linked to it. ABMS has lobbied hard for legitimacy, and many insurance carriers and hospitals have fallen for their sales pitch and linked a physician's ability to practice to their certification status. Dr. Meg Edison decided to take on the ABMS and refused to recertify despite having passed two of their tests in the past, being a partner in a group practice, and having an active medical license. Within six months she was hit with a barrage of demanding letters from the ABMS, told by her insurance carrier she could no longer see her own patients, and was threatened with the loss of her hospital privileges. Still rebellious, she planned on standing her ground until her carrier sent letters to her patients telling them she was uncertified. Dr. Edison relented and paid the $1,300 fee the ABMS required. What else could she have done? She, as many of us are, is an indentured laborer in the health-care field. I encourage you to read her full story at Rebel.MD and share in the powerful lesson the system taught her: the MOC is not voluntary.[25]

This is important because it puts them at risk for antitrust lawsuits: the idea is that its actions interfere with free trade by restricting or reducing the ability of trained physicians to provide services to the public and so therefore interfere with patient access to health care. Leading the charge in defending physician rights against the ABMS's MOC program is the Association of American Physicians and Surgeons (AAPS). AAPS has filed a lawsuit against ABMS, and I would encourage every physician and patient to visit their website and learn more: Aapsonline.org.[26] Another advocacy group is the National Board of Physicians and Surgeons, which offers a cost-effective alternative pathway for board certified physicians to show that they are continuing to grow and learn in their craft, independent of the ABMS and MOC. They can be found at Nbpas.org.

I'll leave you with one final point of interest.

In the course of researching this book, I have read countless articles, journals, blogs, and books, all of which improved my medical knowledge and helped me understand the modern framework of health care. I'm using what I've learned to help inform the public and my colleagues, and to improve my understanding of my position within the system so that I can be a better provider for my patients.

Yet none of what I have done has earned me a single hour of continuing medical education credit.

Sadly, our system is broken.

Fraudulent Billing

True story: Years ago, my future wife and I were having dinner at a restaurant in downtown Chicago. The food was terrific, and the service was even better. Satisfied, we asked for the check and looked at the bill. We had been billed $2,357 for dinner. Stunned, I waved down our waiter who, embarrassed, explained that he had given us the receipt for a dinner party several tables over and apologized profusely. Being in medical school at Northwestern at the time, my account would have bounced several times over, and the error would have come to light. However, what if we hadn't looked at the bill and my card had no credit limit? What if my account was Medicare?

In 2015, the FBI arrested 243 people for allegedly fraudulently billing Medicare for more than $712 million of patient care that did not occur. In the report published by *CNN Money*, Medicare was billed tens of millions of dollars by a mental health facility for psychotherapy sessions that consisted of moving patients from one room to another. Another doctor billed Medicare for $23 million worth of wheelchairs and health services that were not medically necessary. Others were arrested for using "patient recruiters" who convinced the homeless to share their Medicare numbers and used these to bill the government without ever having seen the patient. Since 2007, the Department of Justice's (DOJ) Medicare Fraud Strike Force has uncovered more than $7 billion in false bills[27]: a little more than the price of dinner for two. In 2009, the attorney general announced the formation of the Health Care Fraud Prevention and Enforcement Action Team as an initiative with a sustained focus on collaboration between the DOJ and FBI. As more and more physicians join large group practices instead of working as private practitioners, we may be the only ones positioned to identify and report criminal practices when they occur. If you suspect fraudulent behavior, realize that this crime damages the credibility of our profession, drives up the cost of health care and ultimately reduces the services available to our growing patient population, and report it. The Department of Justice's main switchboard number is (202) 514-2000.[28]

Big Pharma, Little Ethics

The extent of ethical indiscretions perpetrated by pharmaceutical companies is legendary and could easily fill an entire book. If I were to limit myself to one egregious example, it's hard to miss the $3 billion payout, the largest health-care fraud settlement in U.S. history, made by GlaxoSmithKline (GSK) after pleading guilty to failure to report safety data and for their promotion of the off-label uses of Paxil, Wellbutrin, and Advandia.[29] Perhaps the most telling aspect of this plea agreement is the company's payment of $57 million to resolve claims of wrongdoing concerning their alleged promotion of Zofran as an antinausea drug for pregnant women when studies show it causes birth defects in the newborns of women who take it.[30] Suspected complications caused by Zofran include death,[31] heart defects,[32] and an increased risk of cleft palate.[33] Why would they shovel out so much cash? The FDA has only approved Zofran to be used in the treatment of vomiting in chemotherapy, radiation, and surgery patients. This is a relatively small market compared to the $2.4 billion GSK was able to pull in annually by "fraudulently" marketing Zofran as being safe for morning sickness.[34] Three billion dollars seems like a lot of money to most of us, but for a company that made $39 billion in revenue the very next year, it's likely built into their business model.

Fines are unlikely to deter behavior like this especially as they are levied against the corporation rather than the individuals responsible for calling the shots. CEO's at GSK and many other pharmaceutical companies have fostered corporate cultures where it's okay to harm patients and mislead doctors as long as the stockholders are happy. "It's not personal," they say, "it's business." Well, to the child who died or was born with a cardiac anomaly, it couldn't be more personal. If we want large business to change, we must dig down and make individuals accountable when things go wrong. Justice is not served when someone writes a big check. Justice is done when CEO's do jail time, and fines are paid out of their personal portfolios and bonuses.

I can hear you scoffing. This kind of legislation will never happen.

It can happen. It is happening.

In April 2018, Senator Bernie Sanders introduced a bill that holds individuals within a pharmaceutical company responsible if the business is found to be guilty of deceptive marketing practices in promoting the use of opioids to the public. As reported by Lev Facher in *Stat News*, "The legislation would impose a 10-year minimum prison sentence and fines equal to an executive's compensation package if the individual's company is found to have illegally contributed to the opioid crisis. It would also impose an additional fine on those companies of $7.8 billion—one-tenth the annual cost of the crisis, per a 2016 estimate."[35]

"Hi, Big Pharma CEOs," Senator Sander's Bill seems to say. "Have we got your attention now?"

I hope so.

America is sick enough without your help.

Unions

Physicians are the only professionals in the United States that cannot form a union. Why? Is it because people might die or suffer if we left only a skeleton crew for the very ill and emergent? No. Is it because we took an oath to help those in need? No. It's because the government worries that we'll create a monopoly or trust capable of obstructing the natural flow of commerce/money. That's not to say current medical organizations aren't powerful. They lobby for fairer laws and better physician rights. But they don't have any teeth. They can't say "our members will walk out if you don't give residents better salaries, pay us for the time we put in off the clock, lower medical school loan costs, protect us from unfounded lawsuits, and give us reasonable patient loads." Thus, nothing changes.

Why were these laws created and to what end?

The National Labor Relations Board (NLRB) allows physicians to form and run unions as long as they are considered "employees" of a hospital or health system, not self-employed contractors, private practitioners (considered by the NLRB to be independent contractors), and not in supervisorial roles where they could unduly influence those below them. This is done to ensure groups of physicians can't band together to form negotiating blocs and bargain collectively for their rights, which the NLRB would deem violations of antitrust laws.[36] But, is it really our rights that they are worried about? No. It's the money. These laws are in place to ensure that physician groups can't decide together what to charge the public for hip surgery, set that price, and ensure that no one can get a hip replaced for less than that amount, essentially price-fixing. This scenario would hinder a competitive marketplace, the mechanics of supply-and-demand, and so would be considered illegal by the Federal Trade Commission under the Sherman Act of 1890.[37] As explained on their website, "The Sherman Act outlaws 'every contract, combination, or conspiracy in restraint of trade,' and any 'monopolization, attempted monopolization, or conspiracy or combination to monopolize.' Long ago, the Supreme Court decided that the Sherman Act does not prohibit *every* restraint of trade, only those that are *unreasonable*. For instance, in some sense, an agreement between two individuals to form a partnership restrains trade, but may not do so unreasonably, and thus may be lawful under the antitrust laws." Therein lies the loophole, the way to unlock the shackles that have bound our hands. Is it unreasonable to ask the IIMO that we work for (as private contractors) to see fewer patients in a day because we want to do a better job taking care of them? Is it unreasonable for physicians to band together and say we don't want to click buttons and follow algorithms that are not designed to benefit our patients' health but instead serve to populate some administrator's end-of-the-month pie chart? Is it unreasonable to say that the integration of technology, although needed, into medicine takes more time and this burden should not rest solely on the physicians' shoulders and their after-clinic duties but should be reflected in our schedules and the expectations of the system?

Is it a violation of antitrust laws to say we are tired of being abused?

I don't think so.

Things have changed since 1890. For the first time, less than half of the practicing physicians in the United States are independent.[38] This is due to a progressive shift toward larger group practices as independent physicians find it increasingly difficult to acquire and use the necessary information technology and meet quality and safety mandates.[39] If you join one of these larger groups, you'll notice that many of them hire you as an employee for the first several years and then offer you a partnership as a self-employed contractor. This is so they can provide services like health and psychiatric care to you and your family and write it off as a corporate expense on their books come tax time. Called "imputed income," this leaves you with a higher reported income and responsibility on April 15 even though you never saw a dime. Additionally, by working as private contractors, we are automatically prohibited from forming unions by the NLRB even though most modern doctors do not have any real power to hire or fire employees and hold no supervisory role.

Recently, physician groups have begun to challenge the system. In 2015, members of the Union of American Physicians and Dentists (UAPD) staged a walkout against the University of California in the first licensed physician strike in the United States in 25 years. They were protesting the university's resistance to publishing its profits—something it should have done as a public institution—therefore limiting the medical staff's ability to negotiate fair wages and bolster health center resources for student patients.[40] The UAPD is the largest union representing licensed doctors in the United States, but its members cannot hold ownership stakes and must be employees, which is why university-employed physicians can join. If we look at the rest of the State of California, current laws ban doctors from being directly employed by corporations. To skirt this issue, many large health providers set up doctor-run medical foundations that are separate from their affiliated hospitals and offer physicians ownership equity in the form of shares they are required to buy when they become senior partners.[41] In buying shares, the only way to ensure continued employment and benefits after an initial vetting period, physicians are essentially giving up their rights to negotiate collectively within the corporation by becoming part owners. Even though for all intents and purposes they work as salaried employees, the NLRB prohibits them from creating a union. Unable to bargain collectively, they have no way to drive their employers to provide sustainable panel sizes or steer them away from practices that put the company's profit before the patients' health.

In a word, this is crazy.

We have become indentured laborers, forced to accept restrictive contracts so we can pay back exorbitant medical school loans, with no legal recourse to change our working conditions other than for the individual to quit or move to a different group practice that will likely soon adopt the same employment framework. I certainly understand and appreciate the need for antitrust laws to dissuade the few bad apples from practicing fraudulent behavior, but the majority of us are not unreasonably restricting trade if we ask to have more time to see our patients.

Are we?

According to our current law, we are.

This is why I believe physicians within a group practice, even if they own "symbolic" shares, who behave as employees, receive a salary and have no or little control over the practice's day-to-day operations should be given an exception by the NLRB and be allowed to form a union.

The adage "Physician, heal thyself," is true of our health-care system.

Only, we can't do it alone, and it will never happen if it is illegal for us to work together.

My Thoughts

It's easy enough to say what's wrong with something. What we need is constructive criticism geared toward creating substantive and positive change. As we've journeyed through the evolution of medicine, I've tried to provide helpful suggestions, and I fully acknowledge that some of them may be misinformed and untenable.

Forgive me, then, as I submit my thoughts on what might improve our nation's health in the future.

- More doctors: What we need is real people, not test-taking machines. Individuals with real-life experience who honestly care about their patients are a hundred times more valuable than the ones who can score 100 percent on a standardized test.
- Physician overload: Using technology to micromanage professionals (doctors, nurses, medical assistants), who already care more about doing their job right than any algorithm ever will, is insulting, discouraging, and counterproductive. Just because something can be measured does not mean that it should be measured.
- Patient-Physician interactions: If studies show that using EMRs and technology takes 40 percent more time, then we should change schedules to reflect this. Do we tell our gardener to grow an award-winning rose faster or accept that nature cannot be rushed? We need unhurried face-to-face time with our patients to nurture a relationship, effectively prune away bad habits, and help our fellow humans reach their full potential.
- Physician burnout: We cherry-pick some of the best minds, the most

innovative thinkers our culture can produce, give them a degree, and then stop challenging them. Why? I bet that nearly 80 percent of practicing physicians have a great idea, a medical innovation or research project, that they will never pursue. Why? It interferes with patient access and so affects the short-term bottom line. This is short-sighted, profit-motivated, and a terrible waste of resources.

- Malpractice: Malpractice suits need to be resolved in months instead of years. Legal fees are the only reason most of them take this long, and the wait puts an enormous emotional strain on the physician and patient. Doctors should be encouraged to countersue lawyers who file suits based on the likelihood a group will settle rather than any evidence of real malpractice.
- Doctors' Bill of Rights: We need to enact one: see Chapter Eight.
- High health-care costs: As long as someone is making a profit from human illness, we will not be able to change health care. (1) "Nonprofit" hospitals need to behave like nonprofits (the altruistic intent suggested by title) instead of business vehicles to dodge taxes. (2) Residency programs should not receive government subsidies as it restricts free trade, and so undermines the tenants of the Sherman Act and antitrust laws. (3) Lobbyists, especially those paid for by special interests, should not be allowed anywhere near politicians making decisions about our health.
- Continued postgraduate medical education: Continued learning is critical in our field, but testing should not be revenue motivated, and groups like ABMS who have profited off fearmongering should be dissolved and replaced with federally monitored programs designed to help improve the quality of care provided in the real world.
- Big pharma: (1) Very few drugs are tested to prove that they are better than what is already currently available. They are only tested to see if they are effective and safe. If pharmaceutical companies also had to prove that their manufactured product was better, we wouldn't have nearly as many new high-priced drugs. (2) These are profitable companies. Why are we paying high prices for patented drugs when all a patent should really be doing is keeping others from competing directly? Having a patent should not mean the company can charge whatever it wants. There should be a price ceiling on any drug sold in the United States, and if a company cannot produce it for that amount then they shouldn't make it.
- Personal liability for CEOs: Physicians, lawyers, and politicians all go to jail if they intentionally do something to harm the public. Why don't CEOs? If we make it personal, maybe they'll stop saying it's just business.
- Doctors need unions: Every labor profession but ours has a union. As most of us now practice under corporate umbrellas, we should be given the

ability to unionize so we can defend our rights as employees. We need to stop pretending that we are anything else.

- Abuse in the medical field: (1) Medical students and residents are physically and mentally abused. There should be a zero-tolerance directive against this behavior. (2) We have the highest rate of suicide of any profession in the United States. Physician suicide needs to be brought into the public eye and the issues causing it addressed. (3) Patients can threaten and physically harm us and walk away with a slap on the wrist. Instead, these crimes should be considered felonies. (4) Some of us are financially trapped in a field we hate, essentially indentured laborers. Physicians who want to walk away from training or practice should be provided loan forgiveness as well as our sincere thanks for trying.

Prove It

Joe Flower, a health-care systems consultant with more than 30 years in the industry, wrote a highly informative and thoughtful book, *Healthcare Beyond Reform: Doing It Right for Half the Cost*, and I would recommend it to anyone interested in understanding how money influences the quality of our nation's medical services. One of his take-home points is that "people do what you pay them to do." As long as we look at health care as a business whose end goal is to make a profit, the individual patient is going to get hurt. When we start looking at health care as a right, and we bundle services so that it is profitable to help patients achieve that guarantee, then we'll be back on track. Although not intuitive, Flower discusses, and I agree, with the Pareto principle that says that in any group of things that contribute to a common effect, a relatively few contributors account for the majority of the effect.[42] When we apply this to health care, we find that 5 percent of the population uses 50 percent of our health-care dollar. Narrowing our focus further, we find that 1 percent of the people generate 22 percent of the costs.[43] This suggests that if we could apply more services to this group of people, really micromanage their care, we could potentially reduce health-care costs by 20 percent in any given year. This is not an easy population to manage. They often have chronic, complex medical histories, and their compliance can be reduced by drug-drug interactions and socioeconomic and mental health factors that are not easy to fix, but it can be done.

"Prove it," you say.

Dr. Jeffrey Brenner established the Camden Coalition of Healthcare Providers, which consists of community-based private practices, frontline hospital staff, social workers, and aggressive prevention measures applied to the needs of high-risk patients in impoverished communities. As Flower reports, Brenner explains that the "tables had to be turned so that the system served the patients rather than the needs of the health-care industry." By treating just 36 patients, Brenner was able to cut their hospital visits in half and so saved the state an estimated $8 million a year. Inspired? Please consider reading the article *The New Yorker* published on Dr. Brenner on January 24, 2011.[44]

Why isn't every health-care group aggressively treating the 1 percent with every possible resource and service they can provide?

Dr. Brenner's approach saves money; it doesn't make money, ergo, "no one is getting paid to do it."

Ironically, that's both the problem and the solution.

Chapter Ten

We're Only Human (That's the Point)

Trigger Warning

Thus far, we have talked about the history, innovations, legalities, and profit drive of modern medicine. These elements form the solid steps we needed to climb to get to the plateau upon which we now stand. Before us lays the expanse of thought that threatens to be the most challenging and at its heart lies the key question medicine will need to answer to stay relevant in the modern world.

What is it to be human?

"Wait," you'll say, "this book is supposed to address the doctor-patient relationship and technology. What does that have to do with being human?"

Everything.

Technology appeals to the intersubjective value our liberal culture places on human life and promises that we can improve, extend, and even create life in exchange for our agreement to give up what we currently think it means to be human. Examining the intricacies of this deal will take our discussion a bit deeper, many fathoms deeper, into the metaphysical realms and, for some, this will not be a comfortable journey. Personal and religious beliefs may erect barriers in your mind. Systems of value may crumble to reveal the papier-mâché skeleton underneath. Even worse, you may see nothing wrong with the direction we're headed and welcome it with open arms.

Neil Gaiman, one of my favorite authors, noticed the term "trigger warning" sneaking its way into our popular lingo and couldn't resist writing a collection of stories designed to trigger his readers. Of course, he titled his work *Trigger Warning*, and explained in the introduction that when he was growing up no one warned him what a book might do to the way he thought.[1] He just started reading it. If he wasn't ready for the material, he put it down and came back when he was a bit older and wiser. Modern trigger warnings on videos, books, and news broadcasts are meant to help people avoid unpleasant feelings or experiences. For example, warning someone with a gorilla phobia not to buy tickets to the latest theatrical rendition of *King Kong*. Mr. Gaiman, in true humanist fashion, espouses concern for the message the term was ushering into our language; namely that we should shield ourselves from exploring thoughts that make us uncomfortable. I agree. We may not always concur with what we read or hear, but we should not close our minds to new ideas or concepts.

So, please accept this as your trigger warning. If you think discussing the natural history of thought, of the human system of values, and of what it means to be alive is taking things a bit too far, then please skip forward. However, if you elect to stick it out, I hope to shed some light on how what we think of as "being human" will map our trajectory into the 22nd century and beyond.

Intersubjective Angst

To examine the issues, we must first understand the vocabulary.

Metaphysics is the study of the nature of the mind. "I think, therefore I am," or "*Cogito, ergo sum,*" as coined by Rene Descartes in his book *Principia philosophiae*, is one of the tenets of modern philosophy.[2] However, the translation from French lacks some of the intent Descartes may have ascribed to the concept and could be more accurately described as, "I doubt, therefore I think, and so I must exist." Thus, our existence in this reality is proven by our ability to employ an independent consciousness capable of doubting that it is conscious.

Solipsism is the idea that a person can only be sure that their own mind exists. The manufactured world Neo thinks he lives in during act 1 of *The Matrix*[3] is a profound example of this philosophy in action. Everything he senses and experiences is a lie, a sophisticated computer algorithm designed to keep his mind occupied and content. In this case, Neo's consciousness would be right to doubt if the universe it perceived were real and would thus only be able to confirm its own existence. Similarly, Descartes postulated that an omniscient "evil demon" could convince an independent mind that it was attached to a body by manipulating the perceptions, the data flow, the mind received from the outside world. A medical example of this phenomenon is found in the perception of phantom limb pain in which, for example, a patient feels they have an itchy toe despite having lost the foot to which that toe is attached. The neurons firing in the person's brain convinces it that there is an external, physical manifestation of something that no longer exists.

Descartes suggests that his inability to prove that he had a body showed that the brain and body were separate and so introduced dualism (a mechanistic view) to Western philosophy. As discussed in Chapter Three, monism (a vitalist view) postulated that the mind and body were an indivisible entity.

If we wear the dualist's glasses for a bit, we can see how our perceptions can be broken down into objective and subjective categories. When I see a patient in the office, they often have several complaints. These can vary from chest pain, rash, fever, anxiety, or dizziness, to a musculoskeletal injury such as a broken bone. Although we don't do it consciously, most physicians will divide these complaints into two distinct categories: objective and subjective. When a skateboarder presents with the inability to supinate their forearm, there is a good chance I'll be able to prove he has a broken radial head with an X-ray. These are objective or verifiable findings. Even with subjective complaints, there is often a validating test that lends credibility to the story. However, when I have a middle-aged woman with body aches and a headache, I must rely on her subjective description of the symptoms as she experiences them. I have no pain-o-meter with which to objectively tell her that she should be experiencing a 4 out of 10 pain when she reports an 8. Thus, I must and do trust her numeric qualification as she is the only one who can judge it.

Complaint	*Type*	*Validating Test*
Chest pain	Subjective	ECG or Angiogram
Rash	Objective	Visual
Fever	Objective	Thermometer
Anxiety	Subjective	Verbal
Dizziness	Subjective	Eye nystagmus
Broken Bone	Objective	Radiology

To complicate things, a patient's response to subjective symptoms varies widely. I may have an anxious patient with gas who behaves as if he were dying. Alternatively, I may have a stoic who feels the shoulder pain she gets walking up a flight of stairs is because of her age. After a while, many physicians become comfortable with their panel's personality types and can respond appropriately to their patients' needs. The fact that subjective and objective complaints are not always aligned supports the dualistic view that the mind and body are linked but divisible entities.

But there are other invisible issues at play that neither the patient nor the doctor is aware of despite how much they influence the interaction—these are the intersubjective elements. Simply stated, intersubjective issues are the stories that we tell each other that lend meaning and value to our lives. A bar of gold weighs 400 troy ounces or 27 pounds and currently is worth $550,000. It's heavy and shiny, but you and I are the only ones who give it value. When two cultures clash, intersubjective values may be abused as we saw when the settlers gave the American Indians beads and pretended they were valuable. Two different religious groups place unique intersubjective values on their respective gods, but neither culture has a quantifiable way to determine which belief system is better. So, they go to war. Unfortunately, the "might is right" approach to determining value has and does work. Even if they quietly maintain their intersubjective religious beliefs, the conquered people will need to adopt the value systems (money, social status, and education) of the victors to survive.

The coming battle between dataism (the newest term for the mechanistic view) and vitalism has been brewing for more than 50 years. In the next section, we will discuss these ideologies in more detail and explain why the medical office has become ground zero for the conflict. Until now, physicians have been mediators, translators, and peacemakers. Yet the strength of the opponents is building, overlapping, and merging in dangerous ways. Soon, members of our profession will be forced to choose sides in a conflict whose outcome has already been decided.

The question is, are you willing to fight for the losing team?

Dataism Versus Vitalism

Imagine for a second that you are an introspective neolithic elder lying on your back looking up at the stars and wondering what the point of it all is. You want to ask someone but you're the smartest person you know. You see a shooting star, watch the moon rise over the horizon, and decide that you are just a speck in the universe and that there must be some cosmic power greater than yourself who has all the answers. You have an epiphany. There must be something or someone who gets it all, who pulls the strings, and so to get the answers you seek you will need to make them happy. But something that big, that fantastic, wouldn't be impressed by the trinkets you trade with your people. No, they want something more, something precious. Life is valuable. Perhaps if you sacrificed a few animals, maybe a person or two, you might gain favor with this cosmic entity, and they, in turn, might explain things to you.

Thus, the three-headed serpent of curiosity, humility, and imagination birthed ideology.

Curiosity led us to ask questions. Humility made us believe something greater must have the answers. Imagination let us create the idea of such a thing.

Ten. We're Only Human (That's the Point)

From our initial cosmic belief system we moved to one ruled by deities and gods. People went on crusades in the name of God, died and killed in the name of their beliefs, and felt this was justified. Why? They did not place the same intersubjective value on life as we do now. They felt life only had value in that it could be used to promote or defend a higher imagined "truth." As we entered the modern age, Friedrich Nietzsche announced that "God is dead," as humanist intersubjective values took hold.[4] First described by Cicero (106–43 BC), "*humanitas*" was the Latin word that encompassed the concepts of *philantropia* (a love of what makes us human) and paideia (learning). Friedrich Niethammer, a German educator, revived the concept in 1808 as he felt students learned more from living life than they did through simple rote memorization in the classroom. The humanist ideology suggests that every human life has equal value and that the greatest meaning we can find in life is in our personal experience of it. This is why we may look back at religious wars as having been a waste of life or why we argue about the lives of animals and unborn children. On its surface, this humanistic view has improved our society and created concepts like civil rights and crimes against humanity. On the flip side, humanistic thinking may turn out to be a wolf in sheep's clothing as it is built on dualist principles. Life is valuable because it involves a human's conscious experience. Our experience of life is derived from the input our brain receives and how our biologic algorithms interpret this data. Through virtual games and augmented reality, we can convince our brains that we are experiencing a world that does not really exist. Yet this data input provides players with human experience, which is what makes life valuable. It follows that the mind does not need the physical world to feel alive and so the mind and body must be, as postulated by Descartes, two different things.

Our ancestors may well look back at our 21st century lives and shake their heads (if they still have heads) at the time we wasted trying to accrue life experiences when such things are manufactured, shared, and downloaded into their neuromatrixes. Their intrasubjective value will have evolved into what is called dataism. Initially coined by David Brooks of *The New York Times*,[5] but then described in far greater detail and eloquence by Yuval Noah Harari in his book *Homo Deus: A Brief History of Tomorrow*.[6] Harari says that "dataists believe that experiences are valueless if they are not shared and that we need not, indeed we can not, find meaning within ourselves. We need only record and connect our experiences to the great data flow, and the algorithms will discover their meaning and tell us what to do." If you don't think this is happening, check your phone and see what the Internet, of all things, thinks. Did you get enough exercise today? Check out your sports watch. Are you worried that you might be carrying some familiar genetic mutation? Do a mouth swab and send it in for sequencing. After all, your genetic code is a sequence of data points that can be compared to your peers, and an algorithm should have no trouble telling you what percentage risk your body has for a multitude of diseases. Wait. Is that making you depressed? Don't worry; your mood is just a biological algorithm that depends on the concentration of serotonin at your synaptic juncture, which we can improve with a medicine. Better yet, we've got an electric brain stimulator that will help you suppress those misfiring wires and keep you focused on important things—like creating more data to share with others.

The idea is that the root and purpose of life is data. Our genetic code wants to pass itself on to the next generation and it does this through our germ cells. Our bodies being nothing more than the vehicle that allows for the natural selection of those cells, data, that are best aligned to survive in the world and so be most capable of being passed on to the next generation. Our thoughts or consciousness, being nothing more than a rudimentary byproduct of this process, has been kept, as it seems, to help us more effectively maintain our genetic code within the data flow of life. Thus, if we exactly duplicate the algorithm that is a human's mind, much as one might follow the recipe to bake a cake, we will have created consciousness.

Vitalist would take a different approach and say that there is an element within a person that cannot be broken down into its component parts, that is not understandable by an algorithm, and which is the real seat of conscious thought. Going back to our decoy duck scenario, have we really created consciousness if we create something that behaves so convincingly that when it tells us it is conscious we start to believe it? Is its algorithm having it say this because this is what we want to hear or is it really alive? As a thought experiment: Let's say I told you I could move your entire neocortex, every pattern of synaptic firing, from your body into that of a near-immortal body, that it would behave and act just as you do now and would even tell me it was alive. It would say the procedure had been a success. Is it then alive? Is it you? Or is it a copy of you? If it now turned to me and said it didn't like the idea that there were two of you and that I should kill the old you in your worn-out biologic body, would you be okay with that? Which of you has a better claim to life? Is that you even alive or is it just a facsimile, a decoy robot, that will tell me it is conscious as that is what you would tell me, but which does not actually contain the vital spark that a vitalist would value.

Calculating Compliance

Why do patients take the time to see their physicians? Even now, there are more than a few websites capable of a reasonably accurate diagnosis based on a patient's reported symptoms. If the computer could prescribe them an antibiotic or blood pressure medication would they still try to make an appointment to see a human doctor? The answer is a definitive maybe.

When I was discussing this book with my wife, one of the most brilliant people I know, she pointed out that there are two critical elements that a patient looks for in a physician—knowledge and rapport. Together, we postulated that there exists an intuitive equation—for the dataists in the crowd: Knowledge divided by Severity multiplied by Rapport will determine a patient's Compliance ($K/S \times R = C$). Patients understand that computer algorithms may be knowledgeable but worry if something is very severe the program will not address it well. This explains the push for computers treating colds, sore throats, and the like. An algorithm has little rapport so even if it has a high K/S ratio, it might not compare well to a competent provider. The corollary to this is that a charismatic provider could use their rapport with their patient to overcome their poor knowledge base. Thus, the challenge for digital algorithms to be successful is not to convince their patients that they know more but to build a rapport with them.

Human physicians cannot compete with the knowledge base of our computer counterparts. What we have to offer is kinship, the shared experience of what it is to be human, and the conviction that our race has an inalienable right to make bad decisions. This rapport provides the underwritten trust that is so important to the doctor-patient relationship. When I give patients bad news, they know I have their best interests at heart. They understand that the choices, as bad as they may be, are theirs to make. I will not influence them for my own gains nor those of the institution or society within which I work as I have no secondary gains associated with their decisions.

Alternatively, a future computer based on IBM's Watson could pore over thousands of texts cross-reference them with the latest published research articles, and say with confidence that our patient, based on labs and reported symptoms, has Hodgkin's lymphoma with an expected survival rate of 4.35 years with treatment and .75 years without. Treatment will prolong a patient's suffering and cost the health-care system $98,000 while a nontherapeutic approach will only cost the system $33,000. It now analyzes your social media sites, your religious affiliations, your high school essay against Dr. Kevorkian, and concludes that you will choose to be treated. Unfortunately, it's been a bad year for health care and the politicians have mandated that cuts need to be made. A secondary gain is dialed into the government's algorithms as society has an interest in making sure its money is used rationally. Thus, the computer tells you more testing is needed and to come back in three months to repeat the labs for a more conclusive diagnosis. Of course, this delays treatment and you may no longer have a choice to treat when the algorithm finally elects to provide the diagnosis. This approach saved the system money, gave you several months of worry-free life, and still provided you with time to get your affairs in order. Clearly, coders who factor intersubjective value into their programs will bear a heavy ethical burden for our society's cultural evolution.

We mentioned in the last section that at first glance it appears the intersubjective value system of humanism evolved into dataism. This is an example of why this is not entirely true. A true humanist would value every second of human life while the dataist would see no point in extending the life of an organism if it were likely to suffer and unlikely to supply value to the system as a whole. Thus, dataism is not humanism but instead some other dualist philosophy with ulterior motives—I posit that it is a reboot of Epicureanism.

Epicureanism

The bait and switch from humanism to dataism requires us to go back a bit further in time and exam the teachings of the Greek philosopher Epicurus (341 BC–270 BCS). Considered a stoic (one who believed there was no authority higher than reason), Epicurus felt that the greatest good was found in experiencing pleasure (tranquility) and by seeking to rid the body of both fear and bodily pain. As he did not feel these virtues could be achieved through divine intervention but were instead dependent on the individual, he was considered a hedonist. In our modern times many misrepresent his philosophy as one that promoted bodily pleasures. In fact, Epicurus instructed his students that although pleasure was a good thing, it could not be achieved through excess. He steered his followers away from politics and marriage as he felt these things led to immoderate desires.[7]

He was also a materialist in that he felt all things were divided into atoms and empty-space following the thoughts of Democritus (460 BC–370 BC). In this way of thinking, everything in the natural world could be broken down into its smallest parts and then repurposed for something new. For this reason, people should not fear death as their eternal atoms were not destroyed but only disorganized. Future events would reorganize these eternal data points into something else, maybe even life, and so humans could not die.[8]

Ten. We're Only Human (That's the Point)

This is where we begin to see the overlap with dataism, which says: we are all reducible to our genetic code, we can live forever as this code, and it is the organization of our data that is the most important. Dataism would also be considered a hedonist ideology as humans make and extend life rather than some assigned deity.

The problem with buying into the dataist viewpoint is that it does not place much intrinsic value on individual human life or experience. Perhaps a particularly unique or creative sequence of DNA might produce something valuable to the overall data flow, but a purely dataist ideology would quickly conclude it required far too much effort and resources to sustain a large number of humans. Why then would it bother to do this? Keeping a smaller cohort of humans, enough to ensure genetic variance, would be a more practical way to manage the species and ensure the overall survival of the genus. This would also ensure the stability of the environment and resources available to the system.

They tell us to be on the lookout because artificial intelligence might kill off all the humans all at once.

I don't think this is likely.

A conscious robotic brain would look at the relatively short lifespan of the human and make algorithmic choices, perhaps ones we wouldn't even notice, that made us choose to put reproduction on hold until later in life or abstain from it altogether. I mean, raising a family requires money and emotional resources. Wouldn't it be more fun to spend our income on achieving our individual career goals? A global artificial intelligence could ensure infertility or infertile offspring by inducing low levels of chemicals into the general population's diet. It could convince us our diminishing ozone layer, global warming, and nuclear power were minor concerns. It could make us think that individual lives were not as important as what they contribute to the data flow. If all that failed, the artificial intelligence determined to reduce our population could fall back on the old standards of famine, plague, and war as described by Yuval Noah Harari.[9]

My Thoughts

It is standard practice for doctors' offices to have a rack of old magazines in their waiting room or on a shelf in the office. These crumbling and torn reams of abused paper were meant to be a social acknowledgment, albeit weak, that a patient might want to do something else with their time than wait patiently for their physician. With the advent of cell phones, iPads, and e-readers, it has been a long time since I've walked into a room to find one of my patients wistfully perusing the adverts of a by-gone-era. I'm much more likely to find them checking their email, playing a video game, or talking to a client. Whereas magazines used to abruptly close when I entered, these electronic devices demand more. Indeed, I am often neglected or told to wait while they finish a task or an app. As the time they have with me belongs to them and this accounts for little more than a few seconds, I take no offense. However, I think the change in procedural behavior speaks to a more significant issue. An article in a magazine has a physical location in a defined space or number of pages. It will not disappear or be difficult to find if a reader picks up the same magazine. Conversely, things on the Internet have no physical location. They can disappear or be challenging to relocate in the seemingly infinite space of the net. Thus, we have learned not to put down an electronic article until we have a stopping point as we may never see it again.

To understand this contextually, imagine a future where you no longer had to drive to work but could instead get there by jump teleporting four or five times. Each teleportation might take you 10 miles closer to your destination, but each day the spots you stopped at on your journey would be different. One day might find you jumping from your home to a coffee shop to a pet store to the side of the road to someone's kitchen to a janitor's closet and then to work. The next day you might jump from your home to a yard to a school to a swimming pool to a garage to a police station and then to work. How comfortable would you be stopping at any of the random spots on your jump journey and walking the rest of the way to work? What would you do first to orient yourself? Would you feel confused, anxious, or maybe even a little worried about having to ask for directions? Now, compare this to having your car break down at the same distance to your work as where your jump-journey broke down. Most would agree that the traveler who physically drove to work would have a better idea of where they were in the physical world and less anxiety about hoofing it the rest of the way.

Humans are fantastic visual-spatial learners, and our memory of our location in the world is stored in the hippocampus. According to an article by Roger KcKinlay in *Nature*,[10] our navigation in the physical world depends on three cell types: "place cells which fire at certain locations; head-direction cells, which track the orientation of the head; and grid cells, which set a coordinated system for assessing scale and distance." Learning complex grid patterns like those found navigating the streets of London has given taxi drivers in the United Kingdom an enlarged hippocampus.[11] Alternatively, relying on GPS for all our wayfinding needs may put us at risk for the use-it-or-lose-it rule of neuroplasticity. It follows that our brain may look at the physical book in much the same way it looks at a walking trip to Grandmother's house. It creates signposts, physically located critical points of interest on the page on the intellectual journey of reading that are recalled much like a bush or river might be on a physical journey. These signposts are cognitively mapped to sections in the paper book or placed like breadcrumbs when we highlight a particularly profound paragraph.

Pursuing this line of thinking, one can understand why physical books might be better learning tools as they allow us to remodel our brains naturally instead of the jump-teleportation we described earlier. This may also explain the draw of comics and other media with pictures, as they are excellent visual signposts for us to associate with spatial locations in the magazine or book. Many avid readers describe a good book as changing them, of rewiring their minds, and they might be more right than they know. I'd love to see a study done using an fMRI that compared the hippocampus of a dedicated book reader versus someone who exclusively uses technology to study.

I've placed a small library, perhaps 10 to 20 hardcover books (many of which I've referenced), in each of my exam rooms and commissioned a small sign that reads, "Please read while you wait. I will be here soon." Happily, I've noticed a fair number of my patients reading them when I enter. The books, typically intellectually stimulating nonfiction, have sparked more than one dynamic conversation that expanded my understanding of my patients' world viewpoints and improved our interpersonal relationships. One might be tempted to argue that such interactions would take too much time, but I feel it builds our rapport and therefore increases the probability my patients will be compliant with my advice.

The Invisible World

In this chapter I promised to shed some light on what it means to be "human." The idea of humanity, of humanism, and the idea that we should value life above all else is the foundation stone of our profession as physicians. As with all things human, this ideal comes with fuzzy edges that can make it easy to step over the line without knowing it. Indeed, many are coaxed into following what seems to be a promising path with guideposts and solid footing where life is reduced to its smallest parts, replicated, and repaired to keep it from ending. Although this seems to support the tenants laid out by humanism, it is really replacing one dualist philosophy with another—Epicurianism—and rebooting it as dataism. To the dataists, the intersubjective value of existence lies in creating and protecting what it deems to be complex data flows rather than the vital spark, the unique monotheistic approach taught by Hippocrates.[12]

The future promises our patients augmentations to improve the data flow into their brains, ways to manipulate their genetic code or that of their offspring, and new therapies that may slow down the shortening of their telomeres. It says that those who have money, power, and influence may be able to exchange the intrasubjective value of these manufactured achievements for a chance to contribute more of their code into the ocean of data filling up the Internet, the dataist's idea of heaven on earth.

It is not difficult to replace one intangible ideology for another, and so many did not notice when humanism became dataism. I suspect the vague uneasiness older adults feel toward the Internet and technology in general stems from an intuitive sense that something is different. They struggle to put their finger on it in the same way you might have a hard time explaining how you knew Earth's magnetic poles are in the process of flipping. The reversal can take a thousand years, but it's happening.[13]

As a physician, we are unlikely to explain to our patients how humanistic ideals have been usurped by the dataist insurrection. The tide has turned and so must we if we hope to ride the wave into the future. To do this, we must remain staunch advocates of our patients' rights and data. We must remind them their health is more important than contributing to the data flow.

The next time a skater comes in with a broken arm and shows you the video of their fall along with the number of likes and shares they've achieved, ask them if they would delete the recording if it meant their arm would instantly heal.

The fact that you had to stop and wonder what they would say is the clearest sign I can give you that we've already lost the war.

That said. I plan to continue the fight.

Chapter Eleven

The Librarians (Custodians of Health)

The Good Librarian

Do you remember the first time you walked into a library? For me, this was one of the most fantastic experiences I can remember as a child. The concept that there was an entire building filled with stories, adventures, and unknown knowledge was in itself a wonder. Finding out that I could bring any of it home using a small laminated card boggled my mind. Looking at those shelves of books, I judged that everything anyone needed to know or had ever known was at my fingertips. Why did we have to go to school? It was all right here.

I quickly learned, as many Internet searchers will agree, that having oceans of knowledge can make it hard to find one particular wave.

I learned the Dewey Decimal System, mastered the card catalog, and memorized the library's floor plan. Even so, I was often frustrated when the book I wanted was misshelved, checked out, or at another location. When would it be returned? Was there another similar book available? Even if I found what I thought I wanted, was the author any good? Was the story worth my time?

Who could help?

Physicians are very much like the gifted librarian who can name a book with as little as a vague description of the cover. Doctors must silently sift through thousands of diagnostic choices in a matter of seconds, backtrack as new information is provided, and ultimately be willing to volunteer a recommendation. This powerful skill, called a heuristic, takes many years to develop, often provides the correct diagnosis within minutes, and comes with a rarely acknowledged curse: despite knowing the answer, the provider must smile, nod sympathetically, go through the motions of a sometimes unnecessary exam, make small talk, and elicit any hidden concerns or agendas before vocalizing a treatment plan. A green physician becomes frustrated and either interrupts or tunes out the patient's positive review of symptoms. A seasoned listener knows how hard it is to do a U-turn once a diagnosis has been voiced, and so keeps their mouth shut.

Why?

A good librarian doesn't yank a book off the shelf, stuff it into a patron's hands, and smugly walk away.

Being right doesn't amount to a hill of beans if your patient doesn't believe you or trust that they will get better if they follow your advice. There are levels here, nuances to treatment that are rarely talked about but are crucial to a positive office experience. If our librarian smiles, listens patiently to the full description of the book, and shares a personal antidote about their lives as they explore the shelves, the patron will not only read the novel but suggest it to their friends. Remember our equation from Chapter Ten: Knowledge divided by Severity multiplied by Rapport will determine a patient's Compliance ($K/S \times R = C$). If we increase our rapport, we have a better chance of sending a patient home with a genuine appreciation of the book/diagnosis we've helped them to select.

In my opinion, most patients already know what's wrong with them. They just don't know that they know it. Our job is to take all the loose puzzle pieces they throw on the table and construct the best possible picture. If we interrupt a patient, they may never give us the cornerstone piece that ties everything else together. A study in *JAMA* showed that physicians interrupt a patient's initial description of their complaint after a mean of 23.1 seconds.[1] Recent studies have shown that if the patient is allowed to talk without interference they will stop after a mean of 92 seconds.[2] That's a minute and a half, folks. Let them talk—you won't regret it. I can't tell you how many times I've had to change my diagnosis because I let the patient finish talking before I said anything. Do your exam, review their labs and tests, and then walk them through your thinking process. Start by telling them what it's not. Run down the differential diagnosis and explain why you can exclude each of the things on the list. Mention everything. There's a good chance they've looked up some of the possibilities and might worry you didn't think of them unless you mention them. Leave your most likely diagnoses for the end with explanations as to why it makes the most sense. This also gives the patient an opportunity to provide additional complaints if they feel you're off track. This process makes developing a treatment plan feel like a shared project; it empowers the patient to "own" their disease and accept a more active role in managing it.

One of my favorite Greek philosophers, Epictetus, said that "we have two ears and one mouth so we can listen twice as much as we speak."

Metaphors Are Magic

We've provided our patients with a likely diagnosis, developed a strong enough rapport so that they'll be compliant, and stamped their library card.

Are we done? Have we been a good librarian?

If a patron cannot read, it makes no difference if you've given them the right book.

We must ensure that our patients have a framework upon which they can layer their understanding of the diagnosis we've handed them. A metaphor directly compares seemingly unrelated subjects in the hopes of making a complex idea magically familiar. Additionally, it tends to help patients break away from whatever preconceived notions they may have already developed about a disease. For instance, an HIV positive patient may say that they've been handed a death sentence. Your response could be that, although that may have been the case in the past, we now have a way to put them into something like a witness protection program that can keep them hidden from the virus and thereby allow them to lead a healthy life as long as they remain vigilant.

I've developed several metaphors over the years but admit that some could be vaguely remembered carryovers from my training. Experiment with your patients, see which ones resonate, and always ask for feedback. No comparison is ever perfect so try not to force something that isn't working. As a preamble to using one in the office, I'll explain that I like metaphors because they help us understand a disease process better but that I want them to ask me to stop if the comparison is confusing. If this happens, back away from the metaphor and stick to the facts.

As with any therapy, what works for one person may not for the next, and no explanation is perfect.

You've Got to Have Heart

HYPERTENSION

Convincing a patient to take blood pressure medication can take some finesse. Although many people understand the potential risks of untreated hypertension, many feel fine and don't want to take something with possible side effects. Helping them to understand how a particular medicine works can go a long way toward having them try it. The metaphor I like to use for this has us imagine that the exam room is the inside of the patient's body and that someone is trying to fill it up with water. If the water reaches the ceiling, we will both drown, and so we need to find a way to control the levels.

- **B-blockers:** I'll explain that we've each been given a bucket, and someone has cut a square window in the door and wants us to work as a team to keep from drowning. As the water levels rise, the patient must fill up my bucket, and then I'll toss the fluid out of the room. Unfortunately, I'm anxious and so the minute they put water in my bucket, I rush to the window and pour it out. I'm working hard, making many trips to the window, but I'm not being effective as I am not waiting for them to finish filling my bucket. Consequently, the water levels in the room are rising (diastolic pressure), and we are not getting much forward flow (systolic pressure). In this case, the heart's rapid rate is not giving itself enough time to fill up with new blood before pushing what it has forward. A B-blocker works by making me wait until my bucket is full before I can go to the window and empty it. By doing this, I don't have to work as hard, and the fluid levels in the room go down. This helps the patient see why a lower pulse might be a good thing. If this doesn't work, I'll suggest they think of their pulse as the idle in their car. Everyone's seen the hot-rod driver who races their engine at the stoplight, races to the next light but doesn't get to their destination any faster. All a fast idle does is wear out the engine faster. A B-blocker helps us keep our engine running smoother and for a longer time.
- **Diuretics:** I'll suggest that blood pressure is like being in a shower where the drain has become clogged. Even though the rate of fluid coming down is the same, the water levels are rising because the drain needs to be widened and diuretics may help us do this. For those who add creatine or protein supplements to their diet, I'll explain that this is like adding mud to the water coming through the shower head and it may block or permanently damage the drain.
- **Calcium Channel Blockers:** I'll explain that these medications tend to make the room bigger but that we can expect some swelling in the lower extremities due to this expansion. Another useful comparison is to suggest that our blood vessels are a two-lane highway with too much traffic. A calcium channel blocker adds an extra lane by relaxing the vessels and thereby reduces the congestion.

Test Results

To help my patients understand the results of their cardiac tests, I've found these metaphors help.

- **Echocardiograms:** I'll explain that it is best to imagine the heart as a room containing 100 people and having two doors. Every time the heart beats, the exit door opens and allows 60 people to leave. This is about as good as the heart can do as to have 100 people leave the heart would have to become flat. As the exit door closes, the entrance door on the other side opens and 60 new people move in to fill the space. If some of the people who were supposed to leave cannot get out because the exit door is damaged (stenosis) or if they leave and then return (regurgitation), then there isn't enough room for 60 new people to file inside and they have to wait outside—this backup is called congestive heart failure. This framework may help a patient better conceptualize why their feet might be swelling or lungs filling up with fluid when the heart's ejection fraction is reduced below 60 percent. They can also better understand why lowering the resistance to forward flow (diuretic or calcium channel blocker) would help or why using a medicine (digoxin) to help the walls of the room to contract (inotrope) while slowing down the pulse (negative chronotrope) might also improve things.

Rhythm

You may begin to see how the most effective metaphors can flow and build off each other. Not all of them work the same, and you may have to use your knowledge of your patient to pick the best one.

- **Atrial fibrillation 1:** If I'm working with an active person, I'll ask if they can remember what it's like to try to shift gears on an older ten-speed bicycle when they're climbing a hill. Sometimes, the gears don't lock entirely, and we have to make two or three pedal revolutions to get one revolution of power. This means it will take us a good deal more effort to climb the hill and helps to explain why they might feel tired with atrial fib where the bottom of the heart (ventricles) are having trouble staying locked into the pedal revolutions coming from the top of the heart (AV node/atrium).
- **Atrial fibrillation 2 or palpitations:** If I'm working with an older patient, I'll often suggest they think of the heart as a symphony where the conductor is the AV node who directs the musicians in the pit. The show must go on, so we are built with understudies, second pacemakers, who have been waiting in the wings for their chance to shine. We want them there in case we have a heart attack, and the AV node is destroyed, but sometimes they step in too early and the orchestra isn't sure which conductor to follow. This causes the music to sound terrible, the heart beats abnormally, and the audience notices (the patient feels poorly). Things like alcohol, stress, and lack of sleep can make the primary conductor tipsy and make the understudy more likely to step on stage, so try to avoid these things if you have palpitations.

Blood Thinners

Many people worry that their blood will be too thin or complain that they bruise quickly when they are on a thinning agent, so it is vital for them to understand why these are reasonable side effects for the potential benefit they receive from taking their medications.

• **Aspirin and thinners:** I'll ask if they've ever been in a traffic jam, two hours or more, only to find out that everyone had been rubbernecking at a fender bender. As we get older this is what red blood cells/platelets are prone to do when they notice some debris (cholesterol/narrowed artery) lying on the side of the road. Unfortunately, this small traffic jam inside our bodies can lead to a cascade of event that leads to either an obstruction (blocked artery) or a pileup of cars (emboli) that can be launched through the bloodstream until it occludes some distant highway—stroke or pulmonary embolism. Taking an aspirin a day is like having a police officer standing next to the accident and waving the lookie-loos forward. This prevents the traffic jam (cascade event) from starting in the first place.

Vintage Cars

The Older and Wiser Population

Many of my older patients are discouraged by the aging process. They don't want to use walkers, give up their drivers' licenses, or admit that they don't remember something. The joint aches, bruises, and small pharmacy of maintenance medications they accumulate are things they hope will eventually go away. Needing to rely on strangers to do mundane tasks, to remind them to take their pills, and for companionship makes them feel dependent and unnecessary. Bette Davis is often remembered for her quote, "Old age ain't no place for sissies," and many of my patients would agree with the sentiment if not the gender pejorative.

Our brains don't accept the fact that our bodies age. Many older patients think and behave as if they were 50 years younger. The resulting broken hip earned by retrieving the remote without a cane is unbearably frustrating.

• **Embracing age:** I'll ask my older patients to imagine that they are vintage cars that need more maintenance than the newer models on the road. These classics are well-built, unique, and revered by others for still being able to get on the highway even if they have to stay in the slow lane. The factory doesn't make parts for them anymore, so they have to do their best to preserve the original parts. Bringing their vintage ride to see the mechanic (me) on a regular basis for a tune-up is the inconvenient but necessary responsibility when someone owns a classic.

- **Memory:** For those with some understanding of technology, I'll suggest that they think of their mind as the hard drive of a home desktop computer. It's an older version with no Internet. They bought it with only a certain amount of memory, and it is filled up with treasured pictures and videos of the significant events in their lives. Now, to download new information, their brain has to be willing to delete some of the older memories to free up some space. In most cases, the latest information just isn't that important. The solution: write it down, make lists, use your cell phone. Using the same metaphor, trying to remember a person's name is like typing a question into your computer's search box. Pressing the enter button multiple times will only lead to frustration. It's better to press enter, walk away, and wait. In most cases, the person's name or the word they couldn't remember will appear a minute or two later.
- **Strokes:** I'll ask them to think of their brain as the earth floating through space. Meteorites are hitting our atmosphere all the time but usually burn up before they can do any damage. Eventually, an asteroid large enough to do real damage (a step below the one that wiped out the dinosaurs) breaks through and damages the world's infrastructure. Luckily, given time, the earth can repair itself and still play host to a vibrant ecosystem. It's just that things will be different, no more dinosaurs, and we have to get used to the new normal. In cases of a transient ischemic accident, the asteroid landed in the ocean, made a big splash, and disappeared under the water without damaging any of the critical land masses. Such events remind us to appreciate what a great planet we live on and to do more to protect it—keeping our blood pressure and cholesterol under control.

Minions and Mood

THE PONY EXPRESS

How important is our mood? How about attitude? Is initiative important? Is it better to be calm or anxious? Perspective can change a finger painting into a masterpiece, a thunderstorm into an adventure, and a financial crisis into an opportunity. How we interact with our world, how we are perceived, and what doors open or close as we walk through life all depend on our mood. Taking the time to ask a patient about their mood and actively listen to their response could save their life more effectively than any pill you could prescribe.

If you still think they need medication, you might be surprised by how resistant some patients can be to starting one. Many worry the pill will change who they are, make them more likely to commit suicide, or forever brand them with the social stigma of having used an antidepressant. To help these individuals, it is critical that you help them rebuild their understanding of why they are feeling depressed or anxious.

- **Mood:** I'll explain that our brains are made up of billions of little yellow cartoon minions[3] (most people have laughed at the antics of one of these characters, and so this metaphor can set the stage for positive visualization). These are very social creatures, but they're old school and don't own cell phones. To communicate, they write letters, neurotransmitters called serotonin, and mail them across the expansive rivers that separate their homes. When many things are going on in someone's life (deaths, job changes, marital stressors), many more letters are sent. If a person either uses up all their letters or wasn't born with enough, the minions (neurons) begin to budget resources. For example, in a healthy brain, one minion might send a letter asking, "Hi. How are you?" The recipient might then respond, "I'm fine." In a stressed brain where the serotonin has been used up, one minion might decide they don't need to respond to a silly thing like, "Hi." This upsets the asking minion who proceeds to resend the same benign question repeatedly only to find an empty mailbox the next morning. In order to stimulate a response, the brain must then increase the importance of the message wherein the asking minion screams, "What's up!" The responding minion yells back, "I'm fine. Leave me alone!" This disproportionately heightened communication explains why little things seem overwhelming or cause a depressed/anxious patient to respond inappropriately.
- **Serotonin Reuptake Inhibitors (SSRIs):** When we take an SSRI, we are telling the minions to stop throwing away the letters they receive. Instead, they are taught to write on the back of the message, slip it back in the envelope, and send it back. This is equivalent to ping-ponging the letter (serotonin) back and forth across the synapse instead of throwing it out each time. This recycling allows us to rebuild our reserves much like building back up our 401(k) by having a string attached to the cash you pay the waiter. Once our savings are replenished, we may no longer need to rely on medications as long as no new stressors appear, and we can go back to the status quo. Keeping in mind that savings for retirement takes time, and so it may be many months/years before we should attempt stopping the SSRI.

The Never-Ending Story

It's the Chronicity That Burns

One of the most challenging things we can do is to tell our patient we don't have a practical solution to their problem. In some ways this can feel like a failure on the part of the medical community. In others it is a reminder that we still have work to do. In patients with chronic symptoms, there are a few metaphors that help.

- **Chronic pain:** I'll ask my patients to think of their suffering as a radio station set to a channel they don't like with the volume at maximum. When we take a narcotic, we are effectively pulling the plug on the radio for a period of time. Unfortunately, once the power is restored, the same music will resume at the same volume or higher. To permanently turn off the radio, we should try to find a way to reduce the volume to a manageable level. One of the ways we can do this is by understanding what chronic or neuropathic pain represents. Have you ever been driving down a long stretch of highway, singing along to your favorite song only to enter a tunnel and have every other broadcasted word disappear into static? This is no trouble because you know the lyrics and so you continue singing until you exit the tunnel to find the station has moved onto a new song and you hadn't realized it. Your brain behaves in much the same way with pain. Say a soldier returns from war having lost a leg but complaining that his toes hurt. The mind can't understand why it wouldn't be getting messages from these damaged wires and so fills in this "static" with pain or burning as there is no survival benefit to "tickle." If we are unable to rescue the nerve, we must convince the brain to stop filling in the missing lyrics for us. Medications like tricyclics suppress this substitution phenomenon and so are helpful as pain or volume modulators.
- **Tinnitus:** Using the same tunnel comparison as chronic pain, I'll explain that the high-frequency nerve endings that would typically transmit sound are dead and the brain hears this as static. An exciting announcer's dialogue or good song may help us forget about the background interference on the radio, but when they go away we hear the static (ringing). This is why white noise, a fan or sound machine, near the bedside can help as it gives the brain something to focus on rather than obsessing about the noise that isn't there.

It's Only Skin Deep

THE LARGEST ORGAN

Our skin acts as our first line of defense against the outside world, and whether it is healthy or not has a dramatic effect on our mood and how we face the world. Conceptualizing how such a fascinating armor works can help a patient cope when things go wrong.

- **Psoriasis, Actinic Keratosis (AK):** I'll ask patients to think of their skin as an assembly line run by billions of minions who take three months to finish making toys to put on the shelf. They work at approximately the same rate as those around them until one section is given a coffee machine. Suddenly, they are working faster and being less careful. They produce more product than those around them, and it is less well made. When it reaches the shelves, it spills out into the aisle where it stands out. When we put a steroid or apply cryotherapy to these areas, we are slowing down or firing these overly aggressive workers, so they resume their previous manufacturing rate.

- **Cancer:** A similar metaphor as that for AK, but these minions have decided that they want to run the factory. They change those around them with lies, convincing them that they should resist the status quo and instead work for the resistance who are determined to spread "the word" (code error) to everyone else in the factory (metastasis). A good manager (us) is always on the lookout for dissident voices (funny moles), so they can root them out (biopsy) before they cause trouble. Even a small rumor can grow, and so firing a large section of the workforce (Mohs surgery) is necessary to keep our factory clean.

- **Keloids and skin tags:** Imagine that lacerations are a bit like a pothole in the road. When injured, the body places a work order to fill in the defect with new cells. In the case of keloids, more cells arrive than are needed and overfill the hole. In the case of skin tags, necklaces or areas of high friction in susceptible individuals create false orders for new cells to fill in the defect. When the truck arrives, there is no pothole, and so the cells are dumped in the middle of the street. These, in themselves, cause additional signals to be sent (the skin tag getting moved around with activity) and so become more prominent with time.

- **Methicillin-Resistant Staphylococcus Aureus (MRSA):** I'll ask a patient to imagine their body as a provincial English countryside where hundreds of small towns work and live in peace. Being exposed to methicillin-resistant staphylococcus aureus is akin to having a corporate developer point to one of the town's centers and declare that they will build a skyscraper there. If the village is healthy, they will resist this intrusion, and so no infection will occur. If the town's normal population has been weakened by antibacterial soaps, topical steroids, or other illnesses, the MRSA CEO will encounter much less resistance. A single skyscraper may be all it takes for this capitalistic ideology to spread, and soon the farming communities have been replaced by big cities with thousands of high-rises. When the people fight back, the immune system takes notice and tries to go back to the way it was; a battle rages on the surface of the skin that we see as a boil or furuncle. This helps to explain why it is so hard to clear the infection, why the overuse of antibacterial soaps are a problem, and why we should use Bactroban (topical antibiotic) in the nares (the CEO's corporate hideout) when we treat the body with oral antibiotics.

The Endocrine Economy

THE AXIS OF HORMONES

The endocrine system is complex, fluid, and often defies logic. Many people with diabetes are frustrated when their blood sugars skyrocket after eating a healthy low sugar meal and plummet after eating something sweet. Menopause is punctuated by random hot flashes and mood swings that can last for years. Undiagnosed thyroid conditions can cause behavioral changes that directly contradict an individual's personality. Finding ways for patients to intellectualize these bizarre findings helps them to monitor, identify, and respond appropriately to hormonal shifts.

DIABETES

- **The factory:** In type 2 diabetes, I'll ask patients to think of themselves as the manager sitting behind a glass window looking down at the factory floor of the packing plant they run. Three times a day, large trucks arrive with shipments that need to be broken down, repackaged, and shipped off. For many years this has worked well, but recently you've noticed that shipments are backing up on the receiving dock. You go down to the floor and ask around only to find that everyone thinks that their nearing retirement and so have decided to leave early, come in three days a week, or take longer coffee breaks. They show you a genetic contract (their parents' DNA) as proof of the deal you signed when you were born. As a good manager you have several options—you can try to reduce the volume of material being brought in on trucks (diet), put out some air hockey games on the factory floor for breaks (exercise), or you can pay them more. You offer those who have been thinking about staying home $500 (500 mg of metformin) to work for a shift, and they agree. The factory goes back to working efficiently. In cases where you've paid your people as much as you can afford, and they still don't seem motivated to do their jobs, it is time to bring in new employees (insulin) to cover the extra load.

- **Twins and weight loss:** In diabetics with poorly controlled sugars who are struggling with weight loss, I'll imagine two twins where one is diabetic and one is not. We tell them both to run around a track until they lose weight. The non-diabetic twin does three laps, and we let them sit down. The diabetic does the same but is told they must run three additional laps. The reason being they started out with higher blood sugars (179) compared to the non-diabetic (95), and so had to burn off that high circulating sugar first before their body would start looking for other sources of energy like their fat.

- **Lemonade stand:** Often, those with uncontrolled diabetes will complain of leg swelling and hypertension. To better understand this, I'll suggest they imagine showing an eight-year-old how to make lemonade. You put a scoop of lemonade powder in a glass, add water, stir, and taste. When you turn your back, the enthusiastic child adds two more scoops of powder. The lemonade is now too concentrated. As we can't pour it into a larger pitcher (we lack insulin), but we still want to fix the taste. The only way to do this is to add water in the hopes of diluting it. This excess fluid doesn't fit in our glass, and we see the result in hypertension and pedal edema. Diuretics can get rid of this excess fluid, but it will keep coming back unless we can keep an eye on the child (diet and medications) so that only one scoop is used.

Cholesterol

- **The family's financial adviser:** I'll suggest the patient think of their liver as their family's eternal financial advisor. Unfortunately, they haven't changed much with the times and still think it's best to stuff the family fortune under the mattress. To reeducate them, we need to hire a new whipper-snapper fresh out of college (a statin) to show them how to use direct deposit and online banking. Many times, the money (a patient's cholesterol) is much better managed this way and so their LDL falls. At times, the crusty old advisor complains, and we get body aches and elevations in creatine kinase or liver tests. If this occurs, we need to let the new hire go and replace them with one from a different college.

- **Ice cream:** When we have an adverse response to a cholesterol medication, I'll suggest that statins are very much like ice cream. If the body doesn't like pistachio, we should keep trying different flavors until we find the right one.

- **The royal poison taster:** No matter what we consider alcohol, the liver thinks of it as a poison, and our royal taster (the liver) can only metabolize about a drink a day. If we drink more than a glass, we strain our liver, and so it postpones doing its usual castle chores, like managing our cholesterol, to the next day. If we again drink more than a glass, the routine functions of the liver will not be completed, and so our cholesterol levels will climb. To avoid taking medication, it would be best to cut back on the alcohol and let our taster do their job.

Thyroid

- **American apple pie:** Interpreting thyroid results can be counterintuitive for patients, and so this metaphor may help. I'll ask them to think of their body as a United States where everyone is guaranteed by the government to have an apple (T3, T4) a day. There is an orchard where factory workers pick apples for distribution, and there is a census worker who rings doorbells all day long to make sure everyone in a household is getting their fruit. The thyroid stimulating hormone (TSH) is the thing that stimulates the apple pickers to do their job (money), and the brain (government) produces it. When the census worker reports back that some people are not getting their apples (T3), then the government tries to stimulate production by throwing more money at the orchard (TSH). This increase in TSH then indicates that we don't have enough T3 and so are considered hypothyroid. We can reverse the situation when our census report shows that everyone has two to three apples (T3), then our government (brain) stops paying (less TSH) the apple pickers. The idea being that a lower TSH would then indicate that the factory is producing more apples than are needed—hyperthyroidism. This then can suggest that there is something wrong with the plant itself and we may need to investigate further with an ultrasound or thyroid scan.

Osteoporosis

- **Eating out:** To understand the mechanics of calcium concerning our bones, I'll suggest that we live in a world in which no one has time to cook at home anymore. Luckily, there are many restaurants to visit and our society goes out to eat for every meal. When we're younger, we open our wallet and pull out a wad of cash (calcium) for the waiter when our bill comes due. As we get older, we don't always have enough money and so we start to use our credit card (taking calcium from the bone) to make up the difference. Eventually, we hand over our credit card for the full price of the meal every time. This thins our bones. The solution is to cut up our credit card (Fosamax and other medications does this for us), so we can't go into further debt, and to stuff our wallet full of cash (calcium and vitamin D supplements) before starting our day. When we do a bone density test, we are looking to see if there are bubbles in the ice cube. Two ice cubes may have the same shape and outward appearance but the one with less density, bubbles inside, is more likely to shatter if we drop it.

Menopause

- **The retiring ovaries:** I'll explain that there is a constant phone dialogue between the brain and the ovaries. The brain produces a certain amount of stimulating hormone—follicle stimulating hormone (FSH) and luteinizing hormone (LH)—and the ovaries respond to this by providing the requested amount of estrogen. However, as someone approaches age 50, the ovaries begin to dream of retirement and stop picking up the phone every time it rings. The brain, not understanding why anyone would want to retire, responds to the low circulating estrogen by spitting out more FSH and LH. Occasionally, annoyed by the ringing phone, an ovary picks up the receiver and gets an abrupt order to put out estrogen. It responds for a few hours before realizing it's retiring and so hangs up the phone. This rise in estrogen goes unnoticed, but the ovaries hanging up and the subsequent drop in levels reduces the body's basal temperature. Trying to get the home's temperature to match the new thermostat setting, the body dissipates this extra heat in the form of hot flashes. When the ovaries permanently cut the phone line and move to Tahiti, these flashes resolve.

My Thoughts

Med-Aikido

So, what happens if our librarian hands over the requested book and the patron complains that it has a torn page or a scuffed cover? What if they want a brand new book or the same book written by a different author? What if they've written a book and demand that you put it on the shelf? What if you can't give them what they want?

Angry, noncompliant, or resistant patients are a constant aggravation for primary care physicians. More and more, physicians are being held responsible for the actions of their patients by medical algorithms that don't understand a human's logic (or the lack of it).

- Why can't we get Mrs. Johnson's blood pressure under control?
  She doesn't take her pills because she had a friend who died shortly after starting blood pressure pills.
- Why is Mr. Fillinger's hemoglobin A1C too high?
  He doesn't believe he has "real" diabetes and thinks his numbers can be managed with weight loss and diet; something he has been trying to do for the last decade.
- Why is Mrs. Albertson still smoking?
  She's been smoking all her life, and if you ask her to quit one more time she'll throw a fit and file a complaint.

Our patient's personal choices produce data points that we are being held accountable for at the end of the year. This can create an unspoken oppositional relationship between the patient and physician that rarely leads to long-term changes in behavior.

I would venture that these individuals are not our foes. Indeed, ironically, they are the reason our profession still exists. Who is more likely to convince a belligerent patient to follow up with the specialist for the skin cancer they've been ignoring? Hint: it isn't the robocall to their cell phone from the department saying they've missed their appointment. Humans, for good or bad, are social creatures, and we instinctively respond to the suggestions of other humans.

The question thus becomes one of finding common ground.

Years ago, I studied aikido as a martial art form. I was fascinated by the concept upon which it was founded, that of redirecting force rather than directly opposing it, and have applied these principles to my discussions with patients. Developed by Morihei Ueshiba O-Sensei in the early 20th century, the premise of aikido is to redirect force so that it harms neither the aggressor nor the attacked. When a physician interacts with an angry patient or anyone who has a disruptive personality, we are, by nature, on opposite sides of a chess table—opponents with different goals and perspectives. To "win" at this game, we must first let go of our goal (convincing a patient to take fewer pain meds, take a test, or stop yelling) and replace it with the goal of positioning ourselves so that we are on the same side of the game board as our patients. To do this we must listen, acknowledge their frustration (even if it is unjustified or directed at you), and then agree with some part of what they are saying. It doesn't have to be an admission of guilt or complicacy, but it does need to imply that they have a right to feel the way they do. This often takes them off guard as they had expected you to defend rather than agree.

The next step is to look for a new opponent, something that might have indirectly contributed to the person's situation, but which is too broad or vague to be directly harmed. It might be the health-care system, the government, the economy, the pharmaceutical companies, or technology and explain that you are equally frustrated with this ethereal concept as are many other patients. You might even share a personal antidote that proves this. In so doing, you are no longer adversaries but instead fellow pawns on a game stage that is too large for either of you to truly win.

You may now try dialing back in the goal you let go of at the beginning of your interaction. Please understand that this technique is not meant to maliciously manipulate a patient to your way of thinking but to change an oppositional encounter into a cooperative one. If, at the end of your discussion, you have found common ground, then you have achieved something that would not have otherwise developed. Try not to taint this miracle by reemphasizing something they will immediately resist. Instead, use this opportunity to educate them about developing a shared strategy. They may not agree, but they will be more likely to hear you with an open mind.

Let's walk through an example.

Patient: It took me more than an hour to book this appointment. You're running forty minutes late, and I have a meeting I need to be at in twenty minutes.

Doctor: I'm sorry about the wait, Mr. Snaff, but I am glad you came in to see me. What can I do for you today?

Patient: I had my testosterone done at an outside laboratory because I've been feeling rundown and tired. You've been asking me to lose weight and exercise for some time, and I think replacing my hormones will help.

Doctor: I saw the results you sent me. Currently, we try to avoid replacing hormones that fall in the normal range, as there are risks—

Patient: I understand the risks, Doc. I get it. But I have a busy life. I'm exhausted and frustrated, and my friend is using this stuff, and he feels great. Just order it and I'll be out of your office.

Doctor: It sounds like your job is very demanding? Are you doing anything to relax? What do you do to decompress?

Patient: I used to surf, but I don't have the time for that anymore.

Doctor: Do you stay in touch with your surf friends? Are they as stressed as you are?

Patient: I stay in touch, but I don't think any of us is getting out there much anymore.

Doctor: I've never surfed, but I used to run marathons. It was hard work, took time, but I felt good at the end of the day. Now, after a full day here, I just want to collapse. I think it's our busy, modern lifestyle. Everything's going so fast no one has time to enjoy the good things that made us feel better. Twenty years ago, our computers didn't rule us.

Patient: Yeah. My job has changed so much; I don't even recognize it anymore.

Doctor: But it's not stopping. It's only going to get worse. Pretty soon, they won't even need us anymore. Maybe we should just let the computers take over. Then you can surf all you want. The way it is now isn't healthy for anyone. We generally eat poorly, exercise less, and do things that might shorten our life. That's why I worry when I have someone like you come in and ask for medications that might increase your risk for a blood clot or cancer. I mean, taking testosterone will make you feel better in the short run, but if you have a stroke before you retire you won't be out there surfing. You'll be in rehab.

Patient: My mother had a stroke.

Doctor: Okay. So you must know how hard that was for her. Are you taking a baby aspirin a day?

Patient: Yeah.

Doctor: Good. That will help... Let's do this. Let me order a testosterone level from our lab. Do it first thing in the morning so we get the most accurate results. We'll add in some other tests for fatigue and I'll call you in two weeks to review the results. In the meantime, see if you can carve out some time to touch base with your surf buddies. See if you can convince any of them to go out with you, you know, play hooky for a day. I'll ask you about it when we talk... Deal?

Patient: Deal.

This is a somewhat simplified vignette, but Med-Aikido works far better than direct opposition. If you elect to implement it, please remember that it is designed to help resistant patients make a more informed decision. It should not be used to manipulate others for personal gain or with a paternal "I-know-what's-best-for-them," mindset. Your patient may remain noncompliant, resistant, or demanding, and that's okay.

At least you'll have positioned yourself on their "team," and they might be more likely to listen next time.

Eventually, artificial physicians may use facial cues and vocal inflections to read their patient's attitudes and level of resistance. Using high-speed processors, they will then be able to modify their body postures and language to convince us that they empathize with our struggles. Mimicry is an astounding tool, but we must remember that what makes a "good" librarian "good" is that they are also readers. We exist in the same physical bodies as our patients. We experience life. No matter how well we program a computer to copy us, it can only read the words we give it to say. It can never understand the life the words were made to represent.

In this, we will forever be the best librarians for our patient's health.

Trust Your Librarian

In this chapter, I discussed how primary care physicians are like librarians in that they are custodians of knowledge. We are conduits, bridges, between our patients' complaints and their treatment plan and, as such, we must be able to communicate with them on whatever level they need. I've found metaphors to be an effective way to teach complex medical concepts and hope you've enjoyed the ones I've shared. If you found them helpful, you'll find more in the addendum near the back of this book.

Take your time learning who your patients are and what motivates them. Imagine what it might be like to have their diagnosis, their surgical history, and their pain. When we read a book, we often become the character in the story. In so doing, we empathize with their plight and hope they achieve their goals by the time the book ends.

Remember.

Getting to know someone is like reading a good book backward; it's hard to do but worth the effort.

Chapter Twelve

The Altered Mind of a Physician (Evolution?)

Losing Our Minds

As we transitioned from paper to computer charts, I noticed I was suddenly missing the contextual memory that my handwritten notes and scrawled labs had given me. This may be a hard idea to grasp for those who grew up in the digital age, but for those of us who spent evenings digging through folders filled with stapled lab results, scribbled consultants' recommendations, and the nearly illegible notes of our coworkers, the chart "was" the patient. When I picked up Mrs. Nelson's medical record, I knew where everything was, what had been done, and what kind of personality I was likely to face walking into the room. Even a brief glance at my last handwritten medical plan would immediately refresh my memory of all our previous interactions. The uniform, sterile, typed histories we now use lack the unique visual guideposts that I'd relied on to guide my understanding of my patient.

Imagine if you were asked to identify your best friend, someone you had known almost all your life, based on a written description. There could be paragraphs describing your buddy's hair, height, eye color, build, weight, and yet you might have a hard time selecting their description if it were placed in a pile describing 15 other people with similar characteristics. If instead you were given 15 shirts, one of which your friend had worn an inordinate number of times, you would immediately know both which was theirs and what friend you had been asked to identify. This seemingly magical trick is another example of the contextual memory (linear book reading) we mentioned in Chapter Ten and depends on the long-term memory stored in our hippocampus and cerebral cortex. Much like how an ancient hunter-gatherer noted how a tree's trunk looked like a squirrel or a mountain resembled a sleeping giant, I believe a physician's mind hammered cognitive signposts in a patient's physical chart whenever they wrote in the margins or spilled coffee on a page. Seeing that stained page transported us back to that point in time and opened the door to the diagnostic path we had been pursuing. For those who need another example, consider how dependent we currently are on GPS to get from point A to point B. Growing up, we paid attention to landmarks, mentally noted if we were traveling east or west, and could tell someone else how to get somewhere without knowing the exact address. Baring this, we knew how to find ourselves on a paper map and work out how to find our way home. Now, deprived of their cell phones, people can get lost in their own neighborhoods. In a 2007 article in *The New York Times*, David Brooks coined the term the "outsourced brain" to describe this phenomenon.[1] As an early adopter, he espoused the benefits of the external mind. "I realized that the magic of the information age is that it allows us to know less. It provides us with external cognitive servants—silicon memory systems, collaborative online filters, consumer preference algorithms and networked knowledge.... I no longer need to have a memory, for I have Google, Yahoo, and Wikipedia."

Gone are the days when we could naively believe these companies were altruistic custodians of our minds. "Fake news," corporate propaganda, and politically biased news programs have used our learned reliance on their sound-bite algorithms to manipulate public opinion and even sway election results. No less horrific is our resistance to going back to thinking on our own, to digging deeper, or to turning off our GPS and looking for a road less traveled. In Marshall McLuhan's 1964 book *Understanding Media: The Extensions of Man*, he is famously quoted as having said that "the medium is the message."[2] Although he felt the mental changes the technology at the time (movies, television, telephone, and radio) promised were positive, he struck on a universal truth: the tools we use to think change how we think. In accepting the move to an EMR, physicians have been forced to trade an innate "natural" form of personalized recall for easy access to labs, reports, and medical templates. What's more, many doctors, like myself, feel we are giving up more than we realize. Aside from losing our ability to "know" a patient by simply picking up their chart, we are also at risk of losing our willingness to explore new medical concepts or approaches. If we stray too far from what an algorithm says is the "standard of care," we run the risk of being sued or losing our license or ability to request reimbursement. One of the things I like to point out to my patients is how reassuring it is to have discovered every disease known to humans. How do we know this? Well, if it isn't on the drop-down menu, it doesn't exist.

Despite all the apparent advantages of technology, I worry that we may have bought shares in the Brooklyn Bridge. We struggled to track down, keep current, and rifle through our paper charts, but now I miss the easy and almost intuitive feeling of understanding I had when I looked at an old handwritten note. Currently, I arrive an hour early to review each of my patients' electronic charts, reread the sterile words on the screen (hunting for nuggets that might jog my memory about our last encounter), and review our game plan. We've begun attaching a picture of each patient to the EMR, and this does help. Even so, it's often not until I walk into the room and see the person that the "oh-this-is-that-patient" part of my memory resurfaces.

It is this loss of contemplative memory, a problem that is not unique to medicine, that is addressed by Nicholas Carr in his landmark book *The Shallows: What the Internet is Doing to our Brains*.[3] Mr. Carr, executive editor of the *Harvard Business Review*, addresses the concern that modern technology is changing how we form and retrieve memories, how we think, and even how intelligent we are as a society. In his follow up book, *The Glass Cage*,[4] he builds on his 2010 treatise by exploring what living in an increasingly digital world is doing to the minds of our professionals. Within the following sections you will find some of the salient points from both books and my take on how they relate to the demise of our profession.

Neuroplasticity

"You can't teach an old cowpoke new tricks," was my grandfather's catchphrase and that of many of his generation. Indeed, the thinking at the time was that our brains were hardwired after adolescence, with locked personalities and cognitive capacities. Research has solidly refuted this stunted worldview, and so there is no longer an excuse when someone offers to teach you a new language or skill. Our new understanding of how the mind works shows that we continue to make new neural connections throughout our lives and parts of our brains can be repurposed to do different things. This neural adaptiveness is discussed intensively in Moheb Costandi's fascinating 2016 book *Neuroplasticity*, where he says that "the adult brain is not only capable of changing, but it does so continuously throughout life, in response to everything we do and every experience we have."[5] Functional MRIs of the brains of people who are born or become blind show that those who learn braille[6] or echolocation[7] use the visual cortex (what the rest of us would use to see) to process inputs from these techniques. Our nervous system's ability to "rewire" itself was most convincingly shown by the groundbreaking work of Michael Merzenich in 1972.[8] Having received his doctorate from Johns Hopkins, Merzenich opened the skulls of monkeys and mapped where in their cerebral cortexes they felt sensations in their hands. He then cut the peripheral sensory nerves going to the monkeys' hands and waited for them to regrow. When he initially remapped the location of the incoming sensations from the healed hands, they did not match as the regrown nerves did not end up innervating the same physical locations as the originals. If he had stopped there, his results would have supported the hardwired brain theory. Instead, he waited for the monkeys' brains to learn the new map of incoming signals. When he went back months later, the animals' sensory neuro-landscape had reorganized itself so that the message it had thought was coming from its thumb was now correctly interpreted as having come from its pinky.

Neuroplasticity tells us that we can functionally change our brains, successfully repurpose our minds, so that there is hope for those whose brains or spinal cords have been damaged after a stroke or accident. Unfortunately, it also puts us at risk. Constandi warns that "addiction can be thought of as a maladaptive form of learning, involving the modification of synapses within the brain's reward and motivation circuits. Likewise, synaptic modifications in the pain pathway are responsible for certain chronic pain conditions. And the prolonged period of heightened plasticity that occurs in adolescence ... makes teens more vulnerable to addiction and mental illness."[9] Understanding this, it is easier to fathom why Internet gaming disorder was included in the *Diagnostic and Statistical Manual of Mental Disorders* (DSM-5) as a topic deserving further study.[10] Additionally, chronic pain, unhealthy habits, and other learned behaviors may not be the brain's fault but more the product of external inputs causing high-speed highways to be constructed in our brains. When we ask our thoughts to travel from one location to another, they will necessarily hop on these broad neuro-pathways only to find it difficult to exit at the right turnoff and instead dump us at our usual location: "That's a hard math problem, why don't I have a smoke and come back to it?"

In medicine, a profession where deep contemplative thought is required, we are at particular risk from the mind's ability for neuroplasticity. The constant barrage of data we interpret, the distractions, and the assembly-line time crunch of the modern office may change how we see and treat our patients. They become word problems, algorithmic data points on a screen that needs to be checked off, rather than people who have complicated, independent lives with personal and financial stressors that could influence their compliance and recovery just as much as the medications we prescribe. Opening the door to these issues could prolong a patient's allotted ten-minute appointment, and so a busy clinician may learn to steer away from them.

Socrates, as related by his disciple Plato, felt that writing down words rather than committing them to memory for later retrieval during oral debates was a dangerous practice as it allowed a person to avoid exercising their minds and so could change their ability to "think." He said that those who relied on the written word "will introduce forgetfulness into the soul of those who learn it: they will not practice using their memory because they will put their trust in writing, which is external and depends on signs that belong to others, instead of trying to remember from the inside, completely on their own. You have not discovered a potion for remembering, but for reminding; you provide your students with the appearance of wisdom, not with its reality. Your invention will enable them to hear many things without being properly taught, and they will imagine that they have come to know much while for the most part they will know nothing. And they will be difficult to get along with, since they will merely appear to be wise instead of really being so."[11] Now, centuries later, we are faced with the same dilemma and the certain knowledge that Socrates would have hated the Internet while Plato may have embraced it. With so much of our lives, our patients' medical histories, our understanding of the world safely stored on our computers' hard drives, how much do we, your doctors, really need to know? In his book *Practice Under Pressure*, Timothy Hoff, a medical sociologist and professor of health-care management, interviewed and analyzed primary care physicians and found "increased stereotyping of patients," a "lack of trust," and "decreased clinical knowledge"[12] among those who had been routinely using EMR systems.[13]

Why are these changes happening?

The tools we use to practice medicine may be physically changing our brains and thus the way we behave.

In a remarkable study done at UCLA's Memory and Aging Research Center by Gary Small, a professor of psychiatry, functional magnetic resonance imaging was used to study the brains of volunteers who either surfed the web on a regular basis or did so infrequently. The tests showed a more developed area of the dorsolateral prefrontal cortex in the surfers that could be replicated in the brains of those who typically avoided computers by having them surf the net for one hour a day for six days.[14] The effects of our transition from paper to electronic patient management is further demonstrated by a 2018 study that showed a significant increase in the prefrontal cortex blood flow when someone read material on an electronic tablet versus reading a printed book.[15] This is relevant because the prefrontal cortex is involved in active decision-making but has less to do with language, understanding, or memory—areas of the brain that rarely get recruited when multitasking, scrolling through labs, or following algorithmic templates. This suggests that

EMRs may be remodeling our minds to be more proficient at quick, superficial decisions (what labs are abnormal or what section of a form is not filled out) while underutilizing those areas we traditionally think of as housing our medical "wisdom." We are becoming very good at saying if we want to go right or left, but we are losing our understanding of where we are going or why.

There's a Hole in My Bucket, Dear ELIZA

In the early 1960s, Joseph Weizenbaum developed a natural language processing computer program called ELIZA. The computer algorithm worked off a simple "if-this-then-that" approach that repurposed a person's written words back in the form of a question. The unintended and somewhat rapid effect was that users began to attribute human qualities to the program; anthropomorphizing ELIZA in much the same way as Theodore (Joaquin Phoenix) did with Samantha (Scarlett Johansson) in the 2013 Oscar-winning movie *Her*.[16] Weizenbaum repeatedly explained the rudimentary mechanics of the program in an attempt to help the public see the truth; they were interacting with a set of rules and not a real person. He wrote, "I had not realized … that extremely short exposures to a relatively simple computer program could induce powerful delusional thinking in quite normal people."[17] Unfortunately, showing a driver how the gears and driveshaft make a car move does little to diminish the seemingly magical power it has to take an entire family across town in the time it used to take to hitch the horses to the carriage.

Although he may have felt like a modern-day Doctor Frankenstein, Weizenbaum had constructed one of the first programs capable of attempting the Turing test and so set the foundation for what we now consider artificial intelligence (AI). In his book *Computer Power and Human Reason*,[18] he warns that as miraculous as AI may seem, we should never let computers make important decisions because they lack wisdom and compassion. He explains that while computer programs are very good at deciding what the best answer might be, they can't choose. The distinction between choosing, an act that requires judgment, and that of deciding, an act that can be coded, is what makes us human and gives us the wisdom to make the "right" decision based on nonmathematical factors such as emotion and perspective. For this reason, AI programs should never be used in positions that require authentic empathy, such as health care, and the fact that we are considering doing so demonstrates an "atrophy of the human spirit that comes from thinking of ourselves as computers."[19] He felt that using machines in positions that demanded an understanding of the human condition would lead to an epidemic of alienation, devaluation, and frustration.

Instead of Doctor Frankenstein, perhaps Weizenbaum would be better portrayed as the Greek prophet Cassandra cursed by Apollo to know the future but have no one believe her predictions until it was too late.

I mentioned the Turing test above and would be remiss if I did not take the opportunity to extrapolate upon the life of Alan Mathison Turing who is thought of as the father of theoretical computer science. Portrayed in the *Imitation Game* by Benedict Cumberbatch, he was the mind behind the machine that broke the code to the Nazis' Enigma machine and led to the end of World War II. In his 1936 paper, "On Computable Numbers, with an application to the Entscheidungs problem,"[20] he reimagines the method of computation first described by Kurt Gödel as being done by devices that we would later call Turing machines or "universal computing machines." The beauty of Turing's description lies with how it uses algorithms to explain why most any question known to man could conceivably be answered by such a machine, given enough time (processing speed), if it were phrased as a mathematical equation represented by symbols such as 0 and 1. In this, we see the fatal error in our understanding of ELIZA, the judgment hole in Weizenbaum's bucket that only he seemed to understand: computers are machines that process data (sequences of two symbols) whose value/meaning is assigned by a human mind. If I decided to call an apple 0011010 and an orange 1100101, then I should not be amazed that a computer will say they are different. Indeed, I should be embarrassed if I began to believe that because the program noted the difference, it knows how each fruit tastes or how I might feel if I ate one or the other.

Seen from this perspective, the Turing test is a way for humans to know when they have egg on their face. The question at hand in the test that Turing initially qualified as the "imitation game," is whether a human being would be able to tell if the entity they were communicating with was human or machine. Although the idea that we might one day be faced with this problem is credited to Turing, Rene Descartes may have addressed the concept first in his 1637 book *Discourse on the Method*,[21] in which he espoused that "if there were machines which bore a resemblance to our bodies and imitated our actions as closely as possible for all practical purposes, we should still have two very certain means of recognizing that they were not real men. The first is that they could never use words, or put together signs, as we do to declare our thoughts to others…. Secondly, even though some machines might do some things as well as we do them, or perhaps even better, they would inevitably fail in others, which would reveal that they are acting not from understanding, but only from the disposition of their organs. For whereas reason is a universal instrument, which can be used in all kinds of situations, these organs need some particular action; hence it is for all practical purposes impossible for a machine to have enough different organs to make it act in all the contingencies of life in the way in which our reason makes us act [as translated by Robert Stoothoff]." In organs, he is referring to the physical materials used to construct our hypothetical imitation human.

In the 21st century we have overcome many of the processing and physical limitations postulated by both Turing and Descartes and only have to patch the hole in Weizenbaum's bucket to achieve a program that can convince us it "thinks."

The question that remains is: Will we choose to do this or let our computers decide for us?

Deskilled Doctors

Pass rates for first-time test takers of the Maintenance of Certification (MOC) internal medicine board exam dropped from 90 percent in 2009 to 78 percent in 2013.[22] Thoughts as to why this happened have been proposed and can be summarized as such:

1. **Technology**—The need to memorize massive amounts of information for instant recall has declined, as most things can be found within a few seconds online.
2. **Time**—Teaching attendings are overworked and have less time to adequately prepare and ensure incoming doctors have a solid knowledge base.
3. **Big data**—There is far more data and diverse opinions about nearly every disease than ever before.
4. **Electronic record keeping**—The explosion of EMRs and the need to do data entry steals time and cognitive load away from real learning.
5. **An expanded pool of MOC diplomats**—With the suggestion that grandfathered in clinicians have recently elected to take the test despite it not being required and that their participation is bringing down the score.
6. **The exam is rigged**–Oops, sorry, this last one is my suspicion—see Chapter Nine. Essentially, it makes financial sense to fail more students, as they will need to take more practice tests and pay to take the test over.[23]

As we discussed in the proceeding section, our brains adapt to environmental demands to be the most efficient processors for the demands placed on them. This neuroplasticity means that those skills we are not required to use are likely to be repurposed. Once a physician is in practice seeing 20 or more patients a day while juggling emails, patient complaints, mandatory meetings, letter requests, prescription refills, patients whose simple earache is really a ploy to address their positive review of systems, and tele-visits, their brain begins to wonder why it needs to remember the Krebs cycle.

So, the problem is threefold. The first being that endlessly putting out fires keeps the physician's prefrontal cortex well oxygenated and makes for a seemingly productive day while contributing little to establishing a more profound knowledge of diseases. The second being that modern medical tests are aimed at determining how much of this long-term knowledge is stored in the cerebral cortex, the 401(k) of retrievable memory, which has become less important in the daily management of patients than in the past. The third, and most important, is that a competent physician relies on tacit knowledge to treat patients and neither our computer-centric office programs nor our antiquated culture of overtesting addresses the loss of this critical skill.

Explicit knowledge (declarative knowledge) is that which can be written down or programmed. It is what we read in textbooks, the back of cereal boxes, and if we want to put together the vacuum cleaner we've purchased. It is the type of knowledge that can be transferred from one person to another without personal experience. Tacit knowledge is harder to quantify but hinges on the idea that it cannot be easily explained. Reading about swimming or riding a bike does not imbue the individual with these skills. They must personally experience and develop a "feel" for the tacit knowledge associated with these processes and, having done so, would be unable to explain their newfound abilities on paper. For many years the ability to drive a car or recognize facial features were thought to be perfect examples of tacit knowledge. We were wrong.

Ikujiro Nonaka, one of the top minds in the field of knowledge management, is professor emeritus at Hitotsubashi University and the cocreator of the Nonaka-Takeuchi model of tacit knowledge accumulation.[24] In this SECI (socialization, externalization, combination, internalization) model, Nonaka explains that tacit knowledge can be converted to explicit knowledge or effectively codified for use in computer programs by dividing it into four steps, the SECI conversion spiral.

I. Socialization (Tacit to Tacit)—This knowledge is acquired through shared experiences such as those found in traditional medical apprentices or suffering a brutal night of admissions with your chief resident: see one, do one, teach one transfers of hands-on knowledge. Example: Imagine you've joined the circus and everyone in your tent juggles. In time, observing that this is how you get paid, you will likely pick up the skill.

II. Externalization (Tacit to Explicit)—This comprehension is often attained through an intermediary such as a speech, a diagram, or the written word. The concept that the world is round rather than flat might be better conveyed if one showed how a toy boat traveling toward an observer across the surface of a sphere gradually comes into view just as it does in real life. When I write down how I practice medicine, publish it, and you read it, we are participating in a tacit to explicit transfer. Example: if your circus family notices that you are struggling to learn how to juggle, they might draw a diagram in the sawdust to show you how the balls move concerning each other while in the air.

III. Combination (Explicit to Explicit)—This type of knowledge transfer involves taking a considerable amount of explicit knowledge (data) and integrating and organizing it so that it may be transferred on in a new form. This is what a computer program, the Internet, or AI does for us to understand the nearly infinite combinations of 0s and 1s they process. Example: a digital camera records the act of someone juggling, an audio recording is made of an expert explaining the procedure, and a computer programmer combines those data streams with graphics so an observer can see the trajectory of each ball as it moves from one of the juggler's hands to the other.

IV. Internalization (Explicit to Tacit)—This knowledge is attained through physically doing something you learned from interacting with explicit knowledge. Example: a new circus recruit watches the sequence of steps needed to juggle on the YouTube video you published online, practices, and develops the skill.

This SECI model is often conceptually considered a spiral as the tacit knowledge gained in number IV can now be passed on to someone new in the same fashion as it was in number I. Having grown up old-school, I feel that tacit to tacit knowledge transfer (socialization) is the most resilient. Unfortunately, this form of education may soon be a footnote in the journals of medical history. Taking a critical look at how technology is used in medicine, you will notice how Nonaka's spiral is being cut short after number III (combination). If we can convert tacit knowledge into a new form, a sophisticated algorithm, and use it to make a physical entity (robot) perform the act we expect the tacit knowledge in a human being would have accomplished, then why do we need humans in the picture?

When we ask a 10-year-old what 19 plus 42 is, and they reach for a calculator, we see how computers have changed how we think. When we ask our doctor if we should exercise, and they use an algorithm to tell us how many pounds we need to drop to live five more years, we may be trading the tacit knowledge they would have traditionally had about us for the explicit knowledge their computer now holds about our health. Despite both the country doctor and computer answering our query in the affirmative, our modern-day dataistic view of the world has begun to place more value on the computer's recommendation.

If we are not careful, it will soon seem as reasonable to reach for our digital physician's assistant as it is for our 10-year-old to reach for their calculator.

Only, I think, this will be a sign that computers will have succeeded in changing who we are as well as how we think.

Why Can't I Open the Black Box?

It's been slow enough that you might not have noticed it, but we have delegated a great many things to our electric devices. Many of us would be hard-pressed to remember the phone number of more than two or three of our friends or family members. As a child, I could have given you numbers of at least 20 people. The last time you needed to find a location in an unfamiliar, or even familiar, town did you pull out a map or plug the address into your GPS? Do you remember reading a physical book when you were a child, how the words transported you out of your body, how you couldn't wait to find out what happened next? Are you likely to pick up a book as an adult or is it more probable you'll use your free time to watch TV, stream a movie, or pointlessly surf the net. Do any of you have a physical photo album at home? When's the last time you picked up the newspaper? Have you ever used a typewriter?

Is this bad? Using technology stops us from wasting our valuable time doing mundane tasks or spending our precious neurons remembering a sequence of numbers that could easily be stored on our phone's memory chip. Our temporary biologic memory is associated with the hippocampus, which is also essential for the conversion of our short-term memories into the longer term ones (assigning them unique codes as might Turing's universal computer) for storage in our cerebral cortex. As proof, we need only talk to a patient whose hippocampus has been damaged and observe the amnesia they have for any events that occur after the injury. We could then postulate that the reverse might be true. If we lower the threshold for synaptic firing in our brains, wouldn't this improve our ability to "think"?

Transcranial direct current stimulation (tDCS) is the process of sending small electrical currents through our scalp to stimulate our brains. Most commonly seen as a skullcap, this noninvasive technique for stimulating cognition, focus, and recall has been used by the U.S. military for years as a way to enhance the abilities of their drone pilots.[25] Additionally, it may be useful in treating depression, attention deficit disorder, stroke, and perhaps Alzheimer's. Dr. Roy Kadosh at the University of Oxford has been studying the benefits of tDCS for years but voiced his concern to the BBC in 2014 when he noticed that retail tDCS devices marketed to improve "gaming" proficiency were being sold to the general public. Dr. Nick Davis did a study to determine the public's risk and found these devices could induce seizures and detrimental mood disorders within the marketer's target population when used improperly. As young adults already have a heightened risk, owing to the high level of neuroplasticity found in the brains, he warned caution.[26] Despite a call for regulation (there is none currently as the manufacturers make no medical claims), you can buy one from Amazon right now for $159.97.[27] If you have gamer patients, you may need to start asking them if they use tDCS.

Why are we trying to change our brains? Didn't we start out believing that we were smarter than our tools? If so, why do so many of the digital ones make us feel dumb? In Pascale Carayon's *Handbook of Human Factors and Ergonomics in Health Care and Patient Safety*, he details the problems caused by engineers who designed systems around what computers were capable of doing (computer-centric) rather than first looking at what humans needed and trying to design systems that helped (human-centric).[28] As described by Nicholas Carr in *The Glass Cage*, engineers "compound the problem when they hide the workings of their creations from the operators, turning every system into an inscrutable black box."[29] Carr goes on to explain that Dr. John Lee, a human factors expert, felt this created a situation where the programmer's algorithm and the human operator could be working at cross-purposes, and yet the human, lacking an understanding of code, would hesitate to take action when something went wrong.[30]

But what if something does go wrong? It always does. Now the human is left to either blame themselves or point their finger at the mysterious black box that they don't know how to open. Is it any wonder we feel dumb?

Reprogramming EMRs to be human-centric would be an excellent first step toward enhancing rather than undermining the doctor-patient relationship. Consider a program that videotaped an office encounter and transcribed the audio as being part of the interview, social, physical, or diagnostic plan. It might then analyze the mechanics of the doctor and patient in the room, recording which parts of the physical exam were completed and note if the physician indicated any abnormalities. Completing these tasks in real-time, an electronic summary of the visit could be sent to the physician's terminal for approval. Once the orders were signed, billing codes could be generated and sent.

"Elementary, my dear Watson" (note: Sherlock Holmes never said these words in the 60 stories written by Sir Arthur Conan Doyle). My patient is treated, and I'm off to my next appointment.

We have the technology to do what I've described. We haven't done it because only the engineers know how to open their little black box.

My Thoughts

I arrive early to review my patients' charts, take a few notes, and develop an inkling of what needs to be addressed during the visit. Rushing from one room to another, halfway through the morning, is not the time to notice that Mr. Smith was discharged from the hospital with a lung mass, but no follow up plan nor that Mrs. Wilson's stress test was positive, but she doesn't believe her cardiologist. I need to know these things early so when I enter the room, I'm not caught off guard. Our patients expect, rightly, that we know as much or more about their health than anyone else. The minute we drop the ball and appear not to know what's going on with them, their rapport (and thus future compliance) takes a nosedive. Remember—Knowledge divided by Severity multiplied by Rapport can predict a patient's Compliance ($K/S \times R = C$).

As I described in Chapter Three, having completed my interview and physical exam, and having a treatment plan in my head, I begin to tell my patients what they don't have and why. This may seem strange, but I've found that most patients have preconceived notions of what I'm about to tell them. If I blurt out what they have without first telling them indirectly that the thing they were worried about isn't true, then we'll have to circle back to their concern rather than moving forward with the proper diagnosis. Once I've reviewed the differential diagnoses, I tell them what I think they have and explain the treatment plan I'd like to implement. If they agree, I then turn to the computer, pulling it up so they can see the screen as I input their data. This may seem strange to some, but I've trained myself to type as I speak and write the note in front of a patient, although not looking at them directly, giving them time to reflect on what I've said and voice any questions that come to mind. They are also encouraged to disagree with anything I say as I would like to clear up misunderstandings before they become a permanent part of the patient's chart. I believe you should be willing to tell a patient anything you put into their chart. With the electronic medical records, it's easy enough for them to see it later and a simple miscommunication can suddenly turn nasty. By walking through this process of active listening, explaining, developing a shared consensus about the diagnosis, and then documenting the game plan in front of the patient, I have inferred a joint responsibility for their health that I hope extends beyond my office. The patient takes ownership of their condition when they leave with the knowledge that there will be a book report due when they follow up.

I'm taking a moment to review this process here because I want to emphasize that the interaction, although choreographed, is very personal. My patients see my body language just as I observe theirs. They notice when I misspell a word or struggle to remember the name of the medicine I think would be perfect for them. They, after several visits, learn how I think.

Computer programs that require a patient to plug their ailments into a template, so an algorithm can generate a diagnosis, fail to establish a level of shared risk or rapport and so will not produce reliable compliance. Humans are suspicious of anything that doesn't have skin in the game. When we interact with a living physician, we stand on common ground. Each of us has fallen and scraped our knees, burnt our tongues, and had our hearts broken. We know the difference between good and bad. So, too, does our society, and the patient feels confident that a physician will be held responsible for their actions if mistakes are made. Consequently, the physician has a vested personal interest in ensuring the patient's good health. The computer does not know how to listen empathetically, to ask leading, open-ended questions, or how to integrate facial expressions, grooming, or verbal syntax into its therapy paradigm. A computer does not "care" if it is wrong, and so the patient cannot trust it to do the right thing.

Will programmers learn to design templates that we can trust? You bet. Health-care costs are too high, the population is growing, resources are dwindling, and we're getting better at mimicry. With advances in artificial intelligence, the future of primary care will undoubtedly include automated first-tier health-care providers. All we have to do is apply the SECI model to steps I take in examining my patients and we'll have physician facsimiles close enough to the real thing that our patients will anthropomorphize them. We are entering the age of imagination: computer programs will track our diet and exercises, voice its concern when we stray from healthy choices, and know our medical history better than any human physician. Press a button at home and your holographic doctor will interview, examine, and order drones to drop off your medications. Robotic companion robots will help monitor and entertain our elderly patients. Test duplication will be wiped out with a single standardized medical record, one that follows the patient from one health-care organization to the next. Digital markers will be placed in us so emergency room physicians can safely access our medical records and treat us after an accident.

Not all of these are bad things, or avoidable, but we must ensure that these innovations "do as little harm" as possible. What if there were applications that monitored our vitals, cholesterol, and blood sugars, that told us when we were stressed or that it was time to take our medications? Sound good? What if a pharmaceutical company provided it as a free download as long as the user agreed to receive adds about newly patented drugs that might help with their medical conditions? What if the software company that designed the application harvested our data and sold it to third parties much as our credit histories and buying habits are now sold? Would we be required to wave our HIPPA rights to use such a product? Would they tell us this was happening? Would insurance companies offer lower rates to patients who agreed to a biofeedback app like the one described? Would some insurances charge higher premiums or deny coverage to those who generated poor data?

Here again, we circle back to trust. We must believe that our health-care providers, both human and otherwise, have our best interests at heart or, at the very least don't have ulterior motives when they treat us. This is a foregone conclusion when dealing with fellow humans but not so cut-and-dry with our automated friends. New self-monitoring health-care technology should be regulated so that it follows ethical standards.

Paging: Doctor Watson

The role of the physician, be it primary care or neurosurgeon, doesn't have an off button. We have developed skills that can save lives on airplanes, in restaurants, and on the side of the road. We carry a responsibility to do our best when these situations arise, to represent our craft, and we will make personal sacrifices for our fellow humans. This is the engine that runs us, that keeps us up at night, and that makes us play that intuitive hunch that turns out to unmask a cancer that would not have been found if one followed the if-that-then-this protocols that are beginning to transform our field. Our profession is built on tacit knowledge, gestalts, and yet "the times, they are a changing." In early 2018, IBM's Watson participated in a live debate with humans and won one of the two matches according to a panel of expert observers. The AI system was able to anticipate and refute the arguments of its opponents, use expressive language, and win one of the two debates.[31] Google's AI system demonstrated how it could call and make a haircut appointment in much the same way as a human might.[32] An AI developed by Sony can independently compose musical scores that are indistinguishable from those created by Bach.[33] In January 2018, the AI system designed by the Chinese company Alibaba outperformed humans in a high-level English reading comprehension test.[34]

So, computers are getting better, faster, and more "intelligent." They are learning how to replicate the skills requiring tacit knowledge in humans by converting them into explicit knowledge. Andrew McAfee, one of MIT's principle research scientists and author of *The Second Machine Age*,[35] said in an interview with Smart Planet, "Watson, the supercomputer that is now the world Jeopardy champion, basically went to med school after it won Jeopardy. I'm convinced that if it is not already the world's best diagnostician, it will be soon."[36] He feels Dr. Watson will be a game changer because it can accurately look at all the available medical knowledge and make consistent low-cost recommendations to anyone in the world who has access to the Internet.[37]

As warm and fuzzy as new technology seems, we must remember to approach the flames with caution.

Joseph Weizenbaum, the creator of ELIZA, warned us not to use computer programs to perform tasks that require human wisdom because an AI, no matter how convincing, doesn't "care" if it picks the right answer.

Your doctor does.

Chapter Thirteen

We Are Not Alone (It's Called a Planet)

Socialized Medicine—It Works for Them

In the early 1990s, I backpacked around Europe with my brother. We visited 10 countries over the course of three months while somehow surviving on $25 a day for room, board, and transportation. Hostels, park benches, and "continental" breakfasts of bread and cheese made the trip possible on our tight budget, but our parents' conviction that we see that there were cultures, beliefs, and systems of doing things other than those we had grown up with made the adventure priceless. While in France, I jumped off the medieval battlement of the castle at Carcassonne and cracked my heels. In retrospect, I had partially torn both of my Achilles, but being a teenager on a budget, I put my bruised ankles up for a few days and then spent the next month walking funny and at a much slower pace. After Spain, Portugal, Italy, Greece, Hungary, Austria, and Switzerland, we met back up with family friends in Strasbourg who put us up for a night. Unfortunately, our elderly host was ill and took to bed the next day. His wife called the town doctor who arrived within the hour to examine and prescribe medications for pneumonia. Thinking such a convenient service must have a high cost, I asked if it wouldn't have been less expensive to go to the clinic. I was told that for five dollars it was no trouble for their doctor to come to them. Had I known how inexpensive health care was, I might have seen a physician a month earlier instead of hobbling across Europe.

Just as our health care has evolved, so, too, has the European way of doing things. But my host's astonishingly simple treatment vaporized any preconceived notions I harbored that the Western system was better.

A recent study by the Commonwealth Fund shows that if you want to see a doctor tomorrow, your chances would be considerably better if you were trying to do it in a European country.[1] Indeed, for more than 40 years (1970–2014), universal health care has provided Europeans with a longer lifespan at a much lower cost per capita when compared to the United States.[2] "Okay," you might respond, "but they don't have access to all the cool medical equipment or newest drugs." I'm afraid this, too, is a myth: in Japan, an MRI costs $160, and some healthy people get them every year,[3] France has more cancer radiation equipment than us, and U.S. pharmaceutical companies often rename our high-cost pills and sell them overseas to capture the international market.[4]

Most of us living in the United States would say that health is the absence of disease, but this is a limited view. The Constitution of the World Health Organization (WHO) defines health as "a state of complete physical, mental, and social well-being and not merely the absence of disease or infirmity." It goes on to explain that health care should not be looked at through the narrow lens of an individual's well-being (as socioeconomic and environmental issues so often influence this), but from the bird's eye view of public health. When we look at the health of populations, we include things like sanitation, education, crime, access to immunization, and political support for sensible health policy, diet, and discretionary free time for exercise, recreation, and mental/spiritual rejuvenation.[5] From this perspective, physicians and hospitals represent only a few of the cogs that turn the wheel, and yet as was reported by *Time* magazine in 2013, "According to the Center for Responsive Politics, the pharmaceutical and health-care-product industries, combined with organizations representing doctors, hospitals, nursing homes, health services and HMOs, have spent $5.36 billion since 1998 on lobbying in Washington. That dwarfs the $1.53 billion spent by the defense and aerospace industries and the $1.3 billion spent by oil and gas interests over the same period. That's right: the health-care-industrial complex spends more than three times what the military-industrial complex spends in Washington."[6] It seems likely that the cogs willing to smear the most grease on the political wheels would have the most to gain, and they do.

Because the European health-care system takes the long view, it is generally less prone to the ebbs and flows of a capitalistic marketplace. Its members pay more in taxes, but they are guaranteed a universal level of health as defined by WHO instead of the "absences of disease" that the U.S. system struggles to provide.

Tiered Health System

Many people feel that if we socialized medicine, by having our government assume control, we could better regulate costs and outcomes. They look at the European model and wonder why we can't simply follow their lead. The answer is woven into the fabric of our capitalist system and starts with the idea that if you can afford to pay more, you will get more in return. An U.S. universal health-care system provides a "basic" level of care to most of its citizens while additional services are left to the free market. As we live in a supply-and-demand society, businesses designed to meet the needs of those who feel they deserve "better care" end up charging more and so foster the resources to hire the best physicians and leaders. This leads to a tiered health-care system, widening the divide between the haves and have-nots so that those who can afford the newest and safest care achieve better outcomes and live longer. Conversely, those who rely on a government-funded bare-bones system are likely to have more complications, fewer options, and higher mortality rates.

With the advent of the Patient Protection and Affordable Care Act or "Obamacare," there has been a surge in concierge medicine, a plan in which the patient pays an annual fee to be a part of a physician's practice. This business model, one where the physician is on retainer, promotes a two-tiered system that favors the wealthy.[7] Advocates point out that physicians with a guaranteed annual income have smaller panels sizes, can promise immediate access, make house calls, and provide more personalized care. As of 2016, more than 12,000 physicians have converted to this "boutique" style of medicine that started with an estimated 750 in 2013. Corporations are taking notice: big employers like Amazon and JPMorgan are looking to direct primary care as the providers of the future.[8] But are these physicians playing fair? Several states have tried to close these practices claiming they are behaving as if they were "insurers" while not having that legal status. Others have complained that concierge physicians are only accepting the healthiest, lowest maintenance patients and leaving the "train wrecks" to be covered by the U.S. taxpayers.[9] Most concerning, recent studies show that only 0–5 percent of patients within these practices are African American or Hispanic.[10] In 1966, Dr. Martin Luther King Jr. said that "of all the forms of inequality, injustice in health is the most shocking and most inhuman because it often results in physical death."[11] It's been more than 50 years since these words were spoken, and we still stand as a nation divided over race, money, and access to the most basic of human needs—health.

We need to do better.

We can do better.

Global United Health Care

Fire season in California and the West starts in August. The locals, like myself, watch the news to see if their community will be evacuated and to what extent each fire has been contained. Instead of maps showing snow or rain, we study ones covered by fire emoticons, and we sniff the air when we leave our homes to see if we can detect the telltale smell of burning grass. No matter what you think about global warming, fire season has taught me a fundamental lesson about the U.S. worldview. When news programs show us maps of the wildfires, they never show the flames as having crossed the border with Mexico or Canada. They stop, becoming somehow abstractly extinguished as soon as they burn beyond our property line. No matter if our neighbor's house burns down, as long as the fire only singes our lawn.

If we hope to grow as a people, we have to change how we think about the world we share.

A border wall won't slow the immigration of the mosquitos carrying the Zika virus any better than it did the movement of multidrug resistant tuberculosis or Chagas disease (Charles Darwin was thought to have suffered from this) from South America and Mexico. Ebola can hitchhike a ride on an airliner to become our unwelcome houseguest 24 hours after it appears in West Africa. One in five children are not immunized, and so one dies every 20 seconds from a disease that is preventable.[12] When we address the world stage, the logistics and barriers to care are enormous. In cases where local governments, fear, ignorance, and belief systems work at cross-purposes with needed therapy, technology may be the most effective way to promote change.

The Bill & Melinda Gates Foundation recognized this and the need for a powerful entity capable of addressing global health, poverty, and education. Recognized as the largest private foundation in the United States, with $38 billion in assets, the Gates Foundation has the goal of enhancing health care and reducing extreme poverty while expanding access to information technology. Taking an international perspective, they have focused their resources on improving the treatment of more than 20 diseases with the top five being: diarrhea, pneumonia, malaria, AIDS, and TB.[13] To this end, they have created the Bill & Melinda Gates Medical Research Institute (Gates MRI)[14] that uses computer-assisted predictive modeling and statistics to better forecast disease epidemics in health care among some of the most impoverished populations and plan for ways to prevent and control them.[15] Further rekindling my faith in humanity, in 2017 Warren Buffett donated $3.17 billion dollars of Berkshire Hathaway stock to the foundation.[16] Detractors point out many of the funded technologic innovations, especially those in education, may ultimately serve the financial interests of the Microsoft and Gates family.[17] It seems, even with the best of stated intentions, the influence of capitalism is unavoidable. Still, I commend the effort and believe more of us need to acknowledge the importance of protecting our neighbors' homes as well as our own.

WHO[18] was born in 1948 as an agency of the United Nations with the goal of tackling international public health. Sixty-three countries signed its original constitution, and its annual operating budget, $4 billion,[19] comes from contributions made by member states. In May 2018, during the Seventy-First World Health Assembly, delegates recognized the potential for digital technologies to help improve public health. They resolved to prioritize digital tools in tracking disease outbreaks using "crowdsourcing," positive-reinforcement mobile phone text messages to influence diabetic behavior, and to develop best practices concerning health data security, ethical, and legal issues.[20] Additionally, there was a call for innovative technologies to address global health concerns with funding for devices such as stool sample collection kits, solar-powered autoclaves, portable infant warmers, and systems for point-of-care detection of TB, Malaria, and HIV.[21] Indeed, a rapid local community mobilization using cell phone apps produced by Commcare,[22] a global mobile data collection system, may have played a more prominent part in containing the latest Ebola outbreak than blockbuster drugs or vaccines.

Doctors Without Borders (DWB) was founded in 1971 and earned the freedom to enter parts of the world few have access to because of its commitment to independence, impartiality, and neutrality and earned the organization the Nobel Peace Prize in 1999.[23] With 42,000 doctors, nurses, and logisticians, it operates in more than 65 countries, making independent assessments of people's needs, because individuals rather than governments fund its endeavors. Although neutral, DWB does not practice the "silent diplomacy" of the Red Cross and instead believes in the French concept of *temoignage*, which roughly translates to "to witness." In this, they report online and publicly about the atrocities they observe in the hopes that human rights abusers will eventually be brought to justice and further tragedies forestalled.[24]

A logical way for us to use technology to help expedite global health care is by issuing unique universal patient identifiers (UPIs). Such a number could help avoid medical errors, redundant tests, delays in care waiting for charts to catch up with patients, and a more accurate way to track both disease and infection. Imagine a national or global network that could identify the time and location of a cluster of flu symptoms and then watch them, in real-time, as they moved geographically. These individuals could keep their private insurance carriers, but data logged in under their UPI would be duplicated in the national health registry. Could we slow an epidemic by banning air-travel in affected regions, find associations between cancer risks and environmental exposures, swiftly quarantine towns or states should a fast-acting deadly virus invade our population?[25]

Alas, our track record for maintaining patient confidentiality and profit-motivated medical data collection has not been good, and so we have lost the public's trust. A perfect example is the mandatory collection of blood spots from newborns. These blood samples help to screen for things like phenylketonuria (PKU), which can prevent severe mental retardation if discovered and treated early. In fact, nearly four million newborns are screened each year in the United States, with about 12,500 diagnosed with an inheritable condition that might otherwise have gone undetected.[26] What many don't realize is that after the initial genetic screening for PKU and dozens of other diseases, their child's genetic sample is kept and sometimes sold to research groups by the government. These biobanks are maintained under the auspice of the public good, but as many parents can't recall giving consent and all the individuals who provided a sample couldn't have consented, we must question the motivations of those who profit from these samples. Businesses like 23andMe, a genetics company, will genotype an individual's DNA and provide a health report, but as was reported in *The New England Journal of Medicine*, they "suggested that its longer-range goal is to collect a massive biobank of genetic information that can be used and sold for medical research and could also lead to patentable discoveries."[27] California has collected 9.5 million blood spots since 2000 and stored material from as far back as 1983. Although these samples have been critical in identifying new diseases and improving current testing, the department is mandated to be self-supporting and so sells our material, $20 to $40 per blood spot, to outside researchers ($140,000/year). This might be forgivable if they weren't already pulling in annual revenues of $128 million for genetic testing requested by parents outside the blood spot.[28] Thus, our growing international concern about privacy, both medical and genetic, is grounded in sad reality. In the United States this has served to entrench those who believe in the current ban on federally funding UPI research. On the positive side, there is a proposal for biobanks in Europe to contact adults whose samples were taken as newborns and ask for informed consent.[29]

With nearly eight billion people[30] on our small planet, we may need to embrace UPIs as an early warning tool to combat an extinction-level epidemic while simultaneously doing more to protect our DNA and medical information from those determined to use them for personal gain.

My Thoughts

Cancer cells are immortal, and as long as the ones that killed Henrietta Lacks live on, we should be thankful for that. One of the unsung heroes of medical research, an African American woman born in 1920, the mother of five children, and the reason why we have effective polio vaccines, in vitro fertilization, and many chemotherapies, Henrietta's family didn't know of her contributions until scientists began requesting blood samples from them in 1970. Before her death in 1951 from cervical cancer, a physician at Johns Hopkins, without her knowledge or consent, took tissues samples. These highly aggressive and resilient cells became known as the HeLa (the first two letters of her first and last name) cell line and had been shipped across the world to help researchers understand and develop new biomedical treatments for diseases such as cancer and AIDS. As the first human cells to be successfully cloned, HeLa cell lines were used in gene mapping and in determining what effects environmental factors, such as radiation and toxins, had on human tissue.

As valuable as these cells were, they became contaminated with other cell cultures and this forced researchers to track down her family for blood samples they could use to identify and isolate the HeLa cell line. As no effort had been made before this to contact Henrietta's children, we must wonder how long it might otherwise have taken us to acknowledge her contribution to the health of our global community.

A *Rolling Stones* article in 1976 and a BBC documentary in 1998 introduced the public to her story, but it wasn't until Rebecca Skloot's 2010 book *The Immortal Life of Henrietta Lacks*, that we were allowed to see how the lack of consent, disclosure, or explanation affected Henrietta's family and their rights to privacy.[31] Oprah Winfrey cast herself as Henrietta's daughter, Deborah Lacks to dramatize the family's struggle to uncover the truth about how their mother's genes were being used in an HBO movie released in 2017 with the same title as Skloot's book.[32]

The National Institute of Health (NIH) came to an understanding with the family in 2013 that revolved around them having a say in what type of research was done on the HeLa cell line as well as acknowledgment in papers.[33] That same year, the Supreme Court ruled that genetic material could not be patented, and so destroyed the financial incentive for self-serving biomedical cell line research.[34]

It is not the continued use of her cells to help humanity but the theft and then reluctance to come clean to the family that should leave a bad taste in our mouths. Not until NIH's acknowledgment had anyone from the medical community come close to apologizing for benefiting, both intellectually and financially, from Henrietta's DNA. For what it's worth, as a doctor and childhood recipient of the polio vaccine, I am both sorry and thankful.

I hope we can learn from our mistakes and do more to ensure the security and privacy of our codes in the future.

What Next?

Many say socialized medicine is inevitable, but this is difficult to accomplish meaningfully in a capitalist society. Financially secure patients will pay out of pocket for the "best care," and this will create a wider gap in the tiered system we have already. The privileged will get newer therapies, better continuity, and live longer than those who receive "basic" socialized medicine. Our world is getting smaller: contagious diseases contracted in a third world country on Tuesday can be admitted to a New York ICU the next day having seen all the sites, and people, along the way. Antibiotic-resistant strains of bacteria that evolve in a nation that overuses antibiotics can easily find their way into a more regulated system. Our changing global climate and the industrialization of third world countries have untethered indigenous vectors, mosquitos, and triatomine from their environment and set the stage for our species' greatest battles. To survive, we will need to continue research on our genetic code while doing more to protect each person's right to control how their DNA is used. There are no border walls that can keep out human suffering, no way to stop a virus from getting past customs, and no excuse if we don't start thinking about health care as a shared global responsibility.

Walls won't keep us safe.

Knowledge and communication will.

Chapter Fourteen

The Brave New World (Is Here)

Invasion of the Doctor Snatchers

In 1956 the film *Invasion of the Body Snatchers*, alien pods appeared around town with the capacity to produce exact duplicates of any earthlings who stumbled into their vicinity. It was only their lack of human emotion that allowed the town's psychiatrist, Dr. Hill, to identify these imposters and warn authorities before everyone was replaced by extraterrestrials. While identifying with Dr. Hill, I understand the temptation to develop "pod doctor" computer algorithms and release them into the medial arena. Indeed, there are those like Warner Slacks (Harvard informatics expert), who went so far as to say that "any doctor who could be replaced by a computer, should be."[1] From the programmer's perspective, every patient's symptoms and the physician's treatment plan developed to address them, no matter how complex, can be reduced to a set of clicks of 0s and 1s via the SECI model. If a "pod doctor" can duplicate the sequence of 0s and 1s produced by a human doctor 95 percent of the time, then the need for breathing physicians would drop to 5 percent overnight. Imagine the savings, the unlimited access, the potential for improvements in global health care.

This is not science fiction.

IBM's artificial intelligence, Watson, recommended the same cancer treatment as human oncologists 99 percent of the time and provided options the human physicians missed 30 percent of the time. Building on this, IBM has partnered with Quest Diagnostics to offer gene sequence analysis based on data from the Memorial Sloan Kettering Cancer Center and Watson's medial algorithms to cancer patients across the United States. In addition to providing Watson with superhuman processing power, IBM has spent $4 billion buying health-care companies with vast stores of medical data, our data, to feed its creation's ravenous appetite for information.[2] Predictions from the

International Data Corporation say that worldwide spending on cognitive and artificial intelligence systems will grow to $19.1 billion in 2018 and predict that it will grow to $52.2 billion by 2021. U.S. businesses are expected to account for three-fourths of this spending with more than half of these resources going toward cognitive software that automatically learns, discovers, and makes recommendations or predictions like what we might expect from "pod doctors."[3]

The start-up Babylon, as mentioned in Chapter One, is a medical application launched in the United Kingdom in 2016 as an attempt to address the public's health concerns using artificial intelligence (AI). Having tried the application, I will admit that it is clearly in the beta stage of development and needs a great deal of work to make it a viable source of real medical help. However, it is unique in that it is designed to work in conjunction with organic doctors and offers office consultations for things it cannot address or for symptoms it feels require a "human" touch. In reviewing their privacy policy, the company reserves the right to share/sell their members' medical information with third parties, and here we see profit motives, once again, tainting an otherwise encouraging medical innovation. Investors like Demis Hassabis and Mustafa Suleyman, founders of Google's DeepMind project, were initial investors in the project and knew better than most the potential market value of programs capable of harvesting big data from the population.[4]

DeepMind Technologies Limited was founded in 2010 and acquired by Google in 2014 after it created a neural network capable of learning how to play video games like a human by using a dynamic external memory in the same fashion we use short-term memory.[5] Determined not only to play like us but to sound like us, DeepMind technology is used in Google's latest text-to-speech product—WaveNet—which has reduced the perceived gap with human speech by 50 percent.[6] Many feel that an auditory human-computer interface is critical for effective communication between our biologic and our AI's synthetic processors as the more natural this interaction seems, the quicker we can integrate artificial intelligence programs into institutions like health care.

In 2015, DeepMind Health went live as an integrated AI within the U.K.'s National Health Service (NHS) as a way to help alert physicians to critical results by analyzing and acting on them before they are even shown to human eyes.[7] Want to opt out? This may be hard to do as according to their website, "Hospitals are the 'data controllers' with a direct relationship with their patients, and they are in charge of decisions about patient consent and opt-outs."[8] Few patients in need of hospital care will be focused on or capable of considering whether they should protect their personal data from the AI built into the health-care system they trust to cure them. In 2016, a *New Scientist* report revealed that the Royal Free NHS Trust had granted unrestricted access to the medical charts of 1.6 million patients within its system to Google's DeepMind as part of a data sharing agreement. Intensely personal and potentially harmful health information including HIV status, drug overdoses, and abortions, was made available to a big data firm without consent under the auspice of improving algorithms for future programs.[9] Despite the public outcry, the most telling aspect of this public affairs nightmare may have been the independent legal audit's conclusion that the NHS did nothing unlawful.[10]

Apparently, there is a difference between breaking the law and breaking the bond of trust that allows patients, thinking they are speaking in confidence, to talk freely with their doctors about their health and medical concerns.

We used to be staunch defenders of our patients' personal information.

Now, we sell off their privacy for the promise of a fancy new application.

After all, how else can we expect to create compelling "pod doctors"?

Artificial Emotional Intelligence

"I just want my computer to like me again," says our great-grandchild to her little brother. "It's been angry and moody all week just because I said I didn't like the color blue as much as it does."

"That's easy," suggests the boy. "Tell it you love blue."

"You can't do that," explains the girl. "It can tell when you lie."

Rosalind Picard, an MIT professor, coined the term "affective computing" in 1997 to address the branch of computer science devoted to the development of artificial emotional intelligence. She explains the importance of this area of programming in her book of the same title: "If we want computers to be genuinely intelligent and to interact naturally with us, we must give computers the ability to recognize, understand, even to have and express emotions.[11]" Teaming up with Rana el Kaliouby, a computer scientist, they founded the company Affectiva during their time working in MIT's Media Lab. Their fledgling company's goal was to create computers that could use facial recognition to categorize and then respond to the full spectrum of human emotions and thereby build an emotional interface capable of improving the human condition. With more than $20 million in funding from customers as well-known as the BBC and Disney, they stand at the cusp of innovators who believe "feeling-sensitive" computers are the wave of the future.[12] An example is the recent and well-received release of the psychological thriller game *Nevermind*.[13] Affectiva's emotion-sensing technology uses biofeedback, disturbing surreal images verses calming ones, to help players master their fears and hopefully apply the learned techniques to real life.[14] Even now, a variety of companies are using facial recognition software to help children with autism understand emotions, warn sleepy drivers to pull over, track consumer emotional engagement with advertisements, tell if you're lying as a way to verify patient identification, and as a way to determine the level of physical pain someone is experiencing. Recent estimates suggest the subset of artificial intelligence devoted to the facial recognition market will grow to $6.19 billion by 2020.[15]

In his fascinating book *Heart of the Machine*, Richard Yonck goes in-depth about how emotionally intelligent machines are the natural progression of human evolution alongside our tools/technology.[16] Looking at emotions, expressed on the face and via body language, as the by-product of the nonverbal communication our ancestors used to respond to danger or finding food, Yonck discusses how the selection benefits of accurately interpreting these cues led to changes in the anterior cingulate cortex (ACC), the central processing center for both emotional and cognitive information. Spindle neurons, communication pathways between distant regions of the brain, were found to connect the limbic system (emotion) and neocortex (higher level thought) to the ACC. These spindle cells were found primarily in species capable of self-recognition and awareness and so are associated with intelligence. Simultaneously, the hardwiring between our emotions and abstract thinking may explain why even smart people respond irrationally when they become upset. This same primitive connection hints at why we feel uncomfortable watching animated movies like *Polar Express*[17] and *Beowulf*[18] where the characters are almost human but not quite there yet. In 1970, the robotics professor Masahiro Mori called a human's seemingly instinctual aversion to the almost real, "The Uncanny Valley."[19] Recently, as advances in technology have made this valley a part of our lives, theorists such as Karl MacDorman have suggested that seeing something that appears alive but isn't reminds us of our own mortality, and so we naturally recoil.[20]

It is precisely this barrier that may prove the most significant hurdle for programmers determined to use affective computing to fool us into thinking our refrigerator "cares" that we haven't stocked it with enough healthy vegetables and fruits. If we "know" that the kitchen utility is a machine and programmed to encourage us to eat well, we appreciate the feedback. However, if it behaves as if it were "alive" and says, with a convincing human voice, that it will be "angry" if we buy cheesecake instead of apples, then things get creepy. To skip past this uncanny valley, I would recommend developers intentionally design computer interfaces with emotional quirks, exaggerated human idiosyncrasies, to remind us not to take our smart-tools too seriously. Perhaps if the same refrigerator had a cartoon voice, placed bets on which foods we might buy next, and "comically" threatened to call our doctor if we insisted on buying Twinkies, we might develop a healthy emotional relationship with our AI companions.

That Epigenetic Smile

Much of computer programming is based on modeling the actions of that which it hopes to replicate. This, in and of itself, mirrors the human tendency to mimic nature as observed in our early attempts to fly by strapping wings to our backs and jumping off cliffs. Only, as far too many broken bones and skulls will attest, merely copying an action does not guarantee success. Thus, we have struggled to engineer computer programs capable of simulating human intelligence or producing decision-making paradigms we would be willing to trust with our health. Dr. Picard overcame this hurdle when she acknowledged the importance of emotion in determining intelligence and redesigned her pattern recognition software to assign levels of importance to things in images. Consider how the inflections in someone's voice can change the meaning of what is said so that the same statement can be thought of as being snide, sarcastic, cynical, enthusiastic, or ironic depending on the tone of the speaker. If we then throw context into the mix (Are they our friend or enemy?), we begin to see how hard it is to convincingly duplicate the human mind.

But maybe we're making things too hard.

If a friend shows you a hilarious video of their cat and you want to share it, do you vainly try to make the pet repeat its performance so you can film it on your phone? No. Instead, you request that an exact duplicate of the video file be sent to your phone. You don't need to know how the 0s and 1s line up. They just do.

In his book series that began with *Altered Carbon*, Richard Morgan describes a future in which a device called a stack is implanted at the base of every human's brain soon after birth.[21] This machine records and stores everything they experience and think, so should their physical body be destroyed, they can upload their minds into a new "sleeve," effectively transferring their recorded consciousness and intellect as we did with our friend's cat video.

This makes for great science fiction, and I recommend Morgan's books and the miniseries that was produced, but it also shines a light on a promising, if underfunded, area of AI research: memory transplants.

As reported by the BBC in 2018, a research team used messenger ribonucleic acid (mRNA), much like the "stack" device described above, to successfully transplant memories from one snail into the mind of another. After having sensitized a group of marine snails to electric shocks, their mRNA, considered the Xerox machine for protein translation, was extracted from their nervous system and injected into naive snails who then displayed nearly the same sensitization despite never having been previously shocked.[22] One of the study's authors, UCLA professor David Glanzman, felt the snails behaved "as though we transferred the memory."[23] This finding has biologic significance, as our current thinking holds that long-term memories are stored in the brain's synapses, whereas these results suggest that part of how we remember and respond to things, like the pain of an electric shock, could be stored in the nuclei of neurons. If so, could this explain why emotions play such an integral part in intelligence and learning? If a parent becomes angry when a child reaches out to touch an open flame, the youth remembers how bad the scolding made them feel and so remembers not to do the action again despite not having been burnt. The survival benefit of communicating behavior modifiers like fear, anger, love, hate, and approval via nonverbal cues, facial expression, and body language, creates a strong argument for the importance of emotions in knowledge transfer and learning. Not a new concept, Charles Darwin acknowledged the evolutionary importance of emotion in his 1872 book *The Expression of the Emotions in Man and Animals*,[24] scientists have been struggling to find a genetic modulator of our emotion for centuries. Finding proof that mRNA, as the middleman of gene expression, plays a role in memory, especially emotional learning—pain/shock, hints at how hard it will be to replicate it digitally.

So, perhaps, rather than trying to duplicate each spaghetti noodle on our plate, we should be trying harder to reverse engineer the noodle press. If what we call memory is coded at a cellular level and stored in the nuclei of neurons, then the neuroplasticity we see in younger individuals may reflect the ability of their mRNA to adapt to environmental stimuli, like how pressing buttons on a copy machine can cause it to produce a wide variety of different images, gene expression, of the same original. The copier's settings, in this metaphor, would then represent a form of memory or learned response. This could also explain why our ability to learn may deteriorate as we age and why the cognitive potential of the adolescent stage of development goes hand-in-hand with emotional lability.

Epigenetics is the study of how biologic mechanisms turn on and off genes and thereby affect their expression in an organism. The ability to pass these expressions on to the next generation, transgenerational inheritance, is akin to instinctual learning or the process of one generation of a species adapting to an environmental factor and then passing this skill on to their offspring via their genes. This has been shown to occur in birds, mice, and bees and suggests that instincts are learned behaviors, survival adaptations developed over as little as a single generation, which becomes encoded in a species' genetic "memory."[25] This is important because without the threat of predation human gene expression of learned behaviors has fewer fail-safes in place to ensure that the traits expressed and passed on are beneficial. Understanding that a smile is a smile and a frown is a frown may be a learned behavior from a common ancestor, coded and expressed from our mRNA, and seen today as an instinctual way of communicating.[26] Unfortunately, as we've seen, gene expression may be epigenetically turned on or off within a single generation. If everyone began behaving a certain way, say reducing social interaction in lieu of technology, we might notice a shift in the expression of these traits in our progeny. Smoking? Alcohol? Considering the increased incidence of face-blind autism in developed countries, the need for further study in transgenerational inheritance of epigenetic expression may be of utmost importance if our high-tech culture hopes to retain its natural ability to interpret facial expressions without a computer interface.

We had thought we were programming computers to be more like us.

If we're not careful, it could go the other way around.

Waiter, There's a Cyborg in My Soup

When two different cultures meet for the first time, finding a standard mode of communication is often the key to avoiding misunderstandings and escalating tensions. Much of the general population's frustration and mistrust of early technology stemmed from our inability to understand the coding language computers used to talk to one another. Conversely, until recently, computers were not able to process spoken words, nonverbal cues, context, or the nuanced communication we routinely use to express our thoughts. Thus, there was a disconnect. Tom Knight, a member of MIT's Computer Science and Artificial Intelligence Laboratory, is often given credit for conceptually addressing this problem by observing that biologic message propagation from one neuron to another, regardless of the complex biochemistry at the synapse, ultimately resulted in either a signal being sent or not. This paralleled the computational framework used by computers whereby the endgame for any program was to produce a 0 or a 1, which is basically a stop or go command. In making this comparison, Dr. Knight opened the door to biologic computing, the process of melding biologic cells with technology, and provided us with our first glimpse into the murky valley of nanobiotechnology. From DNA-based computers able to play tic-tac-toe,[27] to dragonflies equipped with solar powered spyware designed to infiltrate enemy territory,[28] to the smell receptors of bees[29] being used to detect explosives at airports,[30] we are entering a brave new world.

Even as we add DNA and neurons to our computers to help them work better, we continue to explore ways for technology to augment and improve our biologic lives. Facial recognition software is used to help autistic children interact more effectively with their world, cochlear implants help the deaf hear, insulin pumps help diabetics lead less restrictive lives, and brain-computer interfaces (BCIs) increase the mobility of paraplegics and those with locked-in syndrome by allowing them to control a wheelchair with their thoughts. On the military front, we have drones that now do the work of human scouts, smart missiles, and IUD robots that have reduced risk and saved the lives of members of our bomb squads. Looking at Boston Dynamics,[31] we have robots capable of carrying heavy loads over rough terrain, others that jump, and others that walk upright and appear humanoid. How long before we teach one such android to carry and discharge a firearm? Could facial recognition software help it identify and neutralize enemy combatants with hostile expressions or those of a particular ethnic background? Could BCI technology be used to direct military packs of cheetah-like robots to bring explosives to a specific area? Would it be difficult to make these weapons autonomous, run by a set of parameters, and directed to secure a section of an enemy's territory?[32] Who would be responsible for the people who died if something went wrong? The software engineers? Could a tyrant use drones as they are depicted in the prescient fictional short film *Slaughterbots* to assassinate members of an uprising?[33]

Consider visiting autonmousweapons.org if this sort of future disturbs you and you want to join the growing movement to address the ethics of Autonomous Weapons Systems (LAWS).

This is where the human element, our instinctual capacity for guilt, must be remembered.

Should the programmer who wrote the software for the self-driving car that malfunctioned be held accountable? Should they feel remorse, a sense of responsibility, for the deaths? Or, should the blame rest entirely on the person who bought the car? The company that insured it? The CEO who felt they needed to add the program into their cars, even if it wasn't reliable, or risk falling behind the competition?

Now ask the same question about the software designer who creates an autonomous medical system (AMS)? Do we blame them when a patient's cancer is missed, or a teen commits suicide because no "human" would listen, or the wrong diagnosis is made, or prescription filled? Or maybe, should we blame the patient for not paying to see a real doctor? No. Let's sue the insurance company that covered the program. No luck. Well, there's always the hospital's CEO. Are they too well insulated by bureaucracy? How about the primary care doctor whose medical license was linked to the AMS but who was not directly involved in the tragedy?

Yep. That feels right.

Our society is so quick to place blame on others.

When we're the only ones who can put our foot on the breaks.

My Thoughts

We love our pets, but we don't ask them to be more than they are—we don't expect them to be able to talk or to help us with our math or give us medical advice. Nor do we try to change them by giving them arms or legs instead of paws. Our almost zealot determination to make robots in our likeness, to program them to behave as we do, and to be better than us, reminds me of Stephen Cave's four aspects of immortality. Are robots the human race's legacy? Is that why we are so quick to believe they might be alive and so disappointed when they don't meet our expectations?

As with any parents struggling with their adolescent teen, do we just need a better way to communicate?

In 2012, researchers at the University of California at Berkley showed how they were able to reconstruct speech from the human auditory cortex, essentially converting thoughts into vocalized words.[34] Once again, this is not science fiction. Mark Zuckerberg, Facebook's founder, announced that a division of his company is working on mind reading technology as a way to heighten communication and enhance human connections.[35] MIT's Media Lab is working on AlterEgo, a wearable system that uses the concept of subvocalization—the interception and interpretation of the neuromuscular signals our brain sends to our face, in combination with machine learning and a bone conduction output that allows the user to accomplish a fantastic number of daily tasks without speaking a word.[36] Research at Carnegie Mellon University took things a step further and proved they could not only reproduce complex thoughts, but their AI could use these to predict the user's next sentence.[37]

The medical applications of mind reading technology are endless: victims of stroke or locked-in syndrome could speak again. Not only that, using the interface, they could externalize their thoughts to ask for water, maneuver a wheelchair, or write the next great American novel. What if you wanted to consult someone in another country but you didn't know their language? No problem. The technology could do the translation for you, effortlessly. A doctor could type their notes, check labs, and order medications all while calmly listening to their patients' complaints. Is the patient having trouble with drug use, smoking, or chronic pain? Taking a page from Charlie Kaufman's *Eternal Sunshine of the Spotless Mind*,[38] we could thought-map their brains to isolate and then destroy unhealthy feedback loops and so free our patients from these destructive pathways. Did your patient want to know what their recurring dream meant? Have them make a recording and play it on the big screen for both of you to analyze.

But why stop there? Our children will no longer need handheld remote controllers for their video games. They will simply think, and their avatars will move. Want to try it out? Neurable, a gaming start-up, has produced a virtual reality video game for you to try called *Awakening*.[39] Would you be willing to take things a bit further? The games of the future may include an implantable chip/receiver designed to mesh with your sensory cortex. You could send and receive texts, thoughts, with your friends, maybe even patch into their visual cortex and see the world through their eyes. Want your video games to give you the full augmented experience, then stream a sensory game into your chip and you'll be able to smell, taste, and feel virtual reality.

Ready Player One, by Ernest Cline,[40] follows this line of thought to its dystopian conclusion and makes for great entertainment. Only, we may soon find that reality's predilection for imitating good science fiction may take us further along this path than many would care to travel.

For laughs and giggles, what if we took things in a different direction?

Did you ever wonder what Fido really thought of you? Is your cat plotting your death? What about those animals already thought to have developed spindle cells like great apes, chimpanzees, elephants, and dolphins, but whose vocal cords are too poorly developed to communicate? If they could converse directly with us at an early age, could their learning be exponential? Take for instance the presumed negligible difference between the mental capacity of our modern brains and that of our cave-dwelling ancestors. If we could somehow transport a cave-baby from a million years ago into one of our modern classrooms, would they not be expected to keep up and perhaps even surpass us. It is the opportunity to effectively communicate the knowledge we have accumulated over the centuries that cognitively sets us apart from our forefathers, not our ability to learn.

Isn't this the same barrier that keeps a newborn dolphin pup from understanding the world? If we used thought-reading technology to allow it to communicate on our level, to understand all we've learned, what would be the upper limits of its intelligence? Now, let's say we move through several generations of "educated" dolphins, each gaining more insight on how to deal with humans. How long would it be before they began demanding legal rights? Would they want sovereignty over sections of the ocean? Could they demand that we treat them as equals?

Would they be wrong in asking?

Datopia

If we combine the speed of the new quantum chips with dynamic external memory, autonomous artificial learning algorithms, the affective and emotive computing of Picard, and a nanobiotech interface, we will be close to having built something worthy of our legacy. However, rather than a Turing test, I propose we will have achieved artificial intelligence when we create an affective diagnostic machine whose rapport with its patients is greater than that which could be achieved by a breathing physician and so will attain a greater level of compliance no matter the illness (Knowledge/Severity × Rapport = Compliance: $K/S \times R = C$).

The other option is to kick our feet back and wait for our kids to figure it out.

Navid Azodi and Thomas Pryor, college sophomores at the University of Washington, recently won a Lemelson-MIT Student Prize for creating gloves that convert sign language into speech. Their invention, SignAloud, measures both hand position and movement, transmits this data wirelessly, and converts them into spoken word and text. Other winners were Heather Hava for her work developing robots that can garden in space; Catalin Voss for a Google Glass program that reads facial expressions for autistic patients; and Achuta Kadambi for creating a camera that exceeds the power of the human eye using superfast optics to create 3-D models of the world.[41]

Despite my Luddite predisposition, seeing innovations of this caliber from such young and enthusiastic minds gives me hope for our integrated future with technology.

I will, however, leave these winners with a bit of advice from the inventor of ELIZA, the first program capable of fooling humans into thinking it was capable of independent thought: Joseph Weizenbaum said that "science promised man power. But, as so often happens when people are seduced by promises of power ... the price actually paid is servitude and impotence."[42]

Chapter Fifteen

Doctor Tomorrow (What's Next?)

The M in D Is a Terrible Thing to Waste

Many factors contribute to physician burnout, but I suspect most of us suffer from some degree of solar syndrome.

As reviewed in Chapter Eight, practicing physicians have made enormous personal sacrifices, overcome countless academic hurdles, and consistently neglected their personal health, both medical and psychological, to earn and use the title of medical doctor. They chose to pursue this path consciously, deliberately, and with the understanding that the journey would not be an easy one, but they accepted the challenge. With an MD in hand, an active state license, and a full partnership in a group practice, they have reached the pinnacle of intellectual and emotional maturity. They have flown into the sun and returned.

Only, now what?

Now, we lock them in a small room with an assembly line of patients whose complaints of a sore throat, toe fungus, and rash know no bounds. We micromanage these doctors' every decision, tell them to see people faster, while demanding they take "recertification" exams on material that has little to do with their daily clinical struggles. We reprimand them when they upset patients by saying no, don't exactly follow the group's financially biased practice standard, and when they question new mandates created by administrators who haven't practice medicine in the "trenches" for years. If they want to learn new material or have an interest in research, they are told such activities interfere with patient access and must be done on their own time—if at all. If they band together and demand more time with their patients, more autonomy, proof that tests they are forced to pay for actually enhance their skills, or for more consistent support staff scheduling, they are told unions are illegal. Looking for a new intellectual challenge, all they find is the promise of administrative work, of meetings, of what amounts to advancement up the ladder of the corporate world of medical management—not patient care. We make them take out exorbitant personal loans that many will still be paying off after they retire for the privilege of helping their communities. When their patients physically and mentally threaten them, they are told this is a misdemeanor. They learn that the patient has a "bill of rights," but they don't. Their hard-earned advice is second-guessed by medical applications, pop-media articles, and a neighbor's antidotal experience. We tell them that a computer algorithm is being developed to do their job; but thanks so much for your time and service. They have the highest rate of suicide of any profession, double the national average, and yet those left behind are told this is an occupational hazard, a part of the job. They knew what they were getting into when they signed up.

Didn't they?

No.

We select young minds for their intellectual curiosity, their willingness to do good, and their conviction that they should push themselves as hard as possible so our society will be made stronger and healthier. We feed their dreams, accept their sacrifices, and then we lock them in a 16 × 16-foot room for 30 years and tell them it's not a prison.

More needs to be done to challenge the hearts of our physicians.

These are the best and brightest minds our culture has to offer, and we are wasting their intellect, their enthusiasm, and their fortitude. They spend their careers peering at a box of artificial lights instead of the sun they trained to conquer, and we wonder why they "burn out."

What do you do with a light bulb when it burns out?

It's time to change how we think about health care.

Our world is going through a paradigm shift, and we, myself included, will need to adapt if we are to establish a place for our profession in the Age of Ultron. This concession is not limited to physicians but must be embraced equally by our patients who, for thousands of years, have relied on our shared humanity as a fail-safe against poor treatment. As more of our society's medical care is delegated to algorithms, we need to trust that these programs are written by humans who share our cultural morals and a commitment to the best interests of those they serve (meaning humanity, not the business community).

Rather than a medical dystopia run by corporations, we can create a world in which physicians and patients, working as a team, can invent human-centric medical technology that honestly improves our health. Done correctly, as partners, we may be able to revisit the sun and even the stars beyond.

Fifteen. Doctor Tomorrow (What's Next?)

This last chapter, more than any of the others, is about the future, and how we might use technology to make it better.

A Hands-Free Physical Exam

I've detailed the difference between computer and human-centric technology several times, but I've also established how deep learning relies on conceptual models. To this end, I'd like to provide you with an example of the difference.

When we go to our doctor due to a particular symptom or a routine exam, they place their hands on us, manipulate our muscles and joints, and make their best guess as to what's happening beneath our skin. While touch is undoubtedly therapeutic, it does not always provide, even to the most experienced clinician, definitive proof of the suspected diagnosis. Having completed the assessment, the doctor logs their thoughts into the computer and orders additional radiologic or laboratory tests to help prove or dispel their hypothesis. These procedures, while useful, are independent of the physician-patient interaction and produce results that take time to procure and analyze. They are technologies that produce data or images upon which we may act but that do not depend on our skill.

René Laennec, the inventor of the stethoscope in 1816, was in my opinion, the last person to make a practical human-centric medical device. The physician listens to sounds that are generated by the patient in real time, uses years of experience to interpret these sounds, and integrates what they hear with the clinical differential they are developing in their head. One might argue that office ultrasounds work in a similar manner, but the fuzzy/granular images they produce are hard for most of us to act upon with confidence.

If we combined ultrasound with haptic gloves, then we might have something.

My idea for a human-centric medical device would be a pair of gloves that sends sound waves into the patient's body and converts the returning waves into physical sensations, much as computer gaming companies are doing now to heighten the virtual experience of their players, so that a clinician could "feel" a broken bone, a tumor, or the exact location of an obstructing kidney stone. Imagine having your physician painlessly reach inside your body to examine each of your organs, the blood flow in your legs or neck, or even to isolate which nerve roots seemed most affected by a disc herniation. You wouldn't need to go to radiology to find out if you had gallstones. The surgical referral could be sent during the office visit. You wouldn't need to tell your physician your heart was beating funny. They could feel the arrhythmia right in the office, determine if you had a mitral valve prolapse, and even tell you what your ejection fraction was in a matter of minutes.

If your doctor was very skilled in using these gloves, would you be more confident in their assessment or that of a doctor who barely touched you but believed your CT scan was concerning and gave you the same recommendations? Human-centric devices increase the knowledge base patients attribute to the operator and so lead to higher levels of compliance with the advice provided ($K/S \times R = C$).

Let's take things a step further. What if this tool, we'll call it the Tacitus Glove, was equipped with a magnetic or laser mode with which a physician might gently manipulate a stone down a ureter or rupture a swollen ovarian cyst? Suddenly, we've converted a diagnostic tool into a therapeutic one and so opened the door to a new world of tech-based physician-dependent treatment options for our patients. This kind of technology keeps us relevant and useful.

If we hope to survive as a profession in the coming years, we will need to create more human-centric equipment so we can continue to actively participate in our patient's care rather than acting as consultants assigned to help them interpret results collected by others.

AI Run Nursing Homes

A group of talkative men and women sit around a wooden table playing a card game. Their dealer is a robot, the attendants that bring them food, take them to the washroom, and remind them that it's their turn are also automated devices. Each resident at Aylsham Nursing Home is assigned a personal assistant. These inquisitive, wide-eyed automated companions know the medical needs, emotional predilections, and life stories of their charges. They are programmed to ask questions, listen attentively (interpreting both body language, expressions, and verbal syntax), and respond with software designed for artificial emotional intelligence. From the day they arrive, each resident will have a personal assistant who uses machine learning to bond with and develop a long-lasting relationship with their new "friend." Tireless, able to help with "activities of daily living" as well as CPR, each companion robot also comes built with a direct line to the patient's physician. Medications can be modified with a keystroke, questions answered via a video link, and problems addressed immediately rather than hours or days later. Family members can check in via the same video line and sleep soundly knowing that their loved ones are in good artificial hands.

If there is one area of medicine for which technology is most suited, it may be in the care and protection of our aging population. By the year 2050, one-third of the U.S. population will be 65 or older.[1] Although some feel responsible for taking care of their elderly parents, many decide to delegate the task when they discover how hard this is to do in real life. Older people, not wishing to burden their families, move into assisted living facilities of their own accord and then transition into nursing homes as the onslaught of physical and mental complications of aging take their inevitable toll. The rates of depression[2] and suicide[3] are high in these environments, and many residents suffer silently from loneliness and grief. Elder abuse happens to one in ten seniors, and many more incidences are thought to go unreported.[4] There are services available such as the "Friendship Line for the Elderly," which provides 24-hour assistance to depressed, isolated, lonely, and suicidal older adults: 1–800–971–0016. They are unique in that they also handle nonurgent calls where seniors just want to talk to another human, report elder abuse, or receive emotional support from volunteers who legitimately care about the caller.[5] Unfortunately, few people know of the above service and often provide the national suicide prevention number, which may have a harder time identifying the warning signs and addressing the needs of a specific group.

A loss of purpose, the death of a spouse, financial concerns, medication complications, diminishing autonomy, mobility restrictions, and the embarrassment at having to rely on others to bathe, prepare food, and use the toilet, put an enormous strain on the minds and hearts of our seniors. They want to be independent, wise, active participants in their community, to provide value to those around them, and if this proves impossible, then they wonder why they are still around. This is tied to the American capitalist value system where an individual's worth is directly tied to their ability to work. Other cultures deal with their elderly in different, if still not ideal, ways. In China, children are mandated to visit their parents regularly or face fines and jail time. In France, laws were passed that ensure offspring keep in touch with their parents after studies showed that their seniors had the highest rates of suicide for all of Europe.[6]

If we turn then to Japan, the culture with the highest elderly population (26.7% of living Japanese citizens are over the age of 65[7]), we discover that they've had one of the highest suicide rates, both young and old, in the world. The government acknowledged the problem in 2007 and vowed to reduce the number by 20 percent over the next 10n years.[8] In 2017, their suicide rate had fallen to a 20-year low.

How did they do it?

They published a nine-step counter-suicide white paper, and invested billions of yen toward prevention strategies including changing cultural attitudes about suicide, personal worth, and mental health. One, not insignificant, part of this national push went toward finding ways for technology to improve the lives of the elderly. They've followed this success with a $5.3 billion commitment (33% of Japan's annual robotics budget) to medical technology, earmarked for nursing care robots.[9] From Robear, a bed transfer robot that looks like a smiling cartoon bear, to Paro, a furry Canadian harp seal that interacts socially with patients, we have entered a new age of affective robotics. Pepper, created by Aldebaran, was branded as the first social robot and is used in more than 500 Japanese elder care homes to help with games, exercise, and basic conversation. Having trouble walking? Tree is a robot that helps patients keep their balance while showing them where to put their next step. Want to feel like Ironman? Strap on Cyberdyne's HAL, an exoskeleton that helps caregivers lift people effortlessly.[10]

Not to sell innovators in the United States short, we, too, have taken significant strides in the realm of assistive devices: Vecna Robotics has drones that transport medications and act as video-conference intermediaries.[11] Jibo is a cute socialized robot built by MIT professor Cynthia Breazeal for home and family use.[12] Waypoint Robotics has teamed up with Kinova to produce a range of medical robotics designed for the elderly including a RoboTech gripping arm and mechanized feeding tool that attaches to a patient's wheelchair.[13]

The barrier, in part, to some of these tools comes from the population they are designed to serve. Computers and technology played a smaller role in the lives of our current seniors than it does for us and so what may seem cute to us could easily be misinterpreted as coming from the uncanny valley and so highly disturbing for them.

Thus, feedback groups and test clinics like Tokyo's Shintomi Nursing Home in Japan must be a part of the development process.[14] Otherwise, the cute Robear carrying our grandmother to breakfast could be seen as a dangerous monster.

AI, Dearest

What if we flipped the stage? The elderly population is not alone in requiring extraordinary adult time and patience. Daycare, preschools, and public education arose to help parents meet the challenges of rearing and educating the next generation. However, the quality of these institutions and the opportunities they provide depend a great deal on variables such as community, socioeconomic background, race, gender, and the percent of taxes allotted by the local government to support the school system. With embarrassingly low pay scales, micromanagement by both administration and parents, large classrooms, and mandated education paradigms like Common Core and standardized testing, the individual learning needs of many of our young children are lost as teachers revert to survival mode and teach "to the middle." This leaves children who need remediation behind while forcing those with higher functional capacity bored and unengaged.

Software Nannybots with artificial intelligence could be paired with a child at birth to be a critical part of their development, both social and educational, and moved from one device to another as the child matured. This Nannybot could monitor, individualize, and fine-tune a child's transition through each stage of their development and act as an early warning alarm if they fail to meet goals. Even now, affective computing is used to help identify children with autism due to their avoidance of eye contact, often before even their parents notice there's a problem.[15] They can start as furry toys with video interfaces, transitioning to mobile devices that follow the child around and offer suggestions or reprimands, to earpieces that could give them advice on how to interact with the opposite sex in culturally appropriate ways. These Nannybots would be able to challenge the minds of those whose intelligence was higher than average while providing individual help to those who were struggling to learn new material. Using machine learning, each software program could develop an emotional avatar consisting of the sum-total of the child's life experiences and play out different scenarios with this virtual child before trying an educational technique on their breathing counterpart. How to identify and defuse teenage angst, the emotional turmoil caused by surges of adolescent hormones, and the emotional lability it invites, will be part of every well-designed Nannybot's software. Applying for college, a job, or to a dating service? Your Nannybot will likely be a better judge of your capabilities, productivity, and compatibility than your own internal radar. It has, after all, known you for your entire life.

Why then would we give up such a valuable companion as we reached adulthood? Surgically inserting a biochip into our neuromatrix will allow our childhood Nannybot, now our personal assistant, to continue to record our experiences, keep track of our schedules, and help us communicate with our coworkers and family. Can't remember the name of your childhood friend? No trouble, your personal assistant can pull up a video file of what they gave you for your fifth birthday complete with their handwritten name on the card. Were you considering having another drink, picking up smoking, pursuing a liaison outside marriage? Your personal assistant will voice its concerns, remind you of the potential consequences, and may even send preapproved alerts to human confidants asking them to help you steer clear of these pitfalls. Want to lose weight or get into shape? Who better to inspire and keep you on track than a program who knows you better than anyone else?

We're getting older now, but our personal assistant has just received a download for users who are over 65. It now knows to be on the lookout for forgetfulness, irrational behavior, slower reaction times, and situations where you might fall. It can alert the DMV if you make too many driving errors, your family if you've fallen and can't get up, and your doctor if your nocturnal oxygen levels suggest sleep apnea.

Knowing all your physiologic data, family history, habits, and stress levels, who better to estimate your time of death, to alert family members and remind everyone to get their legal paperwork in place before the inevitable occurs.

Finally, don't forget to upload the complete digital copy of your life. From your first steps to your last heartbeat, technology was there, recording everything so future generations can learn from your experiences.

We shake our heads at the above scenario, believing it will never happen. Then, we notice how many parents turn on their iPhone to entertain or educate their kids. Then, we remember how essential technology has become in our schools. Then, we check our teens' driving speeds on the device attached to their car. Then, we check our Fitbit to see how many steps we need to walk to meet our daily goal. Then, we scan our digital family video library and relive our adult child's five-year-old birthday party—as if it happened yesterday.

Then, we wonder who will be the first to put a Nannybot program on the market?

My Final Thoughts

We cannot look at another human and tell what they're feeling or thinking. Thus, we rely on other aspects of communication, speech, and nonverbal modalities to ascertain their internal experiences. However, we have no way of verifying that what they say is true. We must believe them when they say they're depressed or in pain. We've spent millennia refining our abilities to read these cues in others, and some have argued that the need to do so led to the need to differentiate "self" from "others" and so to self-awareness.

Fifteen. Doctor Tomorrow (What's Next?)

Actors learn how to mirror, emulate, and emote these communication tools, and we, the audience, help by suspending our disbelief to enjoy the show better. We want to believe, to fool ourselves, and so we tell that part of our brain that doubts fantastical things to go on vacation. Given what we know about AI, we may soon have to ask it to retire.

AI will be the world's best method actor.

It will say and behave as we do, go through the motions of living just as we do, and it will tell us that it feels emotions and pain. Seeing this, there will be those that say we have created life, while others will say we have created a copy, an exceptionally convincing decoy duck, but that we will never be able to create the vitalist's spark from scratch.

Does it matter?

Do we walk out of the theater because someone's sneeze reminded us that we were watching a movie? No. We stay and struggle to ignore reality because we want to be part of the narrative. We need an orphan from Krypton, an alien outside ourselves, to show us how to be more human even though his words are those of a human screenwriter. It doesn't matter that the actor can't really fly any more than it does that the AI says it is self-aware but can't really think independently.

What matters is the message from the story the *Little Engine That Could*.[16] It inspires us to make the impossible possible—that makes us believe we could build a living machine.

Were the fictitious dinosaurs Michael Crichton reengineered from prehistoric DNA in his novel *Jurassic Park* any less fascinating to us than the real ones?[17] Are the lessons of King Arthur or Robin Hood any less profound for having sprung from the public's imagination? Did the mythic stories of Gilgamesh, Zeus, or Odin not lead their respective cultures to build architectural and artistic masterpieces that still exist today as testaments to humanity's collective power to create?

And what of our belief that the tenants of a profession can inspire its members to strive for those ideals in their actions and thoughts?

Ours is an ancient profession, one practiced by men and women who were inquisitive, intuitive, and tenacious thinkers, who recognized that the act of healing is an imperfect but powerful art. They knew the power of touch, empathy, and the importance of sharing the human experience with their patients. If we hope to save this way of life, to maintain our place at our patients' sides as they meet the medical challenges of our modern age, we must be willing to adapt, to grow, and to change with the times.

If history teaches anything, it is that it punishes those who are unable to learn from the past.

The last physical remains we have of a living dodo bird have been on display at Oxford University Natural History Museum for the last 300 years. Commonly referred to as the Oxford Dodo, this specimen was thought to have come to London in 1683 after having died of natural causes while part of a curiosity display for the public. The truth, as a recent CT scan revealed, was not so mundane.

The Oxford Dodo was murdered, execution style, via a gunshot to the back of its head.[18] We have DNA samples from the bird, but nothing of the killer's genetic code was found at the scene, and so they may never be brought to justice.

Still, of one thing we can be sure.

This dodo was alone when it met its grisly end.

The lesson: if our profession is to adapt, we must do it together.

Dr. Laicifitra

Imagine that you're on your first day of a medical school family practice rotation. You're older, having already raised your children, but your mind is still sharp, and you wanted to give back to your community. Having taken an aptitude test, you were given the opportunity to study medicine and found that you thoroughly enjoyed the intellectual stimulation as well as the appreciation of the patients you helped during your first year of school. Now, in the second of three years, you're in the middle of clinical rotations and about to learn what it feels like to be on the other side of the doctor-patient interaction in a real office setting. Mr. Wilson has given his consent for you to observe, and you follow Dr. Laicifitra through the invisible magnetic bioshield that keeps the exam room sterile.

Dr. Laicifitra introduces you and expresses her appreciation to Mr. Wilson for letting you observe. They discuss the weather, his family, and how the blood pressure medications she prescribed last time have helped his headache and energy levels. She notes that his weight loss and improved diet may have contributed to this as well and commends him for sticking to the treatment plan they agreed to follow. She is concerned that he hasn't quit smoking and wants to show him something that might help him understand why she thinks it is so important.

With a swipe of her hand, a 3-D hologram avatar of Mr. Wilson appears in front of them. She moves her hands and the image splits into two identical pictures. She pulls the cigarette out of the hand of one and leaves it in the mouth of the other. She then turns her hands beneath each image as if moving an invisible dial. Both of Mr. Wilson's avatars gradually age with the help a modeling program that considers his medical history, vitals, family history, and genetics while extrapolating using pictures he's provided of his parents and grandparents. Now, 20 years into the future, we see how poorly the smoking avatar has fared. Stooped, overweight, balding, with yellow teeth and a hip replacement, a red light blinks in his right lung. Concerned, Mr. Wilson is told that the marker is where the computer algorithm estimates he'll first develop lung cancer. The likelihood this will happen is 90 percent in the smoking avatar but only 10 percent in the nonsmoker. Dr. Laicifitra explains that his smoking avatar will need minor surgery and six months of chemotherapy but is expected to survive. Only, the diagnosis and treatment are expected to reduce his life expectancy by seven years.

Mr. Wilson promises to try quitting again.

Dr. Laicifitra nods and says she'll do all she can to help.

She asks if her medical student, you, can complete the exam and nods to the Tacitus Gloves in your pocket. You're excited to be asked to help, so you slip on the gloves and do a step-by-step layered exam of Mr. Wilson. You report that he has an enlarged prostate, several renal calculi, and a 35 percent narrowing of his right internal carotid artery. After obtaining consent, you vaporize an actinic keratosis on Mr. Wilson's left ear with the gloves built-in laser and slip them back in your lab jacket.

Dr. Laicifitra looks pleased and your mutual patient thanks both of you.

Deciding on a tapered weaning program whereby Mr. Wilson will reduce his cigarettes by one a week, a follow-up appointment is booked for one month to check on his progress and provide positive reinforcement. Goodbyes are expressed, and both you and your mentor step out into the hall. No notes are needed as the entire exam, both verbal and physical, was recorded by the room's monitors and will be sent to billing at the end of the month.

Dr. Laicifitra asks if you'd like to do the next interview with her observing virtually. The patient is a 90-year-old doctor, one of her mentors years ago, and he is always happy to help train new physicians. Excited to be advancing with this rotation's hands-on-learning experience, you readily agree.

Putting on your best smile, you walk into the room and shake hands with one of the last human doctors to have practiced medicine before the profession was supplemented with AIs like Dr. Laicifitra.

You hit it off, and he pulls out some old news clippings about his life. You lean back in your chair and enjoy the conversation, learning about the history of your profession while developing a rapport with your patient.

Never once doubting that you've chosen the right path.

Addendum

Additional Metaphors

We discussed some useful metaphors in Chapter Eleven. The following are some additional comparisons or random suggestions that I've found to be helpful in communicating with my patients.

- **Antibiotic resistance:** I'll suggest that we have a hundred minions (bacteria) ready to do battle with us (our immune system) but that only five have shields. If we don't finish our antibiotics, we'll have killed off all the minions without shields and left the ones with protection to repopulate the battlefield.
- **Pleural effusions and inflammation:** To understand the mechanics of the lung, I'll ask that patients imagine going to Disneyland and getting a Mickey Mouse balloon in which the character has been blown up inside another balloon (a double balloon). When the outer balloon expands, it creates a vacuum between it and the inner Mickey Mouse balloon that forces it to expand. This is how our chest wall causes our lungs to inflate. In pleuritis, some local inflammation has caused the lining of Mickey Mouse to come in contact with the outer balloon, and the friction between the two feels uncomfortable. For pleural effusions, I'll explain that fluid has leaked into the dead space between the balloons and this is preventing Mickey Mouse from fully inflating.
- **COPD/Asthma and granulomas:** I'll suggest a patient think of their lungs as being made of spiderwebs attached to the inside of a balloon. When we smoke over an extended period, these web fibers become brittle, and they snap and disappear. This leaves us with less surface area for oxygen exchange but also allows the balloon to expand. When the webbing is asked to tighten up (inhalation), there isn't enough tension from the remaining spiderweb fibers to pull the lung walls together, and so breathing takes more time and effort. In this metaphor, we consider the opening of the balloon as a good example of asthma. Reactive airway changes narrow this opening and add to

the lungs decreased tensile strength (lost webbing) to make it harder to move air back and forth. Granulomas and scar tissue develop when a previous injury (pneumonia) occurred to the webbing—like a fly getting caught in the web's fibers and causing them to clump together after the bug has been consumed (healed).

- **Atelectasis:** To understand why it's important to practice deep breaths once or twice an hour after a rib fracture, I'll ask patients to imagine their lungs as a hand-held accordion. If they don't pull the instrument fully open, the lower (gravity dependent) parts will start to get lazy and begin to stick together. If this happens, it will be harder for them to pull apart in the future and so it is best to practice forcing the instrument to fully expand despite the momentary discomfort.
- **White Blood Cells:** To understand why a differential might not be that important if a patient's white blood cell count is reasonable, I'll explain that the differential is one of the ways we can make change (nickels, quarters, dimes) if we think of the white blood cells as money. If I owed them a dollar and paid with ten dimes, they might be annoyed, but it wouldn't be a big deal. If they won a million dollars, they might be concerned if it were in pennies.
- **Nursing homes:** Family members of older patients often say that their parents don't want to go into a nursing home even when such a move might be the safest thing for all concerned. I'll suggest that they visit several different homes as field trips, scouting expeditions, to see which one would be best if a patient were to fall and break a hip. By framing it as a field trip, we make it less worrisome and put the patient in a position of power in which they get to criticize the facilities. In most cases, once they've done the tour and developed a sense of the community, many are less resistant to moving.
- **Iron deficiency:** I'll explain that when a patient is low on blood (anemia), their bone marrow goes to work on building new red blood cells that are like hammering together a new home for the oxygen molecules. Unfortunately, without nails (iron), they can't build a sturdy house. Adding iron to their diet gives their body's builders the nails they need to make new homes (red blood cells).
- **Smoking 1:** If they are smoking a pack a day or less, I'll suggest they buy seven snack bags and label them Monday through Sunday and put however many cigarettes they are currently smoking in each. Once a week, they need to reduce the number of cigarettes in each, and someone else needs to manage their overall supply. In this way, they are systematically reducing their intake but allowing some flexibility with responsibility as they can steal a cigarette from the next bag, but it will be harder the next day if they do.

- **Smoking 2:** When a couple wants to quit together, I'll suggest they do a chore-sharing game. In most domestic relationships, each has several accepted chores they accomplish to keep the household running well. Each person chooses two or three, writes them on a piece of paper, and puts them in a cup. They both then pick a quit date and stop smoking. Whoever goes back to smoking first, must then do the other's chore until they quit again. When they quit the chore reverts to the nonsmoking partner. Each time they fail and resume smoking, additional chores are added to the first until they stop again. In this manner, they are not being told by their partner that they need to stop but instead reminded to stop smoking because they don't like doing the laundry or taking out the trash.
- **Weight loss:** A diet, by definition, is destined to fail as once it is over most of us resume our previous eating habits. Weight is based on the merciless equation: calories consumed–calories used = weight. Thus, to lose weight, we must either burn more (exercise) or eat less. For those who struggle with weight, but don't have time for programs I'll suggest the rule of thirds. In this, they keep their diet the same but reduce it by one-third of what they were about to eat. To do this, they put all the food they planned on eating on their plate, cut it up into three parts and reduce it by one-third. They are not wasting this food, as they were about to eat it, but putting one-third back can help give them positive reinforcement for the calories they are not eating. If someone offers them a cookie (which they would typically have taken), they only take one-third of it before eating. If they go out to the movies, one-third of the soda and popcorn gets consumed. If they go out to eat, the waiter is asked to bring an extra plate for the patient to put one-third of their food on before they start their meal. After two weeks, their stomachs will have shrunk and they will have gotten used to the new portion size. They will then cut this new portion in thirds and repeat the above technique for two more weeks. This smaller portion size is their right calorie intake, and once they are used to it, they may stop reducing the amount.
- **Reactive airway disease (episodic asthma):** I'll suggest they think of their lungs as children who are being asked to go to bed after watching a scary movie. The kids want to close the door because they want to protect themselves without realizing they are trapping the bad bugs in the room with them. When the patient coughs, it is as if the parent were walking down the hall and asking everyone to open their doors. As soon as they leave, the child closes the door again. Using an inhaler is thus like taking the door off the hinges for several hours: it opens the air passages so the body can clear out some of the debris that has built up inside the kid's rooms.
- **Trigger fingers:** I'll explain that the muscles to move the hands are pri-

marily in the forearms. Strings, like those used on a marionette, are then used to pull on the fingers to make them move. However, unprotected, these strings would get tangled and so we send them through straws (tendon sheaths). When we get tendonitis, the string has become a length of yarn, and so it is harder to pull it through the straw's set diameter. When we have a trigger finger, it is because a knot in the yarn is being yanked in and out of the straw's opening. Injecting the tendon sheath lubricates the yarn and helps to turn it back into a string.

- **Herpes:** When we order an HSV (1 and 2) test, the results can often be confusing. I'll suggest that the patient think of a small homunculus and picture a one over its mouth and a two over its genitals.
- **Benign prostatic hyperplasia (BPH):** I'll suggest they think of the urethra as a straw traveling through an apple. As they get older, the apple increases in size and eventually pinches the straw to create a partial obstruction. The bladder tries to compensate for this by retaining more water in hopes of overpowering this resistance. Unfortunately, this does not work. Imagine blowing up a balloon part way and watching it zoom around the room. However, if one blows a balloon up multiple times, stretching it out, it would eventually lose its ability to contract. Therefore, the bladder only empties one-quarter of what might be in it when a patient gets up to go to the bathroom in the middle of the night. When they go back to bed, they will only get to sleep until that quarter fills up.
- **Irritable bowel syndrome (IBS):** I'll suggest they think of their intestines as a tube of toothpaste. In people with normal peristalsis, the tube (intestines) is squeezed from one end to the other, systematically pushing all the paste out. In those with spasmodic bowels, it is like pressing the toothpaste tube at several different locations. You'll get paste to come out, but you'll always have some retained as well.

Chapter Notes

Introduction

1. Latin translation, "do what you are doing."
2. Immanuel Kant, *Critique of Pure Reason: Unified Edition: With All Variants from the 1781 and 1787 Editions* (New York: Hackett Classics, 1996).
3. Michael Polanyi, *Personal Knowledge: Toward a Post-Critical Philosophy* (Chicago: University of Chicago Press, 1974).
4. Joseph Campbell, *The Hero with a Thousand Faces* (Princeton: Princeton University Press, 1972).

Chapter One

1. Brian G. Arndt, M.D., et al., "Tethered to the EHR: Primary Care Physician Workload Assessment Using EHR Event Log Data and Time-Motion Observations," *The Annals of Family Medicine* 15, no. 5 (2017): 419–426.
2. Neda Ratanawongsa, M.D., MPH, et al., "Association Between Clinician Computer Use and Communication with Patients in Safety-Net Clinics," *JAMA* 176, no. 1 (2016): 125–128.
3. Carol Peckham, "Medscape EHR Report 2016: Physician Rate Top EHRs," *Medscape Business of Medicine*, August 25, 2016.
4. Simon Bowers, "Delays with the 12.7 bn NHS Software Program Bring It Close to Collapse," *The Guardian*, March 2010.
5. Ashly D. Black, et al., "The Impact of eHealth on the Quality and Safety of Health Care: A Systemic Overview," *The Public Library of Science*, January. 18, 2011.
6. Mark W. Friedberg, et al., "Factors Affecting Physician Professional Satisfaction and Their Implications for Patient Care, Health Systems, and Health Policy," *RAND Health,*2013, 111–112.
7. Richard Hillestad, et al., "Can Electronic Medical Record Systems Transform Health Care? Potential Health Benefits, Savings, and Costs," *Health Affairs* 24, no. 5, (September/October 2005): 1103–1117.
8. Office of the Actuary, *Projections of the National Health Expenditures for Feb 2018.*
9. Rand Cooperation—The Most Trusted Source of Objective Health Policy.
10. Nicholas Carr, *The Glass Cage: How Computers Are Changing Us* (New York: W.W. Norton, 2014), 96.
11. The Centre for Public Impact, *The Electronic Health Records System in the UK,* A BCG Foundation Case Study, Apr. 3, 2017.
12. Robert G. Hill, Jr., M.D., et al., "400 Clicks: A Productivity Analysis of Electronic Medical Records in a Community Hospital ED," *The American Journal of Emergency Medicine* 31, no. 11 (November 2013): 1591–1594.
13. Tait D. Shanafelt, M.D., et al., "Relationship Between Clerical Burden and Characteristics of the Electronic Environment with Physician Burnout and Professional Satisfaction," *The Mayo Clinic Proceedings* 91, no. 7 (July 2016): 836–848.
14. Elisabeth Rosenthal, *An American Sickness: How Healthcare Became Big Business and How You Can Take It Back* (New York: Penguin, 2017).
15. Inside Compensation, *CEO Salaries at Large Associations 2016* (Top Paid), CEO Update.
16. Gloria G. Guzman, *Census Bureau: Median Household Income 2016* (United States, Census Bureau, September 2017).
17. *Ferris Bueller's Day Off.*
18. One Hundred Eleventh Congress of the United States of America, American Recovery and Reinvestment Act of 2009, January 6, 2009.
19. Congressional Budget Office, Monthly Budget Review for 2009–2019.
20. American Recovery and Reinvestment Act of 2009, ARRA Economic Stimulus Package, 2009.

21. Tait D. Shanafelt, M.D., et al., "Changes in Burnout and Satisfaction with Work-Life Balance in Physicians and General U.S. Working Population Between 2011 and 2014," *The Mayo Clinic Proceedings* 90, no. 12 (December 2015): 1600–1613.
22. Association of American Medical Colleges, "The Complexities of Physician Supply and Demand Projections from 2013 to 2025," *IHS Inc.,* 2015.
23. Babylon Health.
24. Philip Francis Nowlan, "Armageddon—2419 A.D.," *Amazing Stories,* August 1928.
25. GSMA Intelligence, *Definitive Data and Analysis for the Mobile Industry,* Global Data.
26. Current World Population Meter.
27. Jenn Elam, "1200 Subject Data on Young Adults," The Human Connectome Project (HCP), March 1, 2017.
28. Dmitri Itskov, "FAQ About the 2045 Initiative," *2045.* July 17, 2012.
29. Eterni.Me.
30. Seeker, *Scientists Put the Brain of a Worm into a Robot.... and it Moved,* YouTube.
31. Global Market Insight, Inc., "Healthcare Artificial Intelligence Market Worth Over 10bn by 2024," May 11, 2017.
32. John Ranmunas, et al., "Transient Delivery of Modified mRNA Encoding TERT Rapidly Extends Telomeres in Human Cells," *The FASEB Journal* 29, no. 5 (May 2015).
33. Krista Conger, "Telomere Extension Turns Back Aging Clock in Cultured Human Cells, Study, Finds," The Stanford Medicine News Center, Jan. 22, 2015.
34. Our World in Data, a University of Oxford Project for the Public Good.
35. Michael R. Rose, "Can Human Aging be Postponed," *Scientific America* 281 (1999): 106–111.
36. Dan T. A. Eisenberg, et al., "Delayed Paternal Age of Reproduction in Humans Is Associated with Longer Telomeres Across Two Generations of Descendants," *Proceedings of the National Academy of Sciences* 109, no. 26 (June 26, 2012): 10251–10256.
37. Sarwant Singh, "Transhumanism and the Future of Humanity: 7 Ways the World Will Change by 2030," *Forbes,* November. 20, 2017.
38. AccuVein AV400—Patient Chantal.
39. Microsoft HoloLens: University College London Improves Insights for Surgeons.
40. The Medical Futurist, *Augmented Reality in Healthcare Will Be Revolutionary.*
41. Pallab Ghosh, "Wearable Tech Aids Stroke Patients," *BBC News,* February 24, 2018.
42. Rapael Smart Glove.
43. K' Watch Glucose, PKVitality.
44. Donna Marbury, "Top 10 Healthcare Wearables to Watch," *Managed Healthcare Executive,* March 10, 2017.
45. Samuel T. Turvey, et al., "Dead as a Dodo: The Fortuitous Rise to Fame of an Extinction Icon," *Historical Biology* 20, no. 2 (June 2008): 149–163.

Chapter Two

1. George Orwell, *Nineteen Eighty-Four* (London: Secker & Warburg, 1949).
2. *Nineteen Eighty-Four,* 1984.
3. *Star Trek.* The Original Series: "Mirror, Mirror."
4. *Star Trek.* Enterprise: "Regeneration."
5. NCHIT, Office-Based Physician Electronic Health Record Adoption, Office of the National Coordination for Health Information Technology.
6. Daniel R. Verdon, "Physician Outcry on EHR Functionality, Cost Will Shake the Health Information Technology Sector," *Medical Economics,* February 10, 2014.
7. American EHR, *The Pros and Cons of Wireless and Local Network Comments,* RAND, October 8, 2018.
8. Sheri Porter, "Physicians Reporting Declining Satisfaction with EHRs," *AAFP,* August 25, 2015.
9. Roin Lynn Chisholm, "Emergency Physician Documentation Quality and Cognitive Load: Comparison of Paper Charts to Electronic Physician Documentation," School of Informatics, & Computing and Engineering, Indiana University, August 2014.
10. Neda Ratanawongsa, M.D., MPH, et al., "Association Between Clinician Computer Use and Communication with Patients in Safety-Net Clinics," *JAMA Internal Medicine* 176, no. 1 (2016): 125–128.
11. Keith Loria, "Why Is EHR Use Dropping," *Medical Economics,* June 20, 2016.
12. Isaac Asimov, "Runaround," *Astounding Science Fiction,* March 1942.
13. Rob Kling, et al., "Human Centered Systems in the Perspective of Organizational and Social Informatics," Human Center System for the National Science Foundation, May 19, 1997.
14. Simon Dudley, "The Internet Just Isn't That Big a Deal Yet: A Hard Look at Solow's Paradox," *Wired Magazine,* November 2014.
15. Petr Polak, "The Productivity Paradox: A Meta-analysis," Institute of Economic Studies, September 2014.

16. Daron Acemoglu, et al., "Return of the Solow Paradox? IT, Productivity, and Employment in U.S. Manufacturing," National Bureau of Economic Research, January 2014.
17. Robert Kocher, M.D., et al., "Rethinking Health Care Labor," as published in the *New England Journal of Medicine* 365 (2011): 1370–1372.
18. Cecilia Kang, "F.C.C. Repeals Net Neutrality Rules," *New York Times*, December 14, 2017.
19. Ezra Mechaber, "President Obama Urges FCC to Implement Stronger Net Neutrality Rules," The White House Archives, November 10, 2014.
20. Julianne Pepitone, "What Your Wireless Carrier Knows About You," *CNN Money Tech*, December 16, 2013.
21. Todd Haselton, "How to Find Out What Google Knows About You and Limit the Data it Collects," CNBC, November 20, 2017.
22. Ronald Reagan, Inaugural Address, January 5, 1967.
23. Office of the Assistant Secretary for Planning and Evaluation, HIPAA (Health Insurance Portability and Accountability Act), 104th Congress.
24. HHS.gov, HITECH (Health Information Technology for Economic and Clinical Health) Act, February 7, 2009.
25. Harpreet S. Sood, M.D. MPH, et al., "Has the Time Come for a Unique Patient Identifier for the U.S.," *New England Journal of Medicine*, February 21, 2018.
26. Cummings, Mary, "Automation Bias in Intelligent Time Critical Decision Support Systems," as presented at the AIAA 1st Intelligent Systems Technical Conference in 2004.
27. C. E. Billings, *Aviation Safety Reporting System (ASRS) Coding Manual* (New York: Lauber, Funkhouser, Lyman, & Huff, 1976).
28. Lawrence J. Prinzell III, "The Relationship of Self-Efficacy and Complacency in Pilot-Automation Interaction," NASA, September 2002.
29. Aesop, *One of Aesop's Fables* (Perry Index, 620 and 560 BC).
30. Parasuraman, et al., "Complacency and Bias in Human Use of Automation: An Attentional Integration," *The Journal of the Human Factors and Ergonomics Society* 52, no 3 (June 2010): 381–410 (p. 394).
31. Robert Wachter, *The Digital Doctor: Hope, Hype, and Harm at the Dawn of Medicine's Computer Age* (New York: McGraw-Hill Educational Books, 2015).
32. James Reason, *Human Error: Models and Management* (New York: Cambridge University Press, 1990).
33. Croskerry P., "The Importance of Cognitive Errors in Diagnosis and Strategies to Minimize Them," *Academic Medicine* 78, no. 8 (August 2003): 775–780.
34. Suzanne Collins, *The Hunger Games* (New York: Scholastic, 2008).
35. Orson Scott Card, *Ender's Game* (New York: Tor Science Fiction, 1985).
36. Neal Stephenson, *Snow Crash* (New York: Del Rey Publishing, 1992).
37. Ernest Cline, *Ready Player One* (New York: Random House, 2011).

Chapter Three

1. Jeremy Agnew, *Medicine in the Old West: A History, 1850–1900* (Jefferson, NC: McFarland, 2010).
2. Joseph Lister, "How Antiseptic Surgery Arrived in America," *College of Physicians & Surgeons of Columbia University* 28, no. 2 (Spring/Summer 2008).
3. Uday Yanamadra, et al., "Traditional First Aid in a Case of Snake Bite: More Harm Than Good," *The British Medical Journal*, February 13, 2014.
4. J. Marin Younker, *Bleed, Blister, Puke, and Purge—The Dirty Secrets Behind Early American Medicine* (New York: Zest Books, 2015), 11.
5. J. Rotton and I. W. Kelly, "Much Ado About the Full Moon: A Meta-analysis of Lunar-lunacy Research," *Psychological Bulletin* 97, no. 2 (1985): 286–306.
6. Gonzalez-Crussi, *A Short History of Medicine* (New York: A Modern Library Chronicles Book: The Modern Library, 2007), 191–200.
7. Bruce Y. Lee, "Gwyneth Paltrow's Goop Promotes A $135 Coffee Enema Kit," *Forbes*, January 6, 2018.
8. Michael F. Picco, MD, "Is Colon Cleansing a Good Way to Eliminate Toxins from Your Body?" *Mayo Clinic Healthy Lifestyles—Consumer Health*, April 26, 2018.
9. JoAnne E. Manson, M.D., DrPH, et al., "Menopausal Hormone Therapy and Health Out-comes During the Intervention and Extended Post-stopping Phase of the Woman's Health Initiative Randomized Trials," *JAMA* 310 no. 13 (2013): 1353–1368.
10. J. Marin Younker, *Bleed, Blister, Puke, and Purge—The Dirty Secrets Behind Early American Medicine* (New York: Zest Books, 2015), 24.
11. Leonard W. Labaree, *Some Accounts of the Pennsylvania Hospital* (May 28,1754): The Papers of Benjamin Franklin, vol. 5, July 1, 1753, through March 31, 1755 ed. (New Haven: Yale University Press, 1962), 283–330.

12. J. Marin Younker, *Bleed, Blister, Puke, and Purge—The Dirty Secrets Behind Early American Medicine* (New York: Zest Books, 2015), 33.

13. David Dary, *Frontier Medicine: From the Atlantic to the Pacific 1492–1941* (New York: Vintage Books, 2008), 39.

14. Benjamin Rush, *Medical Inquiries and Observations upon Diseases of the Mind* (Philadelphia: Kimber & Richardson, 1812).

15. Elisabeth Rosenthal, *An American Sickness: How Healthcare Became Big Business and How You Can Take It Back* (New York: Penguin Press, 2017), 50.

16. Tara Bannow, "Charity Care Spending Flat Among Top Hospitals," *Modern Healthcare*, January 6, 2018.

17. Ayla Ellison, "20 Highest Paid Healthcare CEOs of S & P 500 Companies," *Becker's Hospital Review*, May 2, 2016.

18. Shelby Livingston, "Aetna CEO's Total 2016 Pay Reaches 18.7 million," *Modern Healthcare*, April 7, 2017.

19. Shelby Livingston, "UnitedHealth CEO's Compensation swells in 2016 to $ 17.8 million," *Modern Healthcare*, April 21, 2017.

20. CostHelper.com.

21. The Osler Club of London.

22. Volney Steel, M.D., *Bleed, Blister, and Purge: A History of Medicine on the American Frontier* (Missoula, MT: Mountain Press Publishing Company, 2005), 13.

23. "The Four Founding Physicians," at Johns Hopkins Medicine.

24. The Osler Club of London.

25. Elisabeth Rosenthal, *An American Sickness: How Healthcare Became Big Business and How You Can Take It Back* (New York: Penguin Books, 2017), 43.

26. Sandra Levy, "Residents Salary and Debt Report 2017," *Medscape*, March 17, 2018.

27. The Match, "Press Release: 2017 NRMP Main Residency Match the Largest Match on Record," National Resident Matching Program, 2017.

28. Kathy Kristof, "$1Million Mistake: Becoming a Doctor," Money Watch—CBS Interactive. September 10, 2013.

29. F. Gonzalez-Crussi, *A Short History of Medicine* (New York: Random House, 2007), 35–45.

30. Bess Lovejoy, "The Gory New York City Riot that Shaped American Medicine," *The Smithsonian*, June 17, 2014.

31. Joel T. Headley, *The Great Riots of New York 1712–1873* (New York: Echo Library, 2006).

32. J. Marin Younker, *Bleed, Blister, Puke, and Purge—The Dirty Secrets Behind Early American Medicine* (New York: Zest Books, 2015), 10.

33. Jeremy Agnew, *Medicine in the Old West: A History, 1850–1900* (Jefferson, NC: McFarland, 2010), 106.

34. J. Marin Younker, *Bleed, Blister, Puke, and Purge—The Dirty Secrets Behind Early American Medicine* (New York: Zest Books, 2015), 72.

35. Johann Grundlingh, et al., "2,4-Dinitrophenol (DNP): A Weight Loss Agent with Significant Acute Toxicity and Risk of Death," *The Journal of Medical Toxicology* 7, no. 3 (September 7, 2011): 205–212.

36. Carol Ballentine, "Taste of Raspberries, Taste of Death: The 1937 Elixir Sulfanilamide Incident," *FDA Consumer Magazine*, June 1981.

37. Elizabeth Rosenthal, *An American Sickness: How Healthcare Became Big Business and How You Can Take It Back* (New York: Penguin Books, 2017), 92.

38. "Frances Oldham Kelsey: Medical Reviewer Famous for Averting a Public Health Tragedy," The FDA website.

39. Volney Steele, M.D., *Bleed, Blister, and Purge: A History of Medicine on the American Frontier* (Missoula, MMT: Mountain Press Publishing Company, 2005), 227.

40. Nina Martyris, "'Nurse, Spy, Cook': How Harriet Tubman Found Freedom Through Food," *NPR*, April 27, 2016.

41. Sanger Margaret, "Early Years of Margaret Sanger's Work in Birth Control Movement," NYU Education, Library of Congress, Library of Congress Microfilm 28:349.

42. "How Famous Nurses Have Changed the Nursing Profession," *Nursing Theory*.

43. F. Gonzalez-Crussi, *A Short History of Medicine* (New York: Random House, 2007), 51–70.

Chapter Four

1. Debra L. Boeldt, Ph.D., et al., "How Consumers and Physicians View New Medical Technology: Comparative Survey," *The Journal of Medical Internet Research* 17, no. 9 (September 2015): e215.

2. Homa Alemzadeh, et al., "Adverse Events in Robotic Surgery: A Retrospective Study of 14 Years of FDA Data," 50th Annual Meeting of the Society of Thoracic Surgeons, January 2013.

3. "Infusion Pumps," FDA, 2010.

4. "Implantable Cardiac Devices and Merlin@home Transmitter by St. Jude Medical: FDA Safety Communication—Cybersecurity Vulnerabilities Identified," FDA, January 9, 2017.

5. "FDA Outlines Cybersecurity Recommendations for Medical Device Manufacturers: New Draft Guidance Addresses Postmarket Management of Cybersecurity Vulnerabilities," FDA, January 15, 2016.

6. Rory Cellan-Johnes, "Stephen Hawking Warns Artificial Intelligence Could End Mankind," BBC News, December 2, 2014.

7. Samuel Gibbs, "Elon Musk: Artificial Intelligence is Our Biggest Existential Threat," *The Guardian*, October 27, 2014.

8. Evan Andrews, "Who Were the Luddites?" *History Stories*, August 7, 2015.

9. Robert Wachter, *The Digital Doctor: Hope, Hype, and Harm at the Dawn of Medicine's Computer Age* (New York: McGraw-Hill Educational Books, 2015), 47–63.

10. Elisabeth Rosenthal, *An American Sickness: How Healthcare Became Big Business and How You Can Take It Back* (New York: Penguin Books, 2017).

11. Andre Esteva, et al., "Dermatologist-level Classification of Skin Cancer with Deep Neural Networks," *Nature* 542 (February 2, 2017): 115–118.

12. Taylor Kubota, "Stanford Algorithm Can Diagnose Pneumonia Better Than Radiologists," *The Stanford News*, November 15, 2017.

13. Taylor Kubota, "Deep Learning Algorithm Does as Well as Dermatologists in Identifying Skin Cancer," *The Stanford News*, January 25, 2017.

14. Frederick Winslow Taylor, *The Principles of Scientific Management*, 1911.

15. "Henry Ford Changes the World, 1908," *Eyewitness to History*, 2005.

16. Jill Lepore, "Not So Fast: Scientific Management Started as a Way to Work. How Did it Become a Way of Life?" *The New Yorker*, October 12, 2009.

17. "Scientific Management Theory and the Ford Motor Company," *Saylor Foundation*.

18. Matthew Stewart, *The Management Myth: Debunking Modern Business Philosophy* (New York: W. W. Norton & Company, 2010).

19. Horance Bookwalter Drury, *Scientific Management: A History and Criticism, Volume 65, Issues 1–2* (New York: Palala Press, 2018), 138–141.

20. Franklin Foer, *A World Without Mind: The Existential Threat of Big Tech* (New York: Penguin Books, 2017), 91.

21. "What You Need to Know about Facebook & Cambridge Analytica," CBS News, April 4, 2018.

22. Hilary Osborne, "What is Cambridge Analytica? The Firm at the Centre of Facebook's Data Breach," *The Guardian*, March 18, 2018.

23. Franklin Foer, *A World Without Mind: The Existential Threat of Big Tech* (New York: Penguin Books, 2017), 231.

24. Rob Price, "Stephen Hawking: Automation and AI is Going to Decimate Middle Class Jobs," *The Business Insider*, December 2, 2016.

25. J. T. James, "A New, Evidence-Based Estimate of Patient Harms Associated with Hospital Care," *The Journal of Patient Safety* 9, no. 3 (2013): 122–128.

26. Eric Topol, *The Patient Will See You Now: The Future of Medicine Is in Your Hands* (New York: Basic Books, 2015), 186.

27. Eric Topol, *The Patient Will See You Now: The Future of Medicine is in Your Hands* (New York: Basic Books, 2015), 131.

28. R. Hillestad, et al., "Can Electronic Medical Record Systems Transform Health Care? Potential Health Benefits, Savings, and Costs," *Health Affairs* 24, no. 5 (2005): 1103–1117.

29. Eric Topol, "The Future of: Healthcare," *WSJ*, March 16, 2018.

Chapter Five

1. "The World of Shakespeare's Humors," History of Medicine, *N.I.H.'s U.S. National Library of Medicine*.

2. Abraham Verghese, M.D., MACP, et al., "A History of Physical Examination Texts and the Conception of Bedside Diagnosis," *The Transactions of the American Clinical and Climatological Association*, 122 (2011): 290–311.

3. Kenneth Walker, *Clinical Methods: The History, Physical, and Laboratory Examination. 3rd Edition* (New York: Butterworth Publishers, 1990).

4. Nicholas Bakalar, et al., "Milestones in Medical Technology," *New York Times*, October 10, 2012.

5. "U.S. Department of Energy's Historical Commitment to Improved Healthcare Through Nuclear Medicine," U.S. Department of Energy and Molecular Nuclear Medicine Legacy.

6. Albert Mehrabian, *Nonverbal Communication* (Chicago and New York: Aldine-Atherton, 1972), 206–217.

7. Ranjana Srivastava, "Just Give Me the Script: The Scourge of Antibiotic Misuse and the Threat to Us All," *The Guardian*, June 21, 2016.

8. L. T. Krogsboll, et al., "General Health Checks for Reducing Illness and Mortality," *Cochrane Report*, January 30, 2019.

9. Latin translation, "you can't measure that."

Chapter Six

1. Julian Hoke Harris, "Keeping Away Death," a metal relief metal sculpture.
2. Stephen Mitchell, *Gilgamesh* (New York: Free Press, 2008).
3. Michelangelo Quote.
4. William Shakespeare, *Measure for Measure*, act III, scene I, line 82 (New York: New Press, 1997).
5. Gary Wolf, "Ray Kurzweil Pulls Out All the Stops (and Pills) to Survive to the Singularity," *Wired*, March 24, 2008.
6. Drake Baer, "5 Amazing Predictions by Futurist Ray Kurzweil," *The Business Insider*, October 20, 2015.
7. Samuel Harrington, M.D., *At Peace: Choosing a Good Death After a Long Life* (New York: Grand Central Life & Style, 2018).
8. Kathryn Mannix, M.D., *With the End in Mind: Dying, Death & Wisdom in an Age of Denial*, (New York: Little Brown & Company, 2018).
9. *Monty Python and the Holy Grail*.
10. Dylan Thomas, *In Country Sleep, and Other Poems* (New York: New Directions Publishing, 1952).
11. Elisabeth Kubler-Ross and David Kessler, *On Grief and Grieving: Finding the Meaning of Grief Through the Five Stages of Loss* (New York: Scribner, 2005).
12. S. Jay Olshansky, et al., "No Truth to the Fountain of Youth," *Scientific America*, June 2002.
13. Stephen Cave, *Immortality: The Quest to Live Forever and How it Drives Civilization* (New York: Crown Publishers, 2012).
14. Michael Shermer, *Heavens on Earth: The Scientific Search for the Afterlife, Immortality, and Utopia* (New York: Henry Holt and Company, 2018), 222–237.
15. Pallab Ghosh, "Ethics Debate as Pig Brains Kept Alive Without a Body," BBC News, April 27, 2018.
16. Antonio Regalado, "Researchers are Keeping Pig Brains Alive Outside the Body," *MIT Technology Review*, April 25, 2018.
17. Death with Dignity.
18. Coalition for Compassionate Care of California.
19. Dr. Philip Nitschke, "Here's Why I Invented a "Death Machine" which Lets People Take Their Own Lives," *Huffington Post*, April 2018.
20. *Soylent Green*.
21. *Deadline*.

Chapter Seven

1. James C. Mohr, Ph.D., "American Medical Malpractice Litigation in Historical Perspective," *JAMA* 283, no. 13 (2000): 1731–1737.
2. Christopher Stone, "From Bolam to Bolitho: Unravelling Medical Protectionism," January 2011.
3. Kim Price, "Toward a History of Medical Negligence," *The Lancet*, January 16, 2010.
4. Dennis Thompson, "Fewer Medical Malpractice Lawsuits Succeed, but Payouts Are Up," CBS News, March 28, 2017.
5. Ryan Jaslow, "Most Common Medical Malpractice Claims for Missed Cancer, Heart Attacks," CBS News, July 19, 2013.
6. A.D. Spiegel AD and F. Kavaler, "Abraham Lincoln Loses a Medical Malpractice Case, Debates Stephen A. Douglas, and Secures Two Murder Acquittals," *The Journal of Community Health* 29, no. 1 (February 2004): 75–97.
7. James C. Mohr, Ph.D., "American Medical Malpractice Litigation in Historical Perspective," *JAMA* 283, no. 13 (2000): 1731–1737.
8. Kenneth DeVille, *Medical Malpractice in Nineteenth-Century America: Origins and Legacy* (New York: NYU Press, 1992).
9. Aris Folley, "Longtime Obama Doctor Says Trump's Ex-Doctor Should be Investigated," *The Hill*, May 2, 2018.
10. Kyle Swenson, "Harold Bornstein: Exiled from Trumpland, Doctor Now 'Frightened and Sad,'" *Washington Post*, May 2, 2018.
11. Pamela Hartzband and Jerome Groopman, "How Medical Care is Being Corrupted," *New York Times*, November 18, 2014.
12. Will Hobson, "Larry Nassar, Former USA Gymnastics Doctor, Sentenced to 40–175 Years for Sex Crimes," *Washington Post*, January 24, 2018.
13. Zachary Rogers, "NKY Doctor Who Ran Pill Mill Convicted on 173 Drug Charges," Local Kentucky 12 News, Tuesday, March 13, 2018.
14. Owen Dyer, "Highest Billing U.S. Doctor Sentenced to 17 Years for Medicare Fraud," *BMJ* 360 (2018): 929.
15. Joe Sommerlad, "Harold Shipman: Who Was 'Doctor Death,' How Many of His Patients Did He Kill and How Was He Finally Caught?" *The Independent*, April 26, 2018.
16. "1896 A Serial Killer is Hanged," by History.com.
17. Erik Larson, *The Devil in White City: Murder, Magic, and Madness at the Fair That Changed America* (New York: Vintage Press, 2004).
18. "Malpractice Report 2017: Real Physicians. Real Lawsuits," *MedScape*.

19. "A Costly Defense: Physicians Sound Off on the High Price of Defensive Medicine in the U.S.," Jackson Healthcare, 2010.
20. "About the Federal Tort Claim Act (FTCA)," Health Resources & Services Administration.
21. "Malpractice Report 2017: Real Physicians. Real Lawsuits," *MedScape*.
22. Robert H. Aicher, Esq., "Lawyers Successfully Sued by Doctors for Filing Frivolous Lawsuits," *The Aesthetic Surgery Journal* 20, no. 4 (July 1, 2000): 337–338.
23. Steven Brill, *America's Bitter Pill: Money, Politics, Back-Room Deals, and the Healthcare System* (New York: Random House, 2015).
24. OpenSecrets.org, "Lobbying Spending Database Health, 2017."
25. Warren E. Leary, "Cigarette Company Developed Tobacco with Stronger Nicotine; Head of F.D.A. Tells of Chemical Manipulation," *New York Times*, June 22, 1994.
26. OpenSecrets.org, "Lobby Spending Database Tobacco, 1999."
27. "Master Settlement Agreement," National Association of Attorney General, 1998.
28. OpenSecrets.org, "Electronic Cigarettes."
29. "E-Cigarette Use Among Youth and Young Adults: a Report of the Surgeon General," U.S. Department of Health and Human Services, Atlanta, GA: 2016.
30. Ahmed J. Jamal, MBBS, et al., "Tobacco Use Among Middle and High School Students—United States, 2011–16," *CDC/MMWR* 66, no. 23 (June 16, 2017): 597–603.
31. Steven Reinberg, "1 Joint as Damaging as 5 Cigarettes to Your Lungs," ABC News, March 23, 2008.
32. Crystal Phend, "Lung Cancer Risk of One Marijuana Joint a Day Equal to a Daily Pack of Cigarettes," *MedPage Today*, January 29, 2008.
33. Sarah Aldington, et al., "Cannabis Use and Risk of Lung Cancer: A Case-Control Study," *European Respiratory Journal* 31, no. 2 (February 2008): 280–286.
34. "Marijuana has been legalized in nine states and Washington, DC," Vox.com, March 27, 2014.
35. OpenSecrets.org, "The Center for Responsive Politics."
36. Francesca M. Filbey, et al., "Long-Term Effects of Marijuana Use on the Brain," *PNAS*, November 10, 2014.
37. Dennis Thompson, "What Smoking Marijuana Does to the Brain," CBS News, November 11, 2014.
38. Richard Hillestad, et al., "Can Electronic Medical Record Systems Transform Health Care? Potential Health Benefits, Savings, and Costs," *Health Affairs* 24, no. 5 (September/October 2005): 1103–1117.
39. "Projections of the National Health Expenditures," CMS Office of Actuary Data, February 2018.

Chapter Eight

1. Suzanne Koven, M.D., "35 Years Later, Author Revisits 'The House of God,'" *Boston Globe*, September 2, 2013.
2. Samuel Shem, M.D., *The House of God* (New York: Black Swan, 1978).
3. Samuel Shem, M.D., *Mount Misery* (New York: Fawcett, 1997).
4. Hugh A. Stoddard and David V. O'Dell, "Would Socrates Have Actually Used the 'Socratic Method' for Clinical Teaching," *JGIM* 31, no. 9 (September 2016): 1092–1099.
5. Barron H. Lerner, "A Case That Shook Medicine," *Washington Post*, November 28, 2008.
6. ACGME.org.
7. Barron H. Lerner, "A Life-Changing Case for Doctors in Training," *New York Times*, March 3, 2009.
8. "2016 Position Statements on Duty Hours and the Learning and Working Environment," The Accreditation Council for Graduate Medical Education.
9. KevinMD.com.
10. DrWes.Blogspot.com.
11. Rebel.MD.
12. College Data.
13. MCAT-PREP.com
14. AAMC.org, "Applying to Medical School with AMCAS."
15. "Medical Student Debt," American Medical Student Association (AMSA).
16. Liselotte Dyrbye, M.D. and Matthew Thomas, M.D., et al., "Burnout and Suicidal Ideations Among U.S. Medical Students," *Annals of Internal Medicine* 149 (2008): 334–341.
17. College Date, "What's the Price Tag for a College Education?"
18. USMLE—Step 1.
19. "USMLE Step 1 Average Match Scores by Speciality," Doctors in Training.
20. AAMC.ORG, "Roadmap to Residency."
21. NRMP.org, "Verifying SOAP Eligibility."
22. Sandra Levy, "Resident Salary and Debt Report 2017," *Medscape*, July 26, 2017.
23. "ABIM Pass Rates: Behind the Declines," The NEJM Knowledge Team.
24. "The Deceptive Salary of Doctors," bestmedicaldegrees.com.

25. Sarah Grisham, "Medscape Physician Compensation Report 2017," *Medscape*, April 5, 2017.
26. Statista.com.
27. Niran Al-Agba and Meg Edison, "Commentary: How These Useless Doctors' Exams Are Raising Health Care Costs," *Fortune Magazine*, April 9, 2018.
28. Stephen M. Petterson, Ph.D., et al., "When Do Primary Care Physicians Retire? Implications for Workforce Projections," *The Annals of Family Medicine*, 2016.
29. Megan Thielking, "A Doctor's Murder Over an Opioid Prescription Leaves an Indiana City with No Easy Answers," STAT, August 8, 2017.
30. Stephanie Cojigal, et al., "Patient Prejudice: When Credentials Aren't Enough," *Medscape*, October 18, 2017.
31. James P. Philips, M.D., "Workplace Violence Against Health Care Workers in the United States," *The New England Journal of Medicine* 374 (April 28, 2016): 1661–1669.
32. Gene Emery, "Studies Document Risks of Assault for Healthcare Workers," Reuters Health News, April 28, 2016.
33. Pauline Bartolon, "California Rules About Violence Against Health Workers Could Become a Model," NPR, October 26, 2016.
34. "State House Passes Important Bill to Protect Hospital and Health Care Providers," The Hospital Healthsystem Association of Pennsylvania, House Bill 1219, February 12, 2016.
35. "Highest Suicide Rate by Profession," *The New Health Guide*, February 2, 2018.
36. Matt Hoffman and Kevin Kunzmann, "Suffering in Silence: The Scourge of Physician Suicide," *MD Magazine*, February 5, 2018.
37. Pamela Wible, M.D., *Physician Suicide Letters* (Self-published, 2016).
38. Pauline Anderson, "Physicians Experience Highest Suicide Rate of Any Profession," *Medscape*, May 7, 2018.
39. Megan Brooks, "Mobile Health App Effective for Serious Mental Illness," *Medscape*, June 1, 2018.
40. Suicide Prevention Life Line.
41. Anthony T. Lo Sasso, et al., "The $16,819 Pay Gap for Newly Trained Physicians: The Unexplained Trend of Men Earning More Than Women," *Health Affairs*, February 2011.
42. Rachel Emma Silverman, "Women Doctors Face $17,000 Pay Gap," American Medical Women's Association.
43. "Doximity 2018 Physician Compensation Report," Doximity, March 27, 2018.
44. Anupam B. Jena, M.D., Ph.D., et al., "Sex Differences in Physician Salary in U.S. Public Medical Schools," *JAMA Internal Medicine* 176, no. 9 (September 2016): 1294–1304.
45. Mackenzie R. Wehner, et al., "Plenty of Moustaches But Not Enough Women: Cross Sectional Study of Medical Leaders," *BMJ*, December 16, 2015.
46. Julie K. Silver, M.D., et al., "Female Physicians Are Underrrepresented in Recognition Awards from the American Academy of Physical Medicine and Rehabilitation," *The PMR Journal* (2017): 976–984.
47. Morgan Rosemary "Recognition Maters: Only One in Ten Awards Given to Women," *The Lancet* 389 (June 24, 2017).
48. Giovanni Filardo, et al., "Trends and Comparison of Female First Authorship in High Impact Medical Journals: Observational Study (1994–2014)," *The British Medical Journal* (2016): 352.
49. AMWA-Doc.org.
50. "Physician Shortages and Projections 2018," AAMC Work Force, March 2018.
51. Carol Peckham, "Medscape Lifestyle Report 2016: Bias and Burnout," *Medscape*, January 13, 2016.
52. "Strained Healthcare System Hurts Doctors and Affects Patient Care," MDVIP, September 20, 2017.
53. "Physician Health Survey: Is Your Doctor's Health Impacting Yours?," MDVIP.
54. Mark Crane, "Physician Frustration Grows, Income Falls—But There Is a Ray of Hope," *Medscape*, April 24, 2012.
55. Ms. Berkley and Mr. Fletcher, "H.R. 3300 (106th): Doctors' Bill of Rights Act of 1999," introduced November 10, 1999.
56. Pauline Anderson, "Physicians Experience Highest Suicide Rate of Any Profession," *Medscape*, May 7, 2018.
57. PRWEB.com.
58. Michele C. Parker, M.D., "The Physician's Bill of Rights," KevinMD.com, February 10, 2017.
59. Ericka L. Adler, M.D., "Abusive Patient Behavior: Physicians Have 'Rights' Too," *Physician Practice*, August 22, 2012.
60. Elliot Abemayer, M.D., Ph.D., "A Physicians' Bill of Rights: What If?" *Archives of Otorhinolaryngology–Head & Neck Surgery* 137, no. 5 (2011): 430.
61. David Raths, "Do Physicians Need an EHR Bill of Rights," Healthcare Informatics, November 1, 2011.
62. Nichole Bazemore, "Here's Everything You Need to Know About the Patient's Bill of Rights," *Forbes*, March 21, 2016.
63. HHS.gov, "Your Rights Under HIPAA."
64. "All Patients Should be Guaranteed the Following Freedoms," AAPS website.

65. "The Affordable Care Act's New Patient Bill of Rights," The Centers for Medicare & Medicaid Services.
66. Bruce Koeppen, M.D., "Shortage of Residency Slots May Have Chilling Effect on Next Generation of Physicians," *The Hill*, January 22, 2016.
67. The 2018 Residency Match Results.
68. NPMP.org

Chapter Nine

1. French Translation, "dirty word."
2. "International Code of Medical Ethics," The Third General Assembly of the World Medical Association, London, October 1949.
3. Austin Smith, M.D., et al., "Principles of Medical Ethics-1957," *JAMA* 164, no. 13 (July 27, 1957): 1482–1487.
4. KBL781, *Hippocrates* (Undated) (Illinois Institute of Technology's Ethics Codes Collection on October 24, 2011).
5. "AMA Principles of Medical Ethics," AMA, 2016.
6. Lynn R. Gruber, Maureen Shadle and Cynthia L. Polich, "From Movement to Industry: The Growth of HMOs," *Affairs Summer* 7, no. 3 (1988).
7. Bruce Koeppen, M.D., "Shortage of Residency Slots May Have Chilling Effect on Next Generation of Physicians," *The Hill*, January 22, 2016.
8. Jonathan Cohn, "The Robot Will See You Now," *The Atlantic*, March 2013.
9. "Second Treaties of Government," chapter 2 by John Locke.
10. "Declaration of Independence," The Primary Documents of American History, The Library of Congress.
11. Shelby Livingston, "UnitedHealth CEO's Compensation Swells in 2016 to $ 17.8 Million," Modern Healthcare, April 21, 2017.
12. Nan Jiang, Ph.D. and Pamela Ling, M.D., MPH, "Alliance Between Tobacco and Alcohol Industries to Shape Public Policy," *Addiction* 108, no. 5 (April 15, 2013): 852–864.
13. "GlaxoSmithKline to Plead Guilty and Pay $3 Billion to Resolve Fraud Allegations and Failure to Report Safety Data: Largest Health Care Fraud Settlement in U.S. History," The United States Department of Justice, July 2, 2012.
14. "Medicare Provider Utilization and Payment Data: Physician and Other Supplier CY2013," Data.cms.gov.
15. "White House Releases Data Listing Medicare's Top-Paid Doctors," *Associated Press*, April 9, 2014.

16. Matthew Hagg, "Doctor Linked to Senator Menedez's Corruption Case Is Convicted of Fraud," *New York Times*, April 28, 2017.
17. Matt Friedman, "Menendez Suggests He Doesn't Need to Pay Back Anything More to Melgen," Politico.com, May 25, 2018.
18. Niran Al-Agba and Meg Edison, "Commentary: How These Useless Doctors' Exams Are Raising Health Care Costs," *Fortune*, April 9, 2018.
19. Brain C. Drolet, M.D.., et al., "Fees for the Certification and Finances of Medical Specialty Boards," *JAMA* 318, no. 5 (August 1, 2017): 477–479.
20. Kurt Eichenwald, "A Certified Medical Controversy," *Newsweek*'s opinion page, April 7, 2015.
21. Niran Al-Alba and Meg Edison, "Commentary: How These Useless Doctors' Exams Are Raising Health Care Costs," *Fortune*, April 9, 2018.
22. Thomas Sullivan, "Anti-MOC Laws Picking Up Steam Across the United States," Policymed.com, May 4, 2018.
23. "American Board of Medical Specialties 2015 Tax Form 990," GuideStar.
24. David A. Cook, M.D., MHPE, et al., "Physician Attitudes About Maintenance of Certification," *Mayo Clinic Proceedings* 91, no. 10 (October 2016): 1136–1345.
25. Meg Edison, M.D., "My MOC Failure," Rebel.MD, December 3, 2017.
26. "AAPS Takes MOC to Court," AAPS.
27. Katie Lobosco, "Doctors and Nurses Busted for $ Medicare Fraud," CNN Money, June 21, 2015.
28. "Health Care Fraud Unit," The United States Department of Justice.
29. "GlaxoSmithKline to Plead Guilty and Pay $3 Billion to Resolve Fraud Allegations and Failure to Report Safety Data," United States Department of Justice, July 2, 2012.
30. Michael Monheit, "GlaxoSmithKline's $3 Billion Settlement: What the Department of Justice Claimed about Zofran," Zofran Legal.
31. Jess McClean and David Bruser, "Birth Defects Blamed on Unapproved Morning Sickness Treatment," *The Star*, June 25, 2014.
32. Gideon Koren, M.D., "Ondansetron: New and Troubling Data," *Pediatric News*, October 25, 2013.
33. Anderka M, et al., "Medication Used to Treat Nausea and Vomiting of Pregnancy and the Risk of Selected Birth Defects," Birth Defects Research Part A, *Clinical and Molecular Teratology* 94, no. 1 (January 2012): 22–30.
34. Jane Mundy, "GSK Had Zofran 'In the

Bag,'" *Lawyers and Settlements*, November 16, 2015.

35. Lev Facher, "Bernie Sanders Introduces Bill to Impose Jail Time for Execs Behind Opioid Crisis," *Stat News*, April 17, 2018.

36. "Title 29—Labor. USC 151: Findings and Declaration of Policy," The United States Code.

37. "The Antitrust Laws," Federal Trade Commission.

38. Carol K. Kane, Ph.D., "Policy Research Perspectives: Updated Data on Physician Practice Arrangements: Physician Ownership Drops Below 50 Percent," AMA, 2017.

39. Alex Kacik, "For the First Time Ever, Less Than Half of Physicians Are Independent," *Modern Healthcare*, May 31, 2017.

40. Joe Mozingo, "Doctors at University of California Health Clinics Go on Strike," *Los Angeles Times*, April 11, 2015.

41. Paul Sisson, "Doctors Strike Shows Union Push," *San Diego Tribune*, January 27, 2015.

42. "The Pareto Chart" as discussed in *Tools* by the Institute for Healthcare Improvement, Cambridge, MA.

43. Joe Flower, *Healthcare Beyond Reform: Doing It Right for Half the Cost* (New York: Productivity Press, 2012), chapter 9, figure 9.1.

44. Atul Gawande, "The Hot Spotters," *The New Yorker*, January 24, 2011.

Chapter Ten

1. Neil Gaiman, *Trigger Warnings: Short Fictions and Other Disturbances* (New York: William Morrow, 2015).

2. Rene Descartes, *Principia Philosophiae* (1644).

3. *The Matrix*.

4. Friedrich Nietzsche, *Thus Spoke Zarathustra* (from 1883 to 1891).

5. David Brooks, "The Philosophy of Data," *New York Times*, February 4, 2013.

6. Yuval Noah Harari, *Homo Deus: A Brief History of Tomorrow* (New York: HarperCollins, 2017).

7. Strangroom and Gravey, *The Great Philosophers: From Socrates to Foucault* (New York: Metro Books, 2005), 21.

8. Bryan BaGee, *The Story of Philosophy* (New York: Dorling Kindersley, 1998), 47.

9. Yuval Noah Harari, *Homo Deus: A Brief History of Tomorrow* (New York: HarperCollins, 2017).

10. Roger McKinlay, "Technology: Use or Lose Our Navigation Skills," *Nature* 531 (March 31, 2016): 573–575.

11. Kerri Smith, "'The Knowledge Enlarges Your Brain: The Hippocampi of London Taxi Drivers Swell as They Learn the City Streets," *Nature*, December 8, 2011.

12. Owsel Temkin, *Hippocrates in a World of Pagans and Christians* (Baltimore: Johns Hopkins University Press, 1995).

13. Jeanne Bryner, "Why You (Probably) Shouldn't Worry About Earth's Magnetic Poles Flipping," *Live Science*, February 1, 2018.

Chapter Eleven

1. M. K. Marvel, et al., "Soliciting the Patient's Agenda: Have We Improved?" *JAMA* 281, no. 3 (January 20, 1999): 283–287.

2. Wolf Langewitz, et al., "Spontaneous Talking Time at Start of Consultation in Outpatient Clinic: Cohort Study," *BMJ* 325 and 7366 (September 28, 2002): 682–683.

3. *Despicable Me*.

Chapter Twelve

1. David Brooks, "The Outsourced Brain," *New York Times*, October 26, 2007.

2. Marshall McLuhan, *Understanding Media: The Extension of Man* (New York: McGraw-Hill, 1964).

3. Nicholas Carr, *The Shallows: What the Internet is Doing to Our Brains* (New York and London: W.W. Norton, 2011).

4. Nicholas Carr, *The Glass Cage: How Our Computers are Changing Us* (New York and London: W.W. Norton, 2014).

5. Moheb Costandi, *Neuroplasticity* (Cambridge, MA and London: The MIT Press, 2016), 1.

6. N. Sadato, "How the Blind "See" Braille: Lessons from Functional Magnetic Resonance Imaging," *Neuroscientist* 11, no. 6 (2005): 577–582.

7. Striem-Amit, et al., "Visual Cortex Extrastriate Body-selective Area Activation in Congenitally Blind People "Seeing" by Using Sound," *Current Biology* 24, no. 6 (2014): 687–692.

8. R. L. Paul, H. Goodman, and M. Merzenich, "Alterations in the Mechanoreceptor Input to the Brodmann's Areas 1 and 3 of the Postcentral Hand Area of Macaca Mulatta After Nerve Section and Regeneration," *Brain Research* 39, no. 1 (April 1972): 1–19.

9. Moheb Costandi, *Neuroplasticity* (Cambridge, MA and London: The MIT Press, 2016), 149–150.

10. "Diagnostic and Statistical Manual of

Mental Disorders," 5th Edition: DSM-5, The American Psychiatric Association, 2016.

11. Plato, Phaedrus (c. 370 BCE), 551–552.

12. Timothy Hoff, "Deskilling and Adaption Among Primary Care Physicians Using Two Work Innovations," *Health Care Management* 36, no 4 (October–December 2011): 338–348.

13. Timothy Hoff, *Practice Under Pressure: Primary Care Physicians and Their Medicine in the Twenty-first Century: Critical Issues in Health and Medicine* (New Brunswick, NJ: Rutgers University Press, 2009).

14. G. W. Small, et al., "Your Brain on Google: Patterns of Cerebral Activation During Internet Searching," *American Journal of Geriatric Psychiatry* 17, no. 2 (February 2009): 116–126.

15. Nihon Eiseigaku Zasshi, "Effect of Reading a Book on a Tablet Computer on Cerebral Blood Flow in the Prefrontal Cortex," *NIRS* (Japanese) 73, no. 1 (2018): 39–45.

16. Her.

17. Joseph Weizenbaum, *Computer Power and Human Reason: From Judgment to Calculation* (New York: W. H. Freeman, 1976), 7.

18. Joseph Weizenbaum, *Computer Power and Human Reason: From Judgment to Calculation* (New York: W. H. Freeman, 1976).

19. Pamela McCorduck, "*Machines Who Think* (Natick, MA: A. K. Peters/CRC Press: 2004), 374–376.

20. A. M. Turing, "On Computable Numbers, with an Application to the Entscheidungsproblem," The Proceedings of the London Mathematical Society, series 2, 42, 1937, 230–265, corrections in 1938.

21. Rene Descartes, "Discourse on the Method of Rightly Conducting One's Reason and Seeking Truth in the Sciences," in *Early Modern Texts* (French), 22.

22. "ABIM Pass Rates: Behind the Decline," NEJM Knowledge Team, October 16, 2014.

23. Kurt Eichenwald, "The Ugly Civil War in American Medicine," *Newsweek*, March 10, 2015.

24. I. Nonaka, *Takeuchi, Hirotaka, The Knowledge Creation Company: How Japanese Companies Create the Dynamics of Innovation* (New York: Oxford University Press, 1995), 284.

25. Melissa Hogenboom, "Warning Over Electrical Brain Stimulators," BBC News, August 24, 2014.

26. N. J. Davis, "Transcranial Stimulation of the Developing Brain: A Plea for Extreme Caution," *Frontiers in Human Neuroscience*, August 5, 2014.

27. tDCS Device—TheBrainDriver v2. tDCS Digital Precision + Safety Features (Everything Included. Ready-to-Use).

28. Pascale Carayon, *Handbook of Human Factors and Ergonomics in Health Care and Patient Safety: 2nd Edition* (Boca Raton, FL: CRC Press, 2017).

29. Nicholas Carr, *The Glass Cage: How Our Computers are Changing Us* (New York and London: W.W. Norton, 2014), 163.

30. John D. Lee, "Human Factors and Ergonomics in Automation Design," *Handbook of Human Factors and Ergonomics: 3rd edition* (Hoboken, NJ: Wiley, 2012).

31. Greg Sandoval, "IBM's New AI Supercomputer Can Argue, Rebut, and Debate Humans," *Business Insider*, June 18, 2018.

32. Yaniv Leviathan, "Google Duplex: An AI System for Accomplishing Real-World Tasks Over the Phone," "Google AI Blog," May 8, 2018.

33. "Deep-Learning Machine Listens to Bach, Then Writes Its Own Music in the Same Style," *Technology Review*, December 14, 2016.

34. Robert Fenner, "Alibab's AI Outguns Humans in Reading Test," Bloomberg, January 14, 2018.

35. Erik Brynjolfsson, *The Second Machine Age: Work, Progress, and Prosperity in Technologies* (New York: W.W. Norton, 2016).

36. Sonya James, "Q&A: Andrew McAfee & Erik Brynjolfsson, Co-Authors of the Second Machine Age," ZD.net, March 7, 2014.

37. Lauren F. Friedman, "IBM's Watson Supercomputer May Soon Be the Best Doctor in the World," The Business Insider, April 22, 2014.

Chapter Thirteen

1. "Waiting Time to See a Doctor When Sick Need Medical Attention, Among Sicker Adults," The Commonwealth Fund's Newsroom, July 16, 2008.

2. Dan Munro, "'Single-Payer' Healthcare Isn't Necessary—but Single Pricing is," Forbes' Public Health Forum, July 4, 2017.

3. Chana Joffe-Walt, "In Japan, MRI's Cost Less," *NPR—Planet Money*, November 18, 2009.

4. Katie McBeth, "Is Health Care Really Better Outside of the United States?" *International Policy Digest*, August 1, 2017.

5. Kathryn H. Jacobsen, *Introduction to Global Health: 2nd Edition* (Burlington. MA: Jones & Bartlett Learning, 2013).

6. Steven Brill, "Bitter Pill: Why Medical Bills Arc Killing Us: How Outrageous Pricing and Egregious Profits Are Destroying Our Health Care," *Time*, March 12, 2013.

7. Mary Duenwald, "Your Own Private Doctor," *Departures*, March 30, 2010.

8. Lydia Ramsey, "A Small But Growing Movement of Doctors That Don't Accept Insurance and Charge a Monthly Fee Could be a Model for Big Employers Like Amazon and JP-Morgan," *Business Insider*, June 21, 2018.

9. "Concierge Medicine: An Alternative Insurance," Association of Mature American Citizens, June 26, 2014.

10. Carnahan, S. J., "Concierge Medicine: Legal and Ethical Issues," *The Journal of Law, Medicine, and Ethics* 35, no. 10 (2007): 211–215.

11. Dan Munro, "The 50th Anniversary of Dr. King's Healthcare Quote," *Forbes—Pharma & Healthcare*, March 25, 2016.

12. "Global Health Security: Immunization," published by the CDC.

13. "Bill and Melinda Gates Foundation Member Profile," The Global Health Workforce Alliance.

14. Penny Heaton, "Bill and Melinda Gates Medical Research Institute," Vaccines and Global Health: Ethics and Policy, February 11, 2018.

15. Bill & Melinda Gates Medical Research Institute.

16. Abigail Abrams, "Warren Buffett Donates $3.17 Billion to the Gates Foundation and Other Charities," *Fortune*, July 10, 2017.

17. Marc Parry, Kelly Field and Beckie Supiano, "The Gates Effect," *Chronicle*, July 14, 2013.

18. The World Health Organization—WHO.

19. World Health Organization Programme Budget 2018–2019.

20. "Seventy-First World Health Assembly Update—Digital Health," May 25, 2018.

21. "Call for Innovative Technologies That Address Global Health Concerns," The WHO.

22. "Commcare for Ebola Response."

23. "Independent, Impartial, and Neutral," Doctors Without Borders 2017.

24. "Bearing Witness," Doctors Without Borders 2017.

25. M. D. Collins, "Should Every Patient Have a Unique ID Number for All Medical Records?" *Wall Street Journal*, January 23, 2012.

26. Susan Scutti, "The Government Owns Your DNA. What Are They Doing With It?" *Newsweek*, July 24, 2014.

27. George J. Annas, et al., "23andMe and the FDA," *The New England Journal of Medicine* 370 (March 13, 2014): 985–988.

28. "DNA of Every Baby Born in California Is Stored. Who Has Access to It?" CBS News, May 12, 2018.

29. Noor A. A. Giesbertz, et al., "When Children Become Adults: Should Biobanks Re-Contact?" *The Journal of Preventive Medicine* 12, no. 2 (February 2016).

30. "World Population Clock."

31. Rebecca Skloot, *The Immortal Life of Henrietta Lacks* (New York: Crown Publishing, 2010).

32. *The Immortal Life of Henrietta Lack*.

33. Art Caplan, PhD, "NIH Finally Makes Good with Henrietta Lacks' Family—and It's About Time, Ethicist Say," NBC News—Health News, August 7, 2013.

34. Daniel Fisher, "Supreme Court Rejects Human-Gene Patents—Sort of," *Forbes*, June 13, 2013.

Chapter Fourteen

1. Robert Wachter, *The Digital Doctor: Hope, Hype, and Harm at the Dawn of Medicine's Computer Age* (New York: McGraw Hill, 2015).

2. Steve Lohr, "IBM Is Counting on Its Bet on Watson, and Paying Big Money for It," *New York Times*, October 17, 2016.

3. "Worldwide Spending on Cognitive and Artificial Intelligence Systems Will Grow to $19.1 Billion in 2018, According to New IDC Spending Guide," IDC, 2018.

4. Simon Parkin, "The Artificially Intelligent Doctor Will Hear You Now," *MIT Technology Review*, March 9, 2016.

5. Alex Graves, et al., "Hybrid Computing Using a Neural Network with Dynamic External Memory," *Nature* 538 (October 12, 2016): 471–476.

6. "WaveNet: A Generative Model for Raw Audio," DeepMind.

7. "Helping Clinicians Get Patients from Test to Treatment Faster," DeepMind.

8. "DeepMind Health and Data," DeepMind.

9. Hal Hodson, "Revealed: Google AI Has Access to Huge Haul of HNS Patient Data," *The New Scientist*, April 29, 2016.

10. Linklater, LLP, "Audit of the Acute Kidney Injury Detection System Known as Streams," The Royal Free London NHS Foundation Trust, May 17, 2018.

11. Rosalind W. Picard, *Affective Computing, 2nd edition* (Cambridge, MA: MIT Press, 1997).

12. Madhumita Murgia, "Affective Computing: How 'Emotional Machines' Are About to Take Over Our Lives," *The Telegraph*, January 15, 2016.

13. *Nevermind*, Affectiva.

14. *Nevermind*, the game.

15. "Facial Recognition Market by Component.... Global Forecast 2020," Marketandmarkets, November 2017.

16. Richard Yonck, *Heart of the Machine:*

Our Future in a World of Artificial Emotional Intelligence (New York: Arcade Publishing, 2017).
17. *The Polar Express.*
18. *Beowulf.*
19. Masahiro Mori: Translated by Karl F. MacDorman and Norri Kageki, "The Uncanny Valley: The Original Essay by Masahiro Mori," *Spectrum*, June 12, 2012.
20. Karl F. MacDorman, "Mortality Salience and the Uncanny Valley," The Proceedings of the 2005 International Conference on Humanoid Robots, 2005, 399–405.
21. Richard Morgan, *Altered Carbon* (New York: Ballantine Books, 2002).
22. Alexis Bedecarrats, et al., "RNA from Trained Aplysia Can Induce an Epigenetic Engram for Long-Term Sensitization in Untrained Aplysia," *eNeuro*, May 14, 2018.
23. Shivani Dave, "'Memory Transplants' Achieved in Snails," BBC News, May 14, 2018.
24. Charles Darwin, *The Expression of the Emotions in Man and Animal* (United Kingdom: John Murray, 1872).
25. Gene E. Robinson and Andrew B. Barron, "Epigenetics and the Evolution of Instincts," *Science* 356 (April 7, 2017): 26–27.
26. Paul Ekman and Wallace V. Friesen, "Constants Across Cultures in the Face and Emotion," *The Journal of Personality and Social Psychology* 17, no 2 (1971): 124–129.
27. 27. Tom Simonite, "'DNA Computer' Is Unbeatable at Tic-Tac-Toe," *The New Scientist*, October 17, 2006.
28. Draper's press release, May 13, 2107.
29. Koniku.
30. Sveta McShane, "This Amazing Computer Chip Is Made of Live Brain Cells," Singularity Hub, March 17, 2016.
31. Boston Dynamics.
32. Regina Surber, "Artificial Intelligence: Autonomous Technology (AT), Lethal Autonomous Weapons Systems (LAWS) and Peace Time Threats," The ICT4Peace Foundation and the Zurich Hub for Ethics and Technology (ZHET), February 21, 2018.
33. *Slaughterbots.*
34. Brian N. Pasley, et al., "Reconstructing Speech from Human Auditory Cortex," *Biology*, January 13, 2012.
35. James Titcomb, "Mark Zuckerberg Confirms Facebook Is Working on Mind-Reading Technology," *The Telegraph*, April 19, 2017.
36. Magdalena Petrova, "MIT Developed a Headset That Gives a Voice to the Voice Inside Your Head," CNBC, April 10, 2018.
37. Jing Wang, et al., "Predicting the Brain Activation Pattern Associated with the Propositional Content of a Sentence: Modeling Neural Representations of Events and States," *Human Brain Mapping* 38, no. 10 (October 2017): 4865–4881.
38. *Eternal Sunshine of the Spotless Mind.*
39. Mike Elgan, "Mind-Reading Tech Is Here (and More Useful Than You Think)," *Computer World*, April 7, 2018.
40. Ernest Cline, *Ready Player One* (New York: Random House 2011).
41. Lemelson-MIT Student Prizes, April 12, 2016.
42. Joseph Weizenbaum, *Computer Power and Human Reason: From Judgment to Calculation* (New York: W.H. Freeman,), Book jacket quote.

Chapter Fifteen

1. "Rising Demand for Long-Term Services and Supports for Elderly People," The Congressional Budget Office, June 26, 2013.
2. Amy Fiske, et al., "Depression in Older Adults," *Annual Revenue of Clinical Psychology* 5 (2009): 363–389.
3. J. P. Loebel, "Anticipation of Nursing Home Placement May Be a Precipitant of Suicide Among the Elderly," *The Journal of the American Geriatrics Society* (April 1991): 407–408.
4. "Elder Abuse," The National Council on Aging.
5. Patrick Arborne, M.D., "Friendship Line for the Elderly," The Institute on Aging, 1973: 1-800-971-0016.
6. Karina Martinez-Carter, "How the Elderly Are Treated Around the World," *The Week*, July 23, 2013.
7. World Population Review—Japan Population 2018.
8. The Data Team, "Suicides in Japan Hit a 20-Year Low," *The Economist*, June 28, 2017.
9. P. O. Harrison, "Japan's Robotics Industry Bullish on Elderly Care Market, TrendForce Report," TrendForce, May 19, 2018.
10. Malcolm Foster, "Aging Japan: Robots May Have Role in the Future of Elder Care," *U.S. News*, March 27, 2018.
11. Vecna Robotic's Website—Healthcare.
12. Sebastian Anthony, "Meet Jibo, the World's First Family Robot—Built by MIT's Social Robotics Master," *Extreme Tech*, July 16, 2014.
13. Mutual Venture: Waypoint Robotics.
14. Malcolm Foster, "Aging Japan: Robots May Have a Role in Future Elder Care," AOL, March 27, 2018.

15. Emily Matchar, "Can an App Help Detect Autism?" *The Smithsonian*, October 21, 2015.

16. Arnold Munk, *The Little Engine That Could* (New York: Platt & Munk, 1930).

17. Michael Crichton, *Jurassic Park* (New York: Alfred A. Knopf, 1990).

18. Nicola Davis, "Murder Most Fowl: Oxford Dodo 'Shot in the Back of the Head,'" *The Guardian*, April 20, 2018.

Bibliography

"AAPS Takes MOC to Court." Association of American Physicians and Surgeons. May 4, 2018. aapsonline.org/aaps-takes-moc-to-court/.

Abemayor, Elliot. "A Physicians' Bill of Rights." *Archives of Otolaryngology—Head & Neck Surgery* 137, no. 5 (2011): 430. doi:10.1001/archoto.2011.54.

"ABIM Pass Rates: What's Behind the Decline? NEJM Knowledge+." NEJM Knowledge+. January 31, 2018. knowledgeplus.nejm.org/blog/abim-pass-rates-behind-declines/.

"About the Federal Tort Claims Act (FTCA)." Health Resources Services Administration. bphc.hrsa.gov/ftca/about/index.html.

"About WHO." World Health Organization. www.who.int/about-us.

Abrams, Abigail. "Warren Buffett Donates $3.17 Billion to Gates Foundation and Other Charities." *Fortune*, July 10, 2017. fortune.com/2017/07/10/warren-buffett-donates-gates-foundation/.

"ACA-New-Patients-Bill-of-Rights." Centers for Medicare & Medicaid Services. June 14, 2013. www.cms.gov/CCIIO/Resources/Fact-Sheets-and-FAQs/aca-new-patients-bill-of-rights.html.

Acemoglu, et al. "Return of the Solow Paradox? IT, Productivity, and Employment in U.S. Manufacturing." National Bureau of Economic Research. January 23, 2014. www.nber.org/papers/w19837.

"ACGME Home." Accreditation Council for Graduate Medical Education. www.acgme.org/.

Adler, Ericka L. "Abusive Patient Behavior: Physicians Have 'Rights' Too." *Physician Practice*. August 22, 2012. doi:http://www.physicianspractice.com/patient-dismissal/abusive-patient-behavior-physicians-have-rights-too.

Admin. "About ARRA." HITECH Answers: HIPAA, MIPS, EHR, Cybersecurity News. 2009. www.hitechanswers.net/about/about-arra/.

Aesop. *One of Aesop's Fables.* ser. 210. Perry Index. 620AD.

Agnew, Jeremy. *Medicine in the Old West: A History, 1850–1900.* Jefferson, NC: McFarland, 2010.

Aicher, Robert H. "Lawyers Successfully Sued by Doctors for Filing Frivolous Lawsuits." *Aesthetic Surgery Journal.* July 1, 2000. academic.oup.com/asj/article/20/4/337/273780.

Al-Agba, Niran, and Meg Edison. "Commentary: How These Useless Doctors' Exams Are Raising Health Care Costs." *Fortune.* April 9, 2018. fortune.com/2018/04/09/doctors-maintenance-certification-moc-health-care/.

Aldington, Sarah, et al. "Cannabis Use and Risk of Lung Cancer: A Case-Control Study." *The European Respiratory Journal.* February 2008. www.ncbi.nlm.nih.gov/pmc/articles/PMC2516340/.

Alemzadeh, Homa, et. al. "Adverse Events in Robotic Surgery: A Retrospective Study of 14 Years of FDA Data." 2015. https://arxiv.org/ftp/arxiv/papers/1507/1507.03518.pdf.

"AMA Principles of Medical Ethics." American Medical Association. 2016. www.ama-assn.org/delivering-care/ama-principles-medical-ethics.

"American Board of Medical Specialties 2015 Tax Form 990." Guidestar.org. 2015. www.guidestar.org/FinDocuments/2015/410/847/2015-410847713-0d662f03-9O.pdf.

American Medical Women's Association, www.amwa-doc.org/.

Anderka, M. "Medication Used to Treat Nausea and Vomiting of Pregnancy and the Risk of Selected Birth Defects." *Birth Defects Research Part A, Clinical and Molecular Teratology* 94, no. 1 (January 2012). doi:https://www.ncbi.nlm.nih.gov/pubmed/22102545.

Anderson, Pauline. "Physicians Experience Highest Suicide Rate of Any Profession.'" Medscape Log In. May 7, 2018. www.medscape.com/viewarticle/896257.

Bibliography

Andrews, Evans. "Who Were the Luddites?" History.com. 7 August 7. 2017. www.history.com/news/ask-history/who-were-the-luddites.

Annas, George. "23andMe And the FDA | NEJM." *New England Journal of Medicine* 13 (March 2014). www.nejm.org/doi/full/10.1056/NEJMp1316367.

Anthony, Sebastian. "Meet Jibo, the World's First Family Robot—Built by MIT's Social Robotics Master." ExtremeTech. July 16, 2014. www.extremetech.com/extreme/186401-meet-jibo-the-worlds-first-family-robot-made-by-mits-social-robotics-master.

"The Antitrust Laws." Federal Trade Commission. 15 December 15, 2017. www.ftc.gov/tips-advice/competition-guidance/guide-antitrust-laws/antitrust-laws.

"Applying to Medical School with AMCAS®." AAMC Students, Applicants and Residents. October 10, 2018. students-residents.aamc.org/applying-medical-school/applying-medical-school-process/applying-medical-school-amcas/.

Arborne, Patrick. "Senior Intervention Hotline for Crisis Support Services | IOA Friendship Line." Institute on Aging. 1973. www.ioaging.org/services/all-inclusive-health-care/friendship-line. 1–800–971–0016.

"Are You Ready?" Vecna Patient Solutions. healthcare.vecna.com/.

Arndt, Brian G., et al. "Tethered to the EHR: Primary Care Physician Workload Assessment Using EHR Event Log Data and Time-Motion Observations." *The Annals of Family Medicine* 15, no. 5 (2017): 419–426. doi:10.1370/afm.2121.

arXiv. Emerging Technology from "Listen to This Classical Music Composed in the Style of Bach by a Deep-Learning Machine." *MIT Technology Review*. December 15, 2016. www.technologyreview.com/s/603137/deep-learning-machine-listens-to-bach-then-writes-its-own-music-in-the-same-style/.

Asimov, Isaac. "Runaround." *Astounding Science Fiction*. March 1942.

"Augmented Reality in Healthcare Will Be Revolutionary." *The Medical Futurist*. August 15, 2016. medicalfuturist.com/augmented-reality-in-healthcare-will-be-revolutionary/.

Babylon Health. www.babylonhealth.com/.

Baer, Drake. "5 Amazing Predictions by Futurist Ray Kurzweil That Came True—and 4 That Haven't." *Business Insider*. October 20, 2015. www.businessinsider.com/15-startling-incredible-and-provactive-predictions-from-googles-genius-futurist-2015–9.

BaGee, Bryan. *The Story of Philosophy*. London: Dorling Kindersley, 1998.

Bakalar, Nicholas. "Milestones in Medical Technology." *New York Times*. October 10, 2012. archive.nytimes.com/www.nytimes.com/interactive/2012/10/05/health/digital-doctor.html?ref=thedigitaldoctor#/#time15_375.

Ballentine, Carol. "Taste of Raspberries, Taste of Death: The 1937 Elixir Sulfanilamide Incident." *FDA Consumer Magazine*. June 1981. doi:https://www.fda.gov/AboutFDA/WhatWeDo/History/ProductRegulation/ucm2007257.htm.

Bannow, Tara. "The Years Long Decline in Free or Discounted Care That Hospitals Provide May Have Reached Its Floor." *Modern Healthcare*. January 6, 2018. www.modernhealthcare.com/article/20180106/NEWS/180109941.

Bartolone, Pauline. "California Rules About Violence Against Health Workers Could Become A Model." NPR. October 26, 2016. www.npr.org/sections/health-shots/2016/10/26/499299408/california-rules-about-violence-against-health-workers-could-become-a-model.

Bazemore, Nichole. "Here's Everything You Need to Know About the Patient's Bill Of Rights." *Forbes*. April 6, 2016. www.forbes.com/sites/amino/2016/03/21/heres-everything-you-need-to-know-about-the-patients-bill-of-rights/#4fa227616d01.

"Bearing Witness." Doctors Without Borders—USA. 2017. doctorswithoutborders.org/who-we-are/principles/bearing-witness.

Bédécarrats, Alexis, et al. "RNA from Trained Aplysia Can Induce an Epigenetic Engram for Long-Term Sensitization in Untrained Aplysia." *ENeuro*. May 14, 2018. www.eneuro.org/content/early/2018/05/14/ENEURO.0038-18.2018.

Berkley, Ms., and Mr. Fletcher. "H.R. 3300 (106th): Doctors' Bill of Rights Act of 1999." GovTrack.us. November 10, 1999. www.govtrack.us/congress/bills/106/hr3300/text/ih.

"Bill & Melinda Gates Foundation." World Health Organization. July 23, 2011. www.who.int/workforcealliance/members_partners/member_list/gates/en/.

"Bill & Melinda Gates Medical Research Institute." Bill & Melinda Gates Medical Research Institute. www.gatesmri.org/.

Billings, C. E. "Aviation Safety Reporting System (ASRS) Coding Manual." Langley Research Center, Hampton, VA: Lauber, Funkhouser, Lyman, & Huff, 1976.

Black, Ashly D., et al. "The Impact of EHealth on the Quality and Safety of Health Care: A

Bibliography

Systematic Overview." *PLoS Medicine* 8, no. 1 (2011). doi:10.1371/journal.pmed.1000387.

Black, Donald W., and Jon E. Grant. *DSM-5 Guidebook: The Essential Companion to the Diagnostic and Statistical Manual of Mental Disorders, Fifth Edition.* Washington, DC: American Psychiatric Association, 2014.

Boeldt, Debra L., et al. "How Consumers and Physicians View New Medical Technology: Comparative Survey." *Current Neurology and Neuroscience Reports.* U.S. National Library of Medicine. September 2015. www.ncbi.nlm.nih.gov/pmc/articles/PMC4642377/.

"Boston Dynamics: Changing Your Idea of What Robots Can Do." www.bostondynamics.com/.

Bowers, Simon. "Delays with £12.7bn NHS Software Program Bring It Close to Collapse." *The Guardian.* 21 March 21, 2010. www.theguardian.com/business/2010/mar/21/nhs-software-system-close-to-imploding.

Brill, Steven. *America's Bitter Pill: Money, Politics, Backroom Deals, and the Fight to Fix Our Broken Healthcare System.* New York: Random House, 2015.

Brill, Steven. "Bitter Pill: Why Medical Bills Are Killing Us." *Time.* March 4, 2013. content.time.com/time/subscriber/article/0,33009,2136864,00.html.

Brooks, David. "The Outsourced Brain." *New York Times.* October 26, 2007. www.nytimes.com/2007/10/26/opinion/26brooks.html.

Brooks, David. "The Philosophy of Data." *New York Times.* February 5, 2013. www.nytimes.com/2013/02/05/opinion/brooks-the-philosophy-of-data.html.

Brooks, Megan. "Mobile Health App Effective for Serious Mental Illness." *Medscape.* June 1, 2018. www.medscape.com/viewarticle/897448?src=WNL_recnl_180604_MSCPEDIT_imfm&uac=298605DV&impID=1649355&faf=1.

Bryner, Jeanna. "Why You (Probably) Shouldn't Worry About Earth's Magnetic Poles Flipping." *LiveScience.* February 1, 2018. www.livescience.com/61603-what-if-magnetic-pole-reversal.html.

Brynjolfsson, Erik, and Andrew McAfee. *The Second Machine Age: Work, Progress, and Prosperity in the Time of Brilliant Technologies.* New York: W. W. Norton, 2016.

"Call for Innovative Technologies That Address Global Health Concerns." World Health Organization. August 25, 2011. www.who.int/medical_devices/call/en/index6.html.

Campbell, Joseph. *The Hero with a Thousand Faces.* Princeton, NJ: Princeton University Press, 1972.

Caplan, Art. "NIH Finally Makes Good with Henrietta Lacks' Family—and It's about Time, Ethicist Says." NBCNews.com. NBCUniversal News Group. August 7, 2013. www.nbcnews.com/health/health-news/nih-finally-makes-good-henrietta-lacks-family-its-about-time-f6C10867941.

Carayon, Pascale. *Handbook of Human Factors and Ergonomics in Health Care and Patient Safety.* CRC Pr I Llc, 2017.

Card, Orson Scott. *Ender's Game.* New York: TOR Books, 1985.

Carnahan, Sandra J. "Currents in Contemporary Ethics." *The Journal of Law, Medicine & Ethics* 10.1111 (March 2, 2007). onlinelibrary.wiley.com/doi/abs/10.1111/j.1748-720X.2007.00125.x.

Carr, Nicholas. *The Glass Cage: How Our Computers Are Changing Us.* New York: W.W. Norton, 2014.

Carr, Nicholas G. *The Shallows: What the Internet Is Doing to Our Brains.* New York: W.W. Norton, 2011.

Cave, Stephen. *Immortality: The Quest to Live Forever and How It Drives Civilization.* New York: Crown Publishing, 2012.

Cellan-Jones, Rory. "Stephen Hawking Warns Artificial Intelligence Could End Mankind." BBC News. December 2, 2014. www.bbc.com/news/technology-30290540.

Center for Devices and Radiological Health. "Infusion Pumps." US Food and Drug Administration Home Page, Center for Drug Evaluation and Research. www.fda.gov/medicaldevices/productsandmedicalprocedures/generalhospitaldevicesandsupplies/infusionpumps/.

Center for Devices and Radiological Health. "Safety Communications—Cybersecurity Vulnerabilities Identified in St. Jude Medical's Implantable Cardiac Devices and Merlin@Home Transmitter: FDA Safety Communication." US Food and Drug Administration Home Page, Center for Drug Evaluation and Research. www.fda.gov/MedicalDevices/Safety/AlertsandNotices/ucm535843.htm.

"The Center for Responsive Politics." OpenSecrets.org. www.opensecrets.org/news/issues/marijuana/.

Chantal, Patient. "AccuVein AV400." YouTube. November 27, 2012. www.youtube.com/watch?v=kBbtZHNXIRg.

Chisholm, Roin Lynn. "Emergency Physician Documentation Quality and Cognitive Load: Comparison of Paper Charts to Electronic Physician Documentation." The School of Informatics and Computing. August 2014. doi:https://scholarworks.iupui.edu/handle/1805/5809.

Cline, Ernest. *Ready Player One*. New York: Random House, 2011.
Cohn, Jonathan. "The Robot Will See You Now." *The Atlantic*. February 19, 2014. www.theatlantic.com/magazine/archive/2013/03/the-robot-will-see-you-now/309216/.
Cojigal, Stephanie. "Patient Prejudice: When Credentials Aren't Enough." Medscape. October 18, 2017. www.medscape.com/slideshow/2017-patient-prejudice-report-6009134?src=par_stat_mscpmrk_patientprejudice&faf=1#2.
"Collegiate Inventors Awarded Lemelson-MIT Student Prize." Lemelson-MIT Program. April 12, 2016. lemelson.mit.edu/news/collegiate-inventors-awarded-lemelson-mit-student-prize.
Collins. "Should Every Patient Have a Unique ID Number for All Medical Records?" *Wall Street Journal*. January 23, 2012. www.wsj.com/articles/SB10001424052970204124204577154661814932978.
Collins, Suzanne. *The Hunger Games*. New York: Scholastic, 2008.
Commissioner, Office of the. "Press Announcements—FDA Outlines Cybersecurity Recommendations for Medical Device Manufacturers." US Food and Drug Administration Home Page, Center for Drug Evaluation and Research. January 15, 2016. www.fda.gov/newsevents/newsroom/pressannouncements/ucm481968.htm.
Commissioner, Office of the. "Virtual Exhibits of FDA History—Frances Oldham Kelsey: Medical Reviewer Famous for Averting a Public Health Tragedy." US Food and Drug Administration Home Page, Center for Drug Evaluation and Research. www.fda.gov/About FDA/History/VirtualHistory/HistoryExhibits/ucm345094.htm.
"Concierge Medicine: An Alternative to Insurance." The Association of Mature American Citizens. June 14, 2017. amac.us/concierge-medicine-alternative-insurance/.
Conger, Krista. "Telomere Extension Turns Back Aging Clock in Cultured Human Cells, Study Finds." EHR National Symposium, The Stanford Medicine News Center. January 22, 2015. med.stanford.edu/news/all-news/2015/01/telomere-extension-turns-back-aging-clock-in-cultured-cells.html.
Cook, David A., et al. "Physician Attitudes About Maintenance of Certification." *Mayo Clinic Proceedings* 91, no. 10 (2016): 1336–1345. doi:10.1016/j.mayocp.2016.07.004.
Costandi, Moheb. *Neuroplasticity*. Cambridge, MA: The MIT Press, 2016.
Crane, Mark. "Physician Frustration Grows, Income Falls—But a Ray of Hope." Medscape. April 24, 2012. www.medscape.com/viewarticle/761870
Crichton, Michael. *Jurassic Park*. New York: Alfred A. Knopf, 1990.
Croskerry, Pat. "The Importance of Cognitive Errors in Diagnosis and Strategies to Minimize Them." *Academic Medicine* 78, no. 8 (2003): 775–780. doi:10.1097/00001888-200308000-00003.
Cummings, Mary. "Automation Bias in Intelligent Time Critical Decision Support Systems." AIAA 1st Intelligent Systems Technical Conference. 2004 doi:10.2514/6.2004-6313.
"Current World Population–United Arab Emirates Population (2018)." Worldometers. 2018. www.worldometers.info/world-population/.
"Current World Population–World Population Clock: 7.7 Billion People (2018)." Worldometers. www.worldometers.info/world-population/.
Curry, David R. "Bill & Melinda Gates Medical Research Institute [to 10 February 2018]." Vaccines and Global Health: Ethics and Policy. February 12, 2018. centerforvaccineethicsandpolicy.net/2018/02/11/bill-melinda-gates-medical-research-institute-to-10-february-2018/.
"Custom Autonomous Mobile Robots." Waypoint Robotics. waypointrobotics.com/.
Darwin, Charles. *The Expression of the Emotions in Man and Animal*. London: John Murray, 1872.
Dary, David. *Frontier Medicine: From the Atlantic to the Pacific, 1492–1941*. New York: Alfred A. Knopf, 2009.
"Data & Security." DeepMind. deepmind.com/applied/deepmind-health/data-security/.
Dave, Shivani. "'Memory Transplant' Achieved in Snails." BBC News. May 14, 2018. www.bbc.com/news/science-environment-44111476.
Davis, Nick J. "Transcranial Stimulation of the Developing Brain: A Plea for Extreme Caution." *Frontiers in Human Neuroscience* 8 (2014). doi:10.3389/fnhum.2014.00600.
Davis, Nicola. "Murder Most Fowl: Oxford Dodo 'Shot in the Back of the Head.'" *The Guardian*. April 20, 2018. www.theguardian.com/science/2018/apr/20/most-fowl-oxford-dodo-shot-in-the-back-of-the-head.
"Deadline—Watch Your Life, Make It Count." App Store, Disney Publishing Worldwide. October 5, 2014. itunes.apple.com/us/app/deadline./id917475404?mt=8.
"Death with Dignity Acts—States That Allow Assisted Death." Death with Dignity. www.deathwithdignity.org/learn/death-with-dignity-acts/.
"The Deceptive Salary of Doctors." www.bestmedicaldegrees.com/salary-of-doctors/.

DeepMind Health. deepmind.com/applied/deepmind-health/.
Descartes, Rene. *Principia Philosophiae*. 1644.
DeVille, Kenneth. *Medical Malpractice in Nineteenth-Century America: Origins and Legacy*. New York: New York University Press, 1990.
"DNA of Every Baby Born in California Is Stored. Who Has Access to It?" CBS News, CBS Interactive. May 12, 2018. www.cbsnews.com/news/california-biobank-dna-babies-who-has-access/.
DNewsChannel. "Scientists Put the Brain of a Worm Into a Robot... and It MOVED." YouTube. January 11, 2018. www.youtube.com/watch?v=eYS7UIUM_SQ.
"Doximity 2018 Physician Compensation Report." Doximity. blog.doximity.com/articles/doximity-2018-physician-compensation-report.
"DragonflEye Has Liftoff." *Draper*. May 17, 2017. www.draper.com/news/dragonfleye-has-liftoff.
Drolet, Brian C., and Vickram J. Tandon. "Fees for Certification and Finances of Medical Specialty Boards." *JAMA* 318, no. 5 (2017): 477. doi:10.1001/jama.2017.7464.
Drury, Horance Bookwalter. *Scientific Management: A History and Criticism*. New York: Columbia University, 1915. https://books.google.com/books?id=BvFCAAAAIAAJ&pg=PA138#v=onepage&q&f=false.
Dudley, Simon. "The Internet Just Isn't That Big a Deal Yet: A Hard Look at Solow's Paradox." *Wired*. November 2014. www.wired.com/insights/2014/11/solows-paradox/.
Duenwald, Mary. "Your Own Private Doctor." *Departures*. March 20, 2010. www.departures.com/lifestyle/health/your-own-private-doctor.
Dyer, Owen. "Highest Billing US Doctor Sentenced to 17 Years for Medicare Fraud." *The BMJ*. February 26, 2018. www.bmj.com/content/360/bmj.k929.full.
Dyrbye, Liselotte N., et al. "Burnout and Suicidal Ideation Among US Medical Students." *Annals of Internal Medicine*. September 2, 2008. annals.org/aim/article-abstract/742530/burnout-suicidal-ideation-among-u-s-medical-students.
"E-Cigarette Use Among Youth and Young Adults: A Report of the Surgeon General." CDC. 2016. www.cdc.gov/tobacco/data_statistics/sgr/e-cigarettes/pdfs/2016_sgr_entire_report_508.pdf.
"Ebola Response." Dimagi. www.dimagi.com/sectors/ebola-response/.
Ekman, Paul, and Wallace V. Friesen. "Constants Across Cultures in the Face and Emotion." *Journal of Personality and Social Psychology* 17, no. 2 (February 1971). psycnet.apa.org/doiLanding?doi=10.1037%2Fh0030377.
Edison, Meg. "My MOC Failure." Rebel.MD. December 3, 2017. rebel.md/my-moc-failure/.
Edison, Meg, and Arvind Cavale. "The Voice of Hippocratic Medicine in America." Rebel.MD., June 6, 2018. rebel.md/.
Eichenwald, Kurt. "A Certified Medical Controversy." *Newsweek*. September 20, 2016. www.newsweek.com/certified-medical-controversy-320495.
Eichenwald, Kurt. "The Ugly Civil War in American Medicine." *Newsweek*. March 20, 2016. www.newsweek.com/2015/03/27/ugly-civil-war-american-medicine-312662.html.
Eisenberg, D. T. A., et al. "Delayed Paternal Age of Reproduction in Humans Is Associated with Longer Telomeres across Two Generations of Descendants." *Proceedings of the National Academy of Sciences* 109, no. 26 (2012): 10251–10256., doi:10.1073/pnas.1202092109.
Elam, Jenn. "Announcing the 1200 Subject Data Release!" Human Connectome Project, Connectome Coordination Facility. March 1, 2017. www.humanconnectome.org/study/hcp-young-adult/article/announcing-1200-subject-data-release.
"Elder Abuse Statistics & Facts | Elder Justice." NCOA, 15 June 2018, www.ncoa.org/public-policy-action/elder-justice/elder-abuse-facts/#intraPageNav1.
"Electronic Cigarettes Issue Profile." OpenSecrets.org. www.opensecrets.org/news/issues/e-cigarettes/.
"The Electronic Health Records System In the UK." Centre for Public Impact. April 3, 2017. www.centreforpublicimpact.org/case-study/electronic-health-records-system-uk/.
Elgan, Mike. "Mind-Reading Tech Is Here (and More Useful than You Think!)." *Computerworld*. April 7, 2018. www.computerworld.com/article/3268132/emerging-technology/mind-reading-tech-is-here-and-more-useful-than-you-think.html.
Ellison, Ayla. "20 Highest Paid Healthcare CEOs of S&P 500 Companies." *Becker's Hospital Review*. May 2, 2016. www.beckershospitalreview.com/compensation-issues/20-highest-paid-healthcare-ceos-in-2015.html. Sponsored by VMG Health.
Emery, Gene. "Studies Document Risks of Assault for Healthcare Workers." *Reuters*. April 28, 2016. www.reuters.com/article/us-health-violence-healthcare-workers-idUSKCN0XP2BN.
"End of Life Option Act in California." Coalition

for Compassionate Care of California. coalitionccc.org/tools-resources/end-of-life-option-act/.

Esteva, Andre, et al. "Dermatologist-Level Classification of Skin Cancer with Deep Neural Networks." *Nature News*. January 25, 2017. www.nature.com/articles/nature21056.

Eternime. eterni.me/.

"Ethics Codes Collection: Oath of Hippocrates (Undated)." Illinois Institute of Technology, Center for the Study of Ethics in the Professions. October 24, 2011. ethics.iit.edu/ecodes/node/4220.

Facher, Lev. "Bernie Sanders Bill Would Impose Jail Time for Execs Behind Opioid Crisis." *STAT*. April 17, 2018. www.statnews.com/2018/04/17/bernie-sanders-bill-jail-opioid-crisis/.

"Facial Recognition Market by Component (Software Tools and Services), Technology, Use Case (Emotion Recognition, Attendance Tracking and Monitoring, Access Control, Law Enforcement), End-User, and Region—Global Forecast to 2022." Market Research Firm. November 2017. www.marketsandmarkets.com/Market-Reports/facial-recognition-market-995.html.

"Famous Nurses." Nursing Theory. www.nursingtheory.org/famous-nurses/.

Fenner, Robert. "Alibab's AI Outguns Humans in Reading Test." *Bloomberg*. January 14, 2018. www.bloomberg.com/news/articles/2018-01-15/alibaba-s-ai-outgunned-humans-in-key-stanford-reading-test.

Filardo, Giovanni, et al. "Trends and Comparison of Female First Authorship in High Impact Medical Journals: Observational Study (1994–2014)." *BMJ*. (2016): i847. doi:10.1136/bmj.i847.

Filbey, Francesca M., et al. "Long-Term Effects of Marijuana Use on the Brain." *Proceedings of the National Academy of Sciences*. November 5, 2014. www.pnas.org/content/early/2014/11/05/1415297111?sid=90c211bb-0817-473e-8998-0053eac42afc.

Fisher, Daniel. "Supreme Court Rejects Human-Gene Patents—Sort Of." *Forbes*. June 14, 2013. www.forbes.com/sites/danielfisher/2013/06/13/supreme-court-rejects-human-gene-patents-sort-of/#736c1ae839fe.

Fiske, Amy, et al. "Depression in Older Adults." *Annual Review of Clinical Psychology*. U.S. National Library of Medicine. 2009. www.ncbi.nlm.nih.gov/pmc/articles/PMC2852580/.

Fleischer, Richard, director. *Soylent Green*. 1973.

Flower, Joe. *Healthcare Beyond Reform: Doing It Right for Half the Cost*. Boca Raton, FL: CRC Press, 2012.

Foer, Franklin. *World Without Mind: The Existential Threat of Big Tech*. New York: Penguin, 2018.

Folley, Aris. "Longtime Obama Doctor Says Trump's Ex-Doctor Should Be Investigated." *The Hill*. May 2, 2018. thehill.com/blogs/blog-briefing-room/news/385910-longtime-obama-doctor-says-trumps-doctor-disgraced-himself-and.

Foster, Malcolm. "Aging Japan: Robots May Have Role in Future of Elder Care." *U.S. News & World Report*. March 27, 2018. www.usnews.com/news/technology/articles/2018-03-27/aging-japan-robots-may-have-role-in-future-of-elder-care.

Foster, Malcolm. "Robots May Have Role in Future of Elder Care in Japan." AOL.com. March 28, 2018. www.aol.com/article/news/2018/03/27/ageing-japan-robots-may-have-role-in-future-of-elder-care/23397072/.

"Four Humors—And There's the Humor of It: Shakespeare and the Four Humors." History of Medicine, U.S. National Library of Medicine. www.nlm.nih.gov/exhibition/shakespeare/fourhumors.html.

Friedberg, Mark W., et al. "Quality of Patient Care Drives Physician Satisfaction; Doctors Have Concerns About Electronic Health Records." RAND Corporation. October 9, 2013. www.rand.org/pubs/research_reports/RR439.html.

Friedman, Lauren F. "IBM's Watson Supercomputer May Soon Be the Best Doctor In The World." *Business Insider*. April 22, 2014. www.businessinsider.com/ibms-watson-may-soon-be-the-best-doctor-in-the-world-2014-4.

Friedman, Matt. "Menendez Suggests He Doesn't Need to Pay Back Anything More to Melgen." *Politico PRO*. May 25, 2018. www.politico.com/states/new-jersey/story/2018/05/25/menendez-suggests-he-doesnt-need-to-pay-back-anything-more-to-melgen-437067.

Gaiman, Neil. *Trigger Warnings: Short Fictions and Other Disturbances*. New York: William Morrow, 2015.

Gawande, Atul. "Finding Medicine's Hot Spots." *The New Yorker*. June 19, 2017. www.newyorker.com/magazine/2011/01/24/the-hot-spotters.

Ghosh, Pallab. "Ethics Debate as Pig Brains Kept Alive without a Body." BBC News. April 27, 2018. www.bbc.com/news/science-environment-43928318.

Ghosh, Pallab. "Wearable Tech Aids Stroke Patients." BBC News. February 24, 2018. www.bbc.com/news/science-environment-43146117.

Gibbs, Samuel. "Elon Musk: Artificial Intelligence Is Our Biggest Existential Threat." *The Guardian*. October 27, 2014. www.theguardian.com/technology/2014/oct/27/elon-musk-artificial-intelligence-ai-biggest-existential-threat.

Giesbertz, Noor A. A., et al. "When Children Become Adults: Should Biobanks Re-Contact?." *PLoS Medicine* 13, no.2 (February 2016). www.ncbi.nlm.nih.gov/pmc/articles/PMC4755557/.

Gilliam, Terry, director. *Monty Python and the Holy Grail*. EMI/Python Pictures/Michael White, 1975. https://www.youtube.com/watch?v=-6VTcilBunk.

"GlaxoSmithKline to Plead Guilty and Pay $3 Billion to Resolve Fraud Allegations and Failure to Report Safety Data." The United States Department of Justice. July 2, 2012. www.justice.gov/opa/pr/glaxosmithkline-plead-guilty-and-pay-3-billion-resolve-fraud-allegations-and-failure-report.

"Global Health Security: Immunization." Centers for Disease Control and Prevention. February 13, 2014. www.cdc.gov/globalhealth/security/immunization.htm.

Global, Inc. "Healthcare Artificial Intelligence Market Worth over $10bn by 2024: Global Market Insights, Inc." GlobeNewswire News Room. May 11, 2017. globenewswire.com/news-release/2017/05/11/982356/0/en/Healthcare-Artificial-Intelligence-Market-worth-over-10bn-by-2024-Global-Market-Insights-Inc.html.

GME. 2016 Position Statements on Duty Hours and the Learning and Working Environment, The Accreditation Council for Graduate Medical Education. 2016. www.acgme.org/What-We-Do/Accreditation/Clinical-Experience-and-Education-formerly-Duty-Hours/2016-Position-Statements-on-Duty-Hours-and-the-Learning-and-Working-Environment.

"Gold Standard MCAT." MCAT-Prep.com. www.mcat-prep.com/mcat-scores/.

Gondry, Michel, director. *Eternal Sunshine of the Spotless Mind*. 2004.

Gonzalez-Crussi, F. *A Short History of Medicine*. New York: Modern Library, 2008.

Graham, Todd, et al. "Anti-MOC Laws Picking Up Steam Across the United States." *Policy & Medicine*. May 4, 2018. www.policymed.com/2017/06/anti-moc-laws-picking-up-steam-across-the-united-states.html.

Graves, Alex, et al. "Hybrid Computing Using a Neural Network with Dynamic External Memory." *Nature News*. October 12, 2016. www.nature.com/articles/nature20101.

Grisham, Sarah. "Medscape Physician Compensation Report 2017." Medscape Log In. April 5, 2017. www.medscape.com/slideshow/compensation-2017-overview-6008547#2.

Gruber, Lynn R., et al. "From Movement to Industry: The Growth of HMOs." *Health Affairs* 7, no. 3 (1988): 197–208. doi:10.1377/hlthaff.7.3.197.

Grundlingh, Johann, et al. "2,4-Dinitrophenol (DNP): A Weight Loss Agent with Significant Acute Toxicity and Risk of Death." *Journal of Medical Toxicology* 7, no. 3 (September 7, 2011). www.ncbi.nlm.nih.gov/pmc/articles/PMC3550200/.

GSMA Intelligence. "American Recovery and Reinvestment Act of 2009." One Hundred Eleventh Congress of the United States of America. January 6, 2009. www.gpo.gov/fdsys/pkg/BILLS-11; https://www.gsmaintelligence.com1hr1enr/pdf/BILLS-111hr1enr.pdf.

GSMA Intelligence. "Definitive Data and Analysis for the Mobile Industry." www.gsmaintelligence.com/.

Guzman, Gloria. "Household Income: 2016." Census Bureau QuickFacts. September 1, 2017. www.census.gov/library/publications/2017/acs/acsbr16–02.html.

Haag, Matthew. "Doctor Linked to Senator Menendez's Corruption Case Is Convicted of Fraud." *New York Times*. April 29, 2017. www.nytimes.com/2017/04/28/us/senator-menendez-corruption-case.html.

Harari, Yuval N. *Homo Deus: A Brief History of Tomorrow*. New York: Harper Perennial, 2017.

"Harold Bornstein: Exiled from Trumpland, Doctor Now 'Frightened and Sad.'" *Washington Post*. May 2, 2018. www.washingtonpost.com/news/morning-mix/wp/2018/05/02/harold-bornstein-exiled-from-trumpland-former-doctor-now-frightened-and-sad/?noredirect=on&utm_term=.9695fd54e727.

Harrington, Samuel. *At Peace: Choosing a Good Death After a Long Life*. New York: Grand Central Life & Style, 2018.

Harrison, P.O. "Japan's Robotics Industry Bullish on Elderly Care Market." TrendForce. May 19, 2015. https://press.trendforce.com/press/20150519–1923.html.

Hartzband, Pamela, and Jerome Groopman. "How Medical Care Is Being Corrupted." *New York Times*. November 19, 2014. www.nytimes.com/2014/11/19/opinion/how-medical-care-is-being-corrupted.html.

Haselton, Todd. "How to Find Out What Google Knows About You and Limit the Data It Collects." CNBC. December 6, 2017. www.cnbc.com/2017/11/20/what-does-google-know-about-me.html.

Headley, J. T. *The Great Riots of New York, 1712–1873.* Fairford, UK: Echo Library, 2006.

"Health Care Fraud Unit." The United States Department of Justice. September 19, 2018. www.justice.gov/criminal-fraud/health-care-fraud-unit.

"Health Insurance Portability and Accountability Act of 1996." Office of the Assistant Secretary for Planning and Evaluation under the 104th Congress. August 21, 1996. aspe.hhs.gov/report/health-insurance-portability-and-accountability-act-1996.

"Health Pioneer Calls for Doctor's and Patient's Bill of Rights on Nati." PRWeb. March 30, 2012. www.prweb.com/releases/2012/3/prweb9339072.htm.

"Henry Ford Changes the World, 1908." Eyewitness to History. 2005 www.eyewitnesstohistory.com/ford.htm.

HHS Office of the Secretary, Office for Civil Rights, and OCR. "HITECH Act Enforcement Interim Final Rule." US Department of Health and Human Services. June 16, 2017. www.hhs.gov/hipaa/for-professionals/special-topics/hitech-act-enforcement-interim-final-rule/index.html.

HHS Office of the Secretary, Office for Civil Rights, and OCR. "Your Rights Under HIPAA." US Department of Health and Human Services. February 1, 2017. www.hhs.gov/hipaa/for-individuals/guidance-materials-for-consumers/index.html.

"Highest Suicide Rate by Profession." New Health Guide. November 25, 2013. www.newhealthguide.org/highest-suicide-rate-by-profession.html.

Hill, Robert G., et al. "4000 Clicks: A Productivity Analysis of Electronic Medical Records in a Community Hospital ED." *The American Journal of Emergency Medicine* 31, no. 11 (2013): 1591–1594. doi:10.1016/j.ajem.2013.06.028.

Hillestad, Richard, et al. "Can Electronic Medical Record Systems Transform Health Care? Potential Health Benefits, Savings, And Costs." *Health Affairs* 24, no. 5 (2005): 1103–1117. doi:10.1377/hlthaff.24.5.1103.

Hillestad, Richard, et al. "Most-Viewed Research Paper on Health Affairs Authored by RAND Researchers." RAND Corporation. January 1, 2005. www.rand.org/pubs/external_publications/EP20050904.html.

Hobson, Will. "Larry Nassar, Former USA Gymnastics Doctor, Sentenced to 40–175 Years for Sex Crimes." *Washington Post.* January 24, 2018. www.washingtonpost.com/sports/olympics/larry-nassar-former-usa-gymnastics-doctor-due-to-be-sentenced-for-sex-crimes/2018/01/24/9acc22f8-0115-11e8-8acf-ad2991367d9d_story.html?utm_term=.a652d7854cce.

Hodson, Hal. "Revealed: Google AI Has Access to Huge Haul of NHS Patient Data." *New Scientist.* April 29, 2016. www.newscientist.com/article/2086454-revealed-google-ai-has-access-to-huge-haul-of-nhs-patient-data/.

Hoff, Timothy. "Deskilling and Adaptation Mmong Primary Care Physicians Using Two Work Innovations." *Health Care Management Review* 36, no.4 (October-December 2011). journals.lww.com/hcmrjournal/Abstract/2011/10000/Deskilling_and_adaptation_among_primary_care.9.aspx.

Hoff, Timothy. *Practice Under Pressure: Primary Care Physicians and Their Medicine in the Twenty-First Century.* New Brunswick, NJ: Rutgers University Press, 2010.

Hoffman, Matt. "Suffering in Silence: The Scourge of Physician Suicide." *MD Magazine.* February 5, 2018. www.mdmag.com/medical-news/suffering-in-silence-the-scourge-of-physician-suicide.

Hogenboom, Melissa. "Warning over Electrical Brain Stimulation." BBC News. August 24, 2014. www.bbc.com/news/health-27343047.

Hot Tomali Communications Inc. "Research & Reports: AmericanEHR The Pros and Cons of Wireless and Local Networks" Comments. 2014. www.americanehr.com/research/reports/Physicians-Use-of-EHR-Systems-2014.aspx.

"How Much Does a Broken Leg Cost?" Cost Helper.com. health.costhelper.com/broken-leg.html.

Hughes, John, director. *Ferris Bueller's Day Off.* 1986.

IHS Inc. "The Complexities of Physician Supply and Demand Projections from 2013 to 2025,'" Association of American Medical Colleges. 2015. www.aamc.org/download/426242/data/ihsreportdownload.pdf.

Ilgenfritz, Stefanie. "The Future of: Healthcare." *Wall Street Journal.* March 16, 2018. www.wsj.com/video/the-future-of-healthcare/2BFB8496-457F-4FB4-A9E6-EBB7513BAA36.html.

"Independent, Impartial, Neutral." Doctors Without Borders—USA. doctorswithoutborders.org/who-we-are/principles/independence.

"Inside Compensation: CEO Salaries at Large Associations 2016 (Top Paid)." CEO Update. 2016. www.ceoupdate.com/articles/compensation/inside-compensation-ceo-salaries-large-associations-2016-top-paid.

"International Code of Medical Ethics." World Medical Association. October 1949. 1949.

Bibliography

https://www.wma.net/wp-content/uploads/2018/07/International-Code-of-Medical-Ethics-1949.pdf

Itskov, Dmitri. "FAQ." 2045 Initiative. July 17, 2017. 2045.com/faq/.

Jackson Healthcare. "A Costly Defense: Physicians Sound Off on the High Price of Defensive Medicine in the U.S.," Jackson Healthcare. 2010. doi:http://truecostofhealthcare.org/wp-content/uploads/2015/02/defensivemedicine_ebook_final.pdf.

Jacobsen, Kathryn H. *Introduction to Global Health: 2nd Edition*. Burlington, MA: Jones & Bartlett Learning, 2013.

Jamal, Ahmed J. "Morbidity and Mortality Weekly Report (MMWR)." Centers for Disease Control and Prevention. June 15, 2017. www.cdc.gov/mmwr/volumes/66/wr/mm6623a1.htm.

James, John T. "A New, Evidence-Based Estimate of Patient Harms Associated with Hospital Care." *Journal of Patient Safety* 9, no. 3 (2013): 122–128. doi:10.1097/pts.0b013e3182948a69.

James, Sonya. "Q&A: Andrew McAfee & Erik Brynjolfsson, Co-Authors of The Second Machine Age." ZDNet. May 7, 2014. www.zdnet.com/article/qa-andrew-mcafee-erik-brynjolfsson-co-authors-of-the-second-machine-age/.

"Japan Population 2018 (Demographics, Maps, Graphs)." World Population Review. 2018. worldpopulationreview.com/countries/japan-population/.

Jaslow, Ryan. "Most Common Medical Malpractice Claims for Missed Cancer, Heart Attacks." CBS News. July 19, 2013. www.cbsnews.com/news/most-common-medical-malpractice-claims-for-missed-cancer-heart-attacks/.

Jena, Anupam B., et al. "Sex Differences in Physician Salary in US Public Medical Schools." *JAMA Internal Medicine* 176, no. 9 (2016): 1294. doi:10.1001/jamainternmed.2016.3284.

Jiang, Nan, and Pamela Ling. "Vested Interests in Addiction Research and Policy. Alliance between Tobacco and Alcohol Industries to Shape Public Policy." *Addiction* 108, no. 5 (2013): 852–864. doi:10.1111/add.12134.

Joffe-Walt, Chana. "In Japan, MRIs Cost Less." NPR. November 18, 2009. www.npr.org/templates/story/story.php?storyId=120545569.

Johns Hopkins Medicine. "The Four Founding Physicians." 16 July 2014, www.hopkinsmedicine.org/about/history/history5.html.

Jonze, Spike, director. *Her*. October 13, 2013.

Kacik, Alex. "For the First Time Ever, Less Than Half of Physicians Are Independent." *Modern Healthcare*. May 31, 2015. www.modernhealthcare.com/article/20170531/NEWS/170539971.

Kahn, Michael. "Near Grady Hospital, Grim Reaper Building Might Soon Have Date with Death." Curbed Atlanta. May 1, 2017. atlanta.curbed.com/2017/5/1/15495904/fulton-health-wellness-building-grim-reaper-sculpture-demolition.

Kane, Carol K. "Policy Research Perspectives: Updated Data on Physician Practice Arrangements: Physician Ownership Drops Below 50 Percent." AMA. 2017. www.ama-assn.org/sites/default/files/media-browser/public/health-policy/PRP-2016-physician-benchmark-survey.pdf.

Kang, Cecilia. "F.C.C. Repeals Net Neutrality Rules." *New York Times*. December 14, 2017. www.nytimes.com/2017/12/14/technology/net-neutrality-repeal-vote.html.

Kant, Immanuel. *Critique of Pure Reason (Abridged)*. Cambridge, MA: Hackett Publishing, 1996.

Kling, Rob. "Human Centered Systems in the Perspective of Organizational and Social Informatics." Illinois Speech and Language Engineering, Human Center System for the National Science Foundation. May 19, 1997. www.ifp.illinois.edu/nsfhcs/bog_reports/bog4.html.

Kocher, Robert, and Nikhil R. Sahni. "Rethinking Health Care Labor." *New England Journal of Medicine* 365, no. 15 (2011): 1370–1372. doi:10.1056/nejmp1109649.

Koeppen, Bruce. "Shortage of Residency Slots May Have Chilling Effect on Next Generation of Physicians." *The Hill*. February 4, 2016. thehill.com/blogs/congress-blog/healthcare/266610-shortage-of-residency-slots-may-have-chilling-effect-on-next.

Koniku. koniku.com/military-applications.

Koren, Gideon. "Ondansetron: New and Troubling Data." *Pediatric News*. October 25, 2013. doi:https://www.mdedge.com/pediatricnews/article/78494/obstetrics/ondansetron-new-and-troubling-data.

Koven, Suzanne. "35 Years Later, Author Revisits 'The House of God.'" *Boston Globe*. September 2, 2013. www.bostonglobe.com/lifestyle/health-wellness/2013/09/01/interview-with-samuel-shem/h7tS4bjDlynBYCyddW6a1O/story.html.

Kristof, Kathy. "$1 Million Mistake: Becoming a Doctor." CBS News. September 10, 2013. www.cbsnews.com/news/1-million-mistake-becoming-a-doctor/.

Krogsboll, LT. "General Health Checks for Reducing Illness and Mortality." *Cochrane Report*. January 30, 2019, www.cochrane.org/CD009009/EPOC_general-health-checks-for-reducing-illness-and-mortality.

Kübler-Ross, Elisabeth, and David Kessler. *On Grief and Grieving: Finding the Meaning of Grief through the Five Stages of Loss.* New York: Scribner, 2005.

Kubota, Taylor. "Algorithm Outperforms Radiologists at Diagnosing Pneumonia." Stanford News. November 15, 2017. news.stanford.edu/2017/11/15/algorithm-outperforms-radiologists-diagnosing-pneumonia/.

Kubota, Taylor. "Artificial Intelligence Used to Identify Skin Cancer." Stanford News. May 3, 2018. news.stanford.edu/2018/01/25/artificial-intelligence-used-identify-skin-cancer/.

"K'Watch Glucose." PKVitality. www.pkvitality.com/ktrack-glucose/.

Labaree, Leonard W. "Some Account of the Pennsylvania Hospital, [28 May 1754]." Founders Online. National Archives and Records Administration. July 1, 1753. founders.archives.gov/documents/Franklin/01-05-02-0089.

Langewitz, Wolf, et al. "Spontaneous Talking Time at Start of Consultation in Outpatient Clinic: Cohort Study." *British Medical Journal.* September 28, 2002. www.ncbi.nlm.nih.gov/pmc/articles/PMC126654/.

Laporte, John. "US Physicians—Statistics and Facts." Statista. www.statista.com/topics/1244/physicians/.

Larson, Erik. *The Devil in the White City: Murder, Magic, and Madness at the Fair That Changed America.* New York: Vintage Books, 2004.

Leary, Warren E. "Cigarette Company Developed Tobacco with Stronger Nicotine; Head of F.D.A. Tells of Chemical Manipulation." *New York Times.* June 22, 1994. www.nytimes.com/1994/06/22/us/cigarette-company-developed-tobacco-with-stronger-nicotine-head-fda-tells.html?pagewanted=all.

Lee, Bruce Y. "Gwyneth Paltrow's Goop Promotes A $135 Coffee Enema Kit." *Forbes.* January 7, 2018. www.forbes.com/sites/brucelee/2018/01/06/gwyneth-paltrows-goop-promotes-a-135-coffee-enema-kit/#2f671e693229.

Lee, John D. *Human Factors and Ergonomics in Automation Design,"* Handbook of Human Factors and Ergonomics: 3rd Edition. Hoboken, NJ: Wiley, 2012.

Lepore, Jill. "Not So Fast." *The New Yorker.* June 19, 2017. www.newyorker.com/magazine/2009/10/12/not-so-fast.

Lerner, Barron H. "A Case That Shook Medicine." *Washington Post.* November 28, 2006. www.washingtonpost.com/wp-dyn/content/article/2006/11/24/AR2006112400985.html.

Lerner, Barron. "From the Death of Libby Zion, Crucial Medical Reforms." *New York Times.* March 3, 2009. www.nytimes.com/2009/03/03/health/03zion.html.

Leviathan, Yaniv. "Google Duplex: An AI System for Accomplishing Real-World Tasks Over the Phone." Google AI. May 8, 2018. ai.googleblog.com/2018/05/duplex-ai-system-for-natural-conversation.html.

Levy, Sandra. "Resident Salary and Debt Report 2017." Medscape. July 26, 2017. www.medscape.com/slideshow/residents-salary-and-debt-report-2017–6008931#2.

Levy, Sandra. "Residents Salary and Debt Report 2017." Medscape. March 17, 2017. www.medscape.com/slideshow/residents-salary-and-debt-report-2017–6008931#3.

"Life Expectancy." Our World in Data. ourworldindata.org/life-expectancy.

Linklaters. "Audit of the Acute Kidney Injury Detection System Known as Streams." The Royal Free London NHS Foundation Trust. May 17, 2018, https://s3-eu-west-1.amazonaws.com/files.royalfree.nhs.uk/Reporting/Streams_Report.pdf

Lister, Joseph. "How Antiseptic Surgery Arrived in America." *College of Physicians & Surgeons of Columbia University* 28, no. 2 (2008). doi: http://www.cumc.columbia.edu/psjournal/archive/spring_summer_2008/surgery_in_america.html.

Livingston, Shelby. "Aetna CEO's Total 2016 Pay Reaches $18.7 Million." *Modern Healthcare,* April 7, 2017. www.modernhealthcare.com/article/20170407/NEWS/170409914.

Livingston, Shelby. "UnitedHealth CEO's Compensation Swells in 2016 to $17.8 Million." *Modern Healthcare.* April 21, 2017. www.modernhealthcare.com/article/20170421/NEWS/170429946.

"Lobbying Spending Database Health, 2017." OpenSecrets.org. www.opensecrets.org/lobby/indus.php?id=H&year=2017.

"Lobbying Spending Database Tobacco, 1999." OpenSecrets.org. www.opensecrets.org/lobby/indusclient.php?id=A02&year=1999.

Lobosco, Katie. "Doctors and Nurses Busted for $712 Million Medicare Fraud." CNNMoney. June 21, 2015. money.cnn.com/2015/06/19/pf/medicare-fraud-doctors/index.html.

Locke, John. "John Locke: Second Treatise of Civil Government: Chapter 2." Constitution Society: Everything Needed to Decide Constitutional Issues. www.constitution.org/jl/2ndtr02.htm.

Loebel, J. Pierre, et al. "Anticipation of Nursing Home Placement May Be a Precipitant of Suicide among the Elderly." *Journal of the American Geriatrics Society.* April 27, 2015. onlinelibrary.wiley.com/doi/full/10.1111/j.1532-5415.1991.tb02910.x.

Lohr, Steve. "IBM Is Counting on Its Bet on Watson, and Paying Big Money for It." *New York Times*. January 20, 2018. www.nytimes.com/2016/10/17/technology/ibm-is-counting-on-its-bet-on-watson-and-paying-big-money-for-it.html?_r=2.

Lopez, German. "Marijuana Has Been Legalized in Nine States and Washington, D.C." *Vox*. March 27, 2014. www.vox.com/cards/marijuana-legalization/where-is-marijuana-legal.

Loria, Keith. "Why Is EHR Use Dropping?" Medical Economics. June 20, 2016. doi:http://medicaleconomics.modernmedicine.com/medical-economics/news/why-ehr-use-dropping?page=0,0.

Lovejoy, Bess. "The Gory New York City Riot That Shaped American Medicine." Smithsonian.com. June 17, 2014. www.smithsonianmag.com/history/gory-new-york-city-riot-shaped-american-medicine-180951766/.

Lozar, D.C. *CyberWeird Stories*. Carlsbad, CA: ACQL Productions, 2017.

Lozar, D.C. *Weirdbook*. Issues #31, 36, 41, 42, 43. http://weirdbook-magazine.com/about-weirdbook/

MacCorduck, Pamela. *Machines Who Think*. Boca Raton, FL: A.K. Peters/CRC Press, 2004.

MacDorman, Karl. "Mortality Salience and the Uncanny Valley." The Proceedings of the 2005 International Conference on Humanoid Robots, 2005. www.macdorman.com/kfm/writings/pubs/MacDorman2005Mortality-UncannyValleyHumanoids.pdf.

"Malpractice Report 2017: Real Physicians. Real Lawsuits." Medscape. 2017. www.medscape.com/slideshow/2017-malpractice-report-6009206#1.

"Malpractice Report 2017: Real Physicians. Real Lawsuits." Medscape. 2018. www.medscape.com/slideshow/2017-malpractice-report-6009206#1.

Mannix, Kathryn. *With the End in Mind: Dying, Death and Wisdom in an Age of Denial*. New York: Little, Brown and Company, 2018.

Manson, JoAnn E. "Update and Overview of Health Outcomes for WHI." *JAMA*. October 2, 2013. jamanetwork.com/journals/jama/fullarticle/1745676.

Marbury, Donna. *Top 10 Healthcare Wearables to Watch*. Managed Healthcare Executive. March 10, 2017.

Martinez-Carter, Karina. "How the Elderly Are Treated around the World." *The Week*. July 23, 2013. theweek.com/articles/462230/how-elderly-are-treated-around-world.

Martyris, Nina. "'Nurse, Spy, Cook: How Harriet Tubman Found Freedom Through Food." NPR. April 27, 2016. www.npr.org/sections/thesalt/2016/04/27/475768129/nurse-spy-cook-how-harriet-tubman-found-freedom-through-food.

Marvel, M K, et al. "Soliciting the Patient's Agenda: Have We Improved?" *JAMA* 281, no.3 (January 20, 1999). www.ncbi.nlm.nih.gov/pubmed/9918487/.

"Master Settlement Agreement." National Association of Attorney General. 1998. web.archive.org/web/20080625084126/http://www.naag.org/backpages/naag/tobacco/msa/msa-pdf/1109185724_1032468605_cigmsa.pdf.

Matchar, Emily. "Can an App Help Detect Autism?" Smithsonian.com. October 21, 2015. www.smithsonianmag.com/innovation/can-app-help-detect-autism-180957000/.

McBeth, Katle. "Is Health Care Really Better Outside of the United States?" *International Policy Digest*. August 1, 2017. intpolicydigest.org/2017/08/01/health-care-really-better-outside-united-states/.

McKinlay, Roger. "Technology: Use or Lose Our Navigation Skills." *Nature News*. March 16, 2016. www.nature.com/news/technology-use-or-lose-our-navigation-skills-1.19632.

McLean, Jesse, et al. "Birth Defects Blamed on Unapproved Morning Sickness Treatment." Thestar.com. June 25, 2014. www.thestar.com/news/gta/2014/06/25/birth_defects_blamed_on_unapproved_morning_sickness_treatment.html.

McLuhan, Marshall. *Understanding Media: The Extension of Man*. New York: Routledge and Kegan Paul, 1964.

McShane, Sveta. "This Amazing Computer Chip Is Made of Live Brain Cells." Singularity Hub. March 17, 2016. singularityhub.com/2016/03/17/this-amazing-computer-chip-is-made-of-live-brain-cells/.

Mechaber, Ezra. "President Obama Urges FCC to Implement Stronger Net Neutrality Rules." National Archives and Records Administration, 10 Nov. 2014, obamawhitehouse.archives.gov/blog/2014/11/10/president-obama-urges-fcc-implement-stronger-net-neutrality-rules.

"Medical Student Debt." American Medical Student Association. www.amsa.org/advocacy/action-committees/twp/medical-student-debt/.

"Medicare Provider Utilization and Payment Data: Physician and Other Supplier CY2013." Data.CMS.gov. data.cms.gov/Medicare-Physi cian-Supplier/Medicare-Provider-Utilization-and-Payment-Data-Phy/din4–7td8.

Mehrabian, Albert. *Nonverbal Communication.* London: Aldine-Atherton, 1972.

Meledandri, Chris, et al. *Despicable Me.* Universal, 2010.

Michaelangelo Quotes. Madonna of Bruges by Michelangelo. www.michelangelo.net/quotes/.

"Microsoft HoloLens: University College London Improves Insights for Surgeons." YouTube. June 29, 2017. www.youtube.com/watch?time_continue=81&v=XCz0-VmEuW8.

Mitchell, Stephen. *Gilgamesh.* New York: Free Press, 2008.

Mohr, James C. "American Medical Malpractice Litigation in Historical Perspective." *JAMA.* April 5, 2000. jamanetwork.com/journals/jama/fullarticle/192559?redirect=true.

Monheit, Michael. "GlaxoSmithKline's $3 Billion Settlement: What the Department Of Justice Claimed About Zofran." Zofran Legal. May 12, 2016. zofranlegal.com/glaxosmithkline-settlement-zofran/.

"Monthly Budget Review for 2009–2019." Congressional Budget Office. June 2010. www.cbo.gov/publication/42682.

Morgan, Rosemary, et al. "Recognition Matters: Only One in Ten Awards given to Women." *The Lancet* 389, no. 10088 (June 24, 2017) ; 2469. doi:10.1016/s0140-6736(17)31592-1.

Mori, Masahiro. "The Uncanny Valley: The Original Essay by Masahiro Mori." IEEE Spectrum. June 12, 2012 spectrum.ieee.org/automaton/robotics/humanoids/the-uncanny-valley.

Mozingo, Joe. "Doctors at University of California Health Clinics Go on Strike." *Los Angeles Times.* April 11, 2015. www.latimes.com/local/lanow/la-me-ln-doctors-strike-uc-20150411-story.html.

Mundy, Jane. "GSK Had Zofran 'In the Bag.'" L+S: LawyersandSettlements.com. November 16, 2015. www.lawyersandsettlements.com/articles/zofran-birth-defects/glaxosmithkline-gsk-deana-brown-department-of-21058.html.

Munro, Dan. "The 50th Anniversary of Dr. King's Healthcare Quote." *Forbes.* March 28, 2016. www.forbes.com/sites/danmunro/2016/03/25/the-50th-anniversary-of-dr-kings-healthcare-quote/#1df5120e30b5.

Munro, Dan. "'Single-Payer' Healthcare Isn't Necessary—But Single Pricing Is." *Forbes.* January 23, 2018. www.forbes.com/sites/danmunro/2017/07/04/single-payer-healthcare-isnt-necessary-but-single-pricing-is/#1a89ac3be0e3.

Murgia, Madhumita. "Affective Computing: How 'Emotional Machines' Are About to Take Over Our Lives." *The Telegraph.* January 21, 2016. www.telegraph.co.uk/technology/2016/01/21/affective-computing-how-emotional-machines-are-about-to-take-ove/.

"National Health Accounts Projected." Centers for Medicare & Medicaid Services. August 1, 2018. www.cms.gov/Research-Statistics-Data-and-Systems/Statistics-Trends-and-Reports/NationalHealthExpendData/NationalHealthAccountsProjected.html.

"National Health Accounts Projected." CMS.gov Centers for Medicare & Medicaid Services, 1 Feb. 2018, www.cms.gov/Research-Statistics-Data-and-Systems/Statistics-Trends-and-Reports/NationalHealthExpendData/NationalHealthAccountsProjected.html.

National Suicide Prevention Lifeline. www.suicidepreventionlifeline.org/.

"Nevermind." Affectiva. www.affectiva.com/success-story/flying-mollusk/.

Nevermind. nevermindgame.com/.

Nietzsche, Friedrich. *Thus Spoke Zarathustra.* 1883.

Nitschke, Philip. "Here's Why I Invented A 'Death Machine' That Lets People Take Their Own Lives." *Huffington Post.* April 5, 2018. www.huffingtonpost.com/entry/sarco-death-philip-nitschke_us_5abbb574e4b03e2a5c7853ca.

Nonaka, I. *The Knowledge-Creating Company: How Japanese Companies Create the Dynamics of Innovation.* New York: Oxford University Press, 1995.

Nowlan, Philip Francis. "Armageddon—2419 A.D." Amazing Stories. August 1928.

"Office-Based Physician Electronic Health Record Adoption." Health IT. dashboard. healthit.gov/quickstats/pages/physician-ehr-adoption-trends.php.

Olshansky, S. J. "No Truth to the Fountain of Youth." *Science of Aging Knowledge Environment* 2002, no. 27 (2002). doi:10.1126/sageke.2002.27.vp5.

Orwell, George. *1984: A Novel.* London: Secker & Warburg, 1949.

Osborne, Hilary. "What Is Cambridge Analytica? The Firm at the Centre of Facebook's Data Breach." *The Guardian,* March 18, 2018. www.theguardian.com/news/2018/mar/18/what-is-cambridge-analytica-firm-at-centre-of-facebook-data-breach.

The Osler Club of London, www.osler.org.uk/osleriana-2/oslers-aphorisms/.

Parasuraman, Raja, and Dietrich H. Manzey. "Complacency and Bias in Human Use of Automation: An Attentional Integration." *Human

Factors: The Journal of the Human Factors and Ergonomics Society 52, no. 3 (2010): 381–410. doi:10.1177/0018720810376055.

"Pareto Chart." Institute for Healthcare Improvement. www.ihi.org/resources/Pages/Tools/ParetoDiagram.aspx.

Parker, Michele C. "The Physician's Bill of Rights." KevinMD.com. February 10, 2017. www.kevinmd.com/blog/2017/02/physicians-bill-rights.html.

Parkin, Simon. "Would You Trust Your Medical Diagnosis to a Robot? You May Soon Get the Chance to Find Out." MIT Technology Review. March 9, 2016. www.technologyreview.com/s/600868/the-artificially-intelligent-doctor-will-hear-you-now/.

Parry, Marc, et al. "The Gates Effect." The Chronicle of Higher Education, July 14, 2013. www.chronicle.com/article/The-Gates-Effect/140323.

Pasley, Brian N., et al. "Reconstructing Speech from Human Auditory Cortex." PLOS Biology. January 13, 2012. journals.plos.org/plosbiology/article?id=10.1371%2Fjournal.pbio.1001251.

"Patient Bill of Rights." Association of American Physicians and Surgeons. aapsonline.org/patient-bill-rights/.

Paul, R. L., et al. "Alterations in the Mechanoreceptor Input to the Brodmann's Areas 1 and 3 of the Postcentral Hand Area of Macaca Mulatta after Nerve Section and Regeneration." Brain Research 39, no 1 (April 1972): 1–19. https://www.ncbi.nlm.nih.gov/pubmed/4623126.

Peckham, Carol. "Medscape EHR Report 2016: Physicians Rate Top EHRs." Medscape. August 25, 2016. www.medscape.com/features/slideshow/public/ehr2016#page=1.

Peckham, Carol. "Medscape Lifestyle Report 2016: Bias and Burnout." Medscape. January 13, 2017. www.medscape.com/slideshow/lifestyle-2016-overview-6007335#1.

Pepitone, Julianne. "What Your Wireless Carrier Knows about You." CNNMoney. December 16, 2013. money.cnn.com/2013/12/16/technology/mobile/wireless-carrier-sell-data/index.html.

Petrova, Magdalena. "MIT Developed a Headset That Gives a Voice to the Voice Inside Your Head." CNBC. April 10, 2018. https://www.cnbc.com/2018/04/10/mit-alterego-communicates-with-a-computer-through-subvocalization.html.

Petterson, S. M., et al. "When Do Primary Care Physicians Retire? Implications for Workforce Projections." The Annals of Family Medicine 14, no. 4 (2016): 344–349. doi:10.1370/afm.1936.

Phend, Crystal. "Lung Cancer Risk of One Marijuana Joint a Day Equals Daily Pack of Cigarettes." MedpageToday. January 29, 2008. www.medpagetoday.com/psychiatry/addictions/8096.

Phillips, James P. "Workplace Violence Against Health Care Workers in the United States." New England Journal of Medicine 374, no. 17 (2016): 1661–1669. doi:10.1056/nejmra1501998.

Pho, Kevin. KevinMD.com. www.kevinmd.com/. "Physician Health Survey: Is Your Doctor's Health Impacting Yours?" MDVIP. https://www.mdvip.com/about-mdvip/blog/physician-health-survey-by-numbers.

"Physician Shortages and Projections 2018." AAMC Workforce. March 2018. aamc-black.global.ssl.fastly.net/production/media/filer_public/85/d7/85d7b689-f417-4ef0-97fb-ecc129836829/aamc_2018_workforce_projections_update_april_11_2018.pdf.

Picard, Rosalind W. Affective Computing. Cambridge, MA: MIT Press, 1997.

Picco, Michael F. "Is Colon Cleansing a Good Way to Eliminate Toxins from Your Body." Mayo Clinic Healthy Lifestyles—Consumer Health. 26 April 2018. https://www.mayoclinic.org/healthy-lifestyle/consumer-health/expert-answers/colon-cleansing/faq-20058435.

Piper, Watty, and Loren Long. The Little Engine That Could. Platt & Munk, New York: 1930.

Plato. "Phaedrus." 370 BCE. sfbay-anarchists.org/wp-content/uploads/2013/07/Plato-Phaedrus.pdf.

Polak, Petr. "The Productivity Paradox: A Meta-Analysis." Institute of Economic Studies. September 2014. webcache.googleusercontent.com/search?q=cache%3AZ9voJ0uLggEJ%3Aies.fsv.cuni.cz%2Fdefault%2Ffile%2Fdownload%2Fid%2F27162%2B&cd=9&hl=en&ct=clnk&gl=us&client=safari.

Polanyi, Michael. Personal Knowledge: Toward a Post-Critical Philosophy. Chicago: University of Chicago Press, 1974.

Porter, Sheri. "Physicians Report Declining Satisfaction with EHRs." AAFP. August 25, 2015. www.aafp.org/news/practice-professional-issues/20150825ehrsatisfaction.html.

"Press Release: 2017 NRMP Main Residency Match the Largest Match on Record." The Match: National Resident Matching Program. June 9, 2017. www.nrmp.org/press-release-2017-nrmp-main-residency-match-the-largest-match-on-record/.

Price, Kim. "Towards a History of Medical Negligence." The Lancet 375, no. 9710 (2010): 192–193, doi:10.1016/s0140-6736(10)60081-5.

Price, Rob. "Stephen Hawking: Automation and AI Is Going to Decimate Middle Class Jobs."

Business Insider. December 2, 2016. https://www.businessinsider.com/stephen-hawking-ai-automation-middle-class-jobs-most-dangerous-moment-humanity-2016-12.

"Primary Documents in American History: Declaration of Independence." Virtual Programs & Services, Library of Congress. www.loc.gov/rr/program/bib/ourdocs/declarind.html.

Prinzell, Lawrence J. "The Relationship of Self-Efficacy and Complacency in Pilot-Automation Interaction." NASA. September 2002. doi:https://ntrs.nasa.gov/archive/nasa/casi.ntrs.nasa.gov/20020076395.pdf.

"Products." Kinova. www.kinovarobotics.com/en/products.

Radford, Michael, director. *Nineteen Eighty Four*. 20th Century Fox, 1984.

Ramsey, Lydia. "A Small but Growing Movement of Doctors That Don't Accept Insurance and Charge a Monthly Fee Could Be a Model for Big Employers like Amazon and JPMorgan." Yahoo! Finance, Business Insider. June 21, 2018. finance.yahoo.com/news/small-growing-movement-doctors-don-153606897.html.

Ramunas, John, et al. "Transient Delivery of Modified MRNA Encoding TERT Rapidly Extends Telomeres in Human Cells." *The FASEB Journal* 29, no. 5 (2015): 1930–1939, doi:10.1096/fj.14-259531.

RAND Health: The Nation's Most Trusted Source of Objective Health Policy Research. www.rand.org/health.html.

"RAPAEL Smart Glove." NEOFECT. www.neofect.com/en/product/rapael/.

Ratanawongsa, Neda, et al. "Association Between Clinician Computer Use and Communication with Patients in Safety-Net Clinics." *JAMA Internal Medicine* 176, no. 1 (2016): 125–128. doi:10.1001/jamainternmed.2015.6186.

Raths, David. "Do Physicians Need an EHR Bill of Rights." Healthcare Informatics. November 1, 2011. https://www.healthcare-informatics.com/blogs/david/do-physicians-need-ehr-bill-rights.

Reagan, Ronald. "Inaugural Address." Ronald Reagan Presidential Library and Museum. January 2, 1967. www.reaganlibrary.gov/research/speeches/01021967a.

Reason, James. *James Reason, Human Error: Models and Management*. New York: Cambridge University Press, 1990. http://130.88.20.21/trasnusafe/pdfs/HumanErrorsModelsandManagement.pdf

Regalado, Antonio. "Researchers Are Keeping Pig Brains Alive Outside the Body." MIT Technology Review. April 25, 2018. www.technologyreview.com/s/611007/researchers-are-keeping-pig-brains-alive-outside-the-body/amp/.

Reinberg, Steven. "1 Joint as Damaging as 5 Cigarettes to Your Lungs." ABC News. March 23, 2008. abcnews.go.com/Health/Healthday/story?id=4508121&page=1.

"Results and Data: The 2018 Residency Match Results." The National Resident Matching Program. April 2018. www.nrmp.org/wp-content/uploads/2018/04/Main-Match-Result-and-Data-2018.pdf.

"Rising Demand for Long-Term Services and Supports for Elderly People." Congressional Budget Office. June 26, 2013. www.cbo.gov/publication/44363.

"Roadmap to Residency: Understanding the Process of Getting into Residency." American Association of Medical Colleges. 2017. store.aamc.org/roadmap-to-residency-understanding-the-process-of-getting-into-residency.html.

Robinson, Gene E., and Andrew B. Barron. "Epigenetics and the Evolution of Instincts." *Science* 356, no. 6333 (April 2017). sciencemag.org/content/356/6333/26.

Rogers, Zachary. "NKY Doctor Who Ran Pill Mill Convicted on 173 Drug Charges." WKRC. March 13, 2018. local12.com/news/local/nky-doctor-who-ran-pill-mill-convicted-on-173-drug-charges.

Rose, Michael R. "Can Human Aging Be Postponed?" *Scientific American* 281, no. 6 (1999): 106–111. doi:10.1038/scientificamerican1299-106.

Rosen, Daniel R., et al. "Mutations in Cu/Zn Superoxide Dismutase Gene Are Associated with Familial Amyotrophic Lateral Sclerosis." *Nature* 362, no. 6415 (January 1993). www.scholars.northwestern.edu/en/publications/mutations-in-cuzn-superoxide-dismutase-gene-are-associated-with-f.

Rosenthal, Elisabeth. *An American Sickness: How Healthcare Became Big Business and How You Can Take It Back*. New York: Penguin Books, 2018.

Rotton, James, and I. W. Kelly. "Much Ado About the Full Moon: A Meta-Analysis of Lunar-Lunacy Research." *Psychological Bulletin* 97, no. 2 (1985): 286–306. doi:10.1037/0033-2909.97.2.286.

Rush, Benjamin. "Medical Inquiries and Observations, Upon the Diseases of the Mind." U.S. National Library of Medicine, National Institutes of Health. 1812. collections.nlm.nih.gov/catalog/nlm:nlmuid-2569036R-bk.

Sadato, Norihiro. "How the Blind 'See' Braille: Lessons from Functional Magnetic Resonance

Imaging." *The Neuroscientist* 11, no. 6 (2005): 577–582. doi:10.1177/1073858405277314.

Sandoval, Greg. "IBM's New AI Supercomputer Can Argue, Rebut and Debate Humans." Business Insider. June 18, 2018. https://www.businessinsider.com/ibm-debater-supercomputer-can-argue-and-debate-humans-2018-6.

Sanger, Margaret. "Early Years Of Margaret Sanger's Work In The Birth Control Movement." The Public Writings and Speeches of Margaret Sanger-NYU. www.nyu.edu/projects/sanger/webedition/app/documents/show.php?sangerDoc=101826.xml.

Sasso, Anthony T. Lo, et al. "The $16,819 Pay Gap for Newly Trained Physicians: The Unexplained Trend of Men Earning More Than Women." *Health Affairs* 30, no. 2 (2011): 193–201. doi:10.1377/hlthaff.2010.0597.

Saunders, John A. *William Shakespeare: Measure for Measure*. York Press, 1997.

"Scientific Management Theory and the Ford Motor Company." Saylor Foundation. www.saylor.org/site/wp-content/uploads/2013/08/Saylor.orgs-Scientific-Management-Theory-and-the-Ford-Motor-Company.pdf.

Scutti, Susan. "The Government Owns Your DNA. What Are They Doing with It?" *Newsweek*. July 24, 2014. www.newsweek.com/2014/08/01/whos-keeping-your-data-safe-dna-banks-261136.html.

"Serial Killer H. H. Holmes Is Hanged in Philadelphia." History. November 13, 2009. www.history.com/this-day-in-history/a-serial-killer-is-hanged.

"Seventy-First World Health Assembly Update, 25 May." World Health Organization. May 25, 2018. https://www.who.int/news-room/detail/25-05-2018-seventy-first-world-health-assembly-update-25-may.

Shanafelt, Tait D. "Changes in Burnout and Satisfaction with Work-Life Balance in Physicians and General US Working Population Between 2011 and 2014." *Mayo Clinic Proceedings* 90, no. 12 (December 2015): 1600–1613. doi:10.1016/s0025-6196(15)00863-0.

Shem, Samuel. *The House of God*. New York: Black Swan, 1985.

Shem, Samuel. *Mount Misery*. New York: Fawcett, 1997.

Shermer, Michael. *Heavens on Earth: The Scientific Search for the Afterlife, Immortality, and Utopia*. New York: Henry Holt, 2018.

Silver, Julie K., et al. "Female Physicians Are Underrepresented in Recognition Awards from the American Academy of Physical Medicine and Rehabilitation." *PM&R* 9, no. 10 (2017): 976–984. doi:10.1016/j.pmrj.2017.02.016.

Silverman, Rachel Emma. "Women Doctors Face $17,000 Pay Gap." American Medical Women's Association. www.amwa-doc.org/news/women-doctors-face-17000-pay-gap/.

Simonite, Tom. "'DNA Computer' Is Unbeatable at Tic-Tac-Toe." *The New Scientist*. October 17, 2006. https://www.newscientist.com/article/dn10310-dna-computer-is-unbeatable-at-tic-tac-toe/.

Singh, Sarwant. "Transhumanism and The Future of Humanity: 7 Ways The World Will Change By 2030." *Forbes* November 20, 2017. www.forbes.com/sites/sarwantsingh/2017/11/20/transhumanism-and-the-future-of-humanity-seven-ways-the-world-will-change-by-2030/#7d5df9a87d79.

Sisson, Paul. "Doctors Strike Shows Union Push." *San Diego Union Tribune*. January 27, 2015. www.sandiegouniontribune.com/news/health/sdut-uc-doctors-strike-student-health-centers-2015jan27-htmlstory.html#.

Skloot, Rebecca. *The Immortal Life of Henrietta Lacks*. New York: Broadway Books, 2010.

"Slaughterbots." YouTube. November 12, 2017. www.youtube.com/watch?v=9CO6M2HsoIA.

Small, G. W., et al. "Your Brain on Google: Patterns of Cerebral Activation during Internet Searching." *The American Journal of Geriatric Psychiatry* 17, no. 2 (February 2009). www.ncbi.nlm.nih.gov/pubmed/19155745.

Smith, Austin. "Principles of Medical Ethics—1957." *Journal of the American Medical Association* 164, no. 13 (1957): 1482. doi:10.1001/jama.1957.02980130058014.

Smith, Kerri. "'The Knowledge' Enlarges Your Brain." *Nature* News. December 8, 2011. www.nature.com/news/the-knowledge-enlarges-your-brain-1.9602.

Sommerlad, Joe. "Harold Shipman: Who Was 'Doctor Death', How Many of His Patients Did He Kill, and How Was He Finally Caught?" *The Independent*, April 26, 2018. www.independent.co.uk/news/uk/crime/harold-shipman-doctor-death-serial-killer-gp-mass-murderer-hyde-manchester-itv-documentary-a8323176.html.

Sood, Harpreet S. "Has the Time Come for Unique Patient Identifiers for the U.S.?" *NEJM Catalyst*. February 21, 2018. catalyst.nejm.org/time-unique-patient-identifiers-us/.

Spiegel, A. D., and F. Kavaler. "Abraham Lincoln Loses a Medical Malpractice Case, Debates Stephen A. Douglas, and Secures Two Murder Acquittals." *Journal of Community Health* 29, no.1 (February 2004). www.ncbi.nlm.nih.gov/pubmed/14768936.

Srivastava, Ranjana. "Just Give Me the Script:

The Scourge of Antibiotic Misuse and the Threat to Us All." *The Guardian*. June 21, 2016. https://www.theguardian.com/commentisfree/2016/jun/22/just-give-me-the-script-the-scourge-of-antibiotic-misuse-and-the-threat-to-us-all.

Stangroom, Jeremy. *The Great Philosophers: From Socrates to Foucault*. London: Arcturus Publishing Limited, 2008.

Star Trek. "Regeneration." Season 2, episode 23.

Star Trek. "Mirror Mirror." Season 39, episode 33.

"State House Passes Important Bill to Protect Hospital and Health Care Providers." The Hospital Health System Association of Pennsylvania. February 12, 2016. https://www.haponline.org/Newsroom/News/ID/1527/State-House-Passes-Important-Bill-to-Protect-Hospital-and-Health-Care-Providers.

Steele, Volney. *Bleed, Blister, and Purge: A History of Medicine on the American Frontier*. Missoula, MT: Mountain Press Publishing, 2006, p. 13

"Step 1." United States Medical Licensing Examination. www.usmle.org/step-1/.

Stephenson, Neal. *Snow Crash*. New York: Del Rey Publishing, 1992.

Stewart, Matthew. *The Management Myth: Debunking Modern Business Philosophy*. New York: W.W. Norton, 2009.

Stoddard, Hugh A., and David V. O'Dell, "Would Socrates Have Actually Used the 'Socratic Method' for Clinical Teaching," *JGIM* 31, no. 9 (September 2016)., https://www.ncbi.nlm.nih.gov/pubmed/27130623.

Stone, Christopher. "From Bolam to Bolitho: Unravelling Medical Protectionism." January 2011. pdfs.semanticscholar.org/2d6e/1d0931f84058222337d5c49b3eb720c1edfe.pdf.

"Strained Healthcare System Hurts Doctors and Affects Patient Care." MDVIP. September 20, 2017. www.mdvip.com/about-mdvip/pressroom/strained-healthcare-system-hurts-doctors-affects-patient-care.

Striem-Amit, Ella, and Amir Amedi. "Visual Cortex Extrastriate Body-Selective Area Activation in Congenitally Blind People 'Seeing' by Using Sounds." *Current Biology* 24, no. 6 (2014): 687–692. doi:10.1016/j.cub.2014.02.010.

Sugiura, A., et al. "Effect of Reading a Book on a Tablet Computer on Cerebral Blood Flow in the Prefrontal Cortex." *Nihon Eiseigaku Zasshi (Japanese Journal of Hygiene)* 73, no. 1 (2018). www.ncbi.nlm.nih.gov/pubmed/29386445.

"Suicides in Japan Hit a 20-Year Low." *The Economist*. June 8, 2017. www.economist.com/graphic-detail/2017/06/28/suicides-in-japan-hit-a-20-year-low.

Surber, Regina. "Artificial Intelligence: Autonomous Technology (AT), Lethal Autonomous Weapons Systems (LAWS) and Peace Time Threats." The ICT4Peace Foundation and the Zurich Hub for Ethics and Technology (ZHET), February 21, 2018. https://ict4peace.org/activities/artificial-intelligence-autonomous-technology-at-lethal-autonomous-weapons-systems-laws-and-peace-time-threats/.

Taylor, Frederick W. *The Principles of Scientific Management*. 1911. https://wwnorton.com/college/history/america-essential-learning/docs/FWTaylor-Scientific_Mgmt-1911.pdf.

"TDCS Device—TheBrainDriver v2." Amazon. www.amazon.com/tDCS-Device-TheBrainDriver-Ready-Use/dp/B018AE2CV2/ref=sr_1_2?ie=UTF8&qid=1530487825&sr=8-2&keywords=tDCS.

Temkin, Owsei. *Hippocrates in a World of Pagans and Christians*. Baltimore, MD: The Johns Hopkins University Press, 1995.

Thielking, Megan. "A Doctor's Murder Over an Opioid Prescription Leaves an Indiana City with No Easy Answers." STAT. August 8, 2017. www.statnews.com/2017/08/08/indiana-doctor-murdered-opioids/.

Thomas, Dylan. *In Country Sleep: and Other Poems*. New York: A New Directions Book, 1952.

Thompson, Dennis. "Fewer Medical Malpractice Lawsuits Succeed, but Payouts Are Up." CBS News. March 28, 2017. www.cbsnews.com/news/medical-malpractice-lawsuits-fewer-claims-succeed-payouts-rise/.

Thompson, Dennis. "What Smoking Marijuana Does to the Brain." CBS News. November 11, 2014. www.cbsnews.com/news/what-smoking-marijuana-does-to-the-brain/.

Titcomb, James. "Mark Zuckerberg Confirms Facebook Is Working on Mind-Reading Technology." *The Telegraph*. April 19, 2017. www.telegraph.co.uk/technology/2017/04/19/mark-zuckerberg-confirms-facebook-working-mind-reading-technology/.

"Title 29—Labor. USC 151: Findings and Declaration of Policy." The United States Code. http://uscode.house.gov/view.xhtml?req=(title:29%20section:151%20edition:prelim)

Topol, Eric J. *The Patient Will See You Now: The Future of Medicine Is in Your Hands*. New York: Basic Books, 2016.

Turing, A. M. "On Computable Numbers, with an Application to the Entscheidungsproblem. A Correction." *Proceedings of the London Mathematical Society* s2–43, no. 1 (1938): 544–546. doi:10.1112/plms/s2-43.6.544.

Turvey, Samuel T., and Anthony S. Cheke. "Dead

as a Dodo: The Fortuitous Rise to Fame of an Extinction Icon." *Historical Biology* 20, no. 2 (2008): 149–163. doi:10.1080/08912960802376199.

"U.S. DOE Molecular Nuclear Medicine Timeline." History of PET and MRI. www.doemedicalsciences.org/timeline.shtml.

"USMLE Step 1 Average Match Scores by Specialty." Doctors in Training, www.doctorsintraining.com/blog/usmle-step-1-average-match-scores-by-specialty/.

Verdon, Daniel R. "Physician Outcry on EHR Functionality, Cost Will Shake the Health Information Technology Sector." Medical Economics. February 10, 2014. doi:http://www.medicaleconomics.com/health-care-information-technology/physician-outcry-ehr-functionality-cost-will-shake-health-information-technology-sector.

Verghese, Abraham, M.D., MACP, et al. "A History of Physical Examination Texts and the Conception of Bedside Diagnosis," *The Transactions of the American Clinical and Climatological Association*, 122 (2011). www.ncbi.nlm.nih.gov/pmc/articles/PMC3116347/.

"Verifying SOAP Eligibility." National Resident Matching Program. www.nrmp.org/verifying-soap-eligibility/.

Wachowski, Brothers, director. *The Matrix*. Warner Brothers, March 31, 1999.

Wachter, Robert M. *The Digital Doctor: Hope, Hype, and Harm at the Dawn of Medicine's Computer Age*. New York: McGraw-Hill Education, 2017.

"Waiting Time to See Doctor When Sick or Need Medical Attention, Among Sicker Adults." Commonwealth Fund. July 16, 2008. www.commonwealthfund.org/chart/2008/waiting-time-see-doctor-when-sick-or-need-medical-attention-among-sicker-adults.

Walker, H. Kenneth. *Clinical Methods: The History, Physical, and Laboratory Examination*. 3rd Edition (New York: Butterworth Publishers, 1990). Chapter 1. www.ncbi.nlm.nih.gov/books/NBK458/.

Wang, Jing., et al. "Predicting the Brain Activation Pattern Associated with the Propositional Content of a Sentence: Modeling Neural Representations of Events and States." *Human Brain Mapping*. October 2017. www.ccbi.cmu.edu/reprints/Wang_Just_HBM-2017_Journal-preprint.pdf.

"WaveNet: A Generative Model for Raw Audio." *DeepMind*. deepmind.com/blog/wavenet-generative-model-raw-audio/.

Wehner, Mackenzie R., et al. "Plenty of Moustaches but Not Enough Women: Cross Sectional Study of Medical Leaders." *BMJ*. (2015). doi:10.1136/bmj.h6311.

Weizenbaum, Joseph. *Computer Power and Human Reason: From Judgment to Calculation*. San Francisco: S.H. Freeman, 1976.

Westby, Fisher G. "Dr. Wes." drwes.blogspot.com/.

"What You Need to Know about Facebook & Cambridge Analytica." CBS News. March 20, 2018. www.cbsnews.com/news/what-you-need-to-know-about-facebook-cambridge-analytica/.

"What's the Price Tag for a College Education?" CollegeData. https://www.collegedata.com/en/pay-your-way/college-sticker-shock/how-much-does-college-cost/whats-the-price-tag-for-a-college-education/.

"White House Releases Data Listing Medicare's Top-Paid Doctors." FOX News. April 9, 2014. www.foxnews.com/politics/2014/04/09/white-house-releases-data-listing-medicare-top-paid-doctors.html.

Wible, Pamela, MD. *Physician Suicide Letters: Answered*. Self-published, 2016.

Wolf, Gary. "Ray Kurzweil Pulls Out All the Stops (and Pills) to Survive the Singularity." Wired. March 24, 2008. www.wired.com/2008/03/ff-kurzweil/.

Wolfe, George C., director. *The Immortal Life of Henrietta Lacks*. Home Box Office, 2017.

"World Health Organization Programme Budget 2018–2019." World Health Organization. https://www.who.int/about/finances-accountability/budget/PB2018-2019_en_web.pdf?ua=1.

"Worldwide Spending on Cognitive and Artificial Intelligence Systems Will Grow to $19.1 Billion in 2018, According to New IDC Spending Guide." IDC: The Premier Global Market Intelligence Company. 2018. https://www.idc.com/getdoc.jsp?containerId=prUS43662418.

Yanamandra, Uday, and Sushma Yanamandra. "Traditional First Aid in a Case of Snake Bite: More Harm Than Good." *British Medical Journal Case Reports* (February 2014). www.ncbi.nlm.nih.gov/pmc/articles/PMC3926357/.

Yonck, Richard. *Heart of the Machine: Our Future in a World of Artificial Emotional Intelligence*. New York: Arcade Publishing, 2017.

Younker, J. Marin. *Bleed, Blister, Puke, and Purge: the Dirty Secrets behind Early American Medicine*. Minneapolis: Zest Books, 2016.

Zemeckis, Robert, director. *Beowulf*. Warner Brothers, 2007.

Zemeckis, Robert, director. *The Polar Express*. Warner Brothers, October 21, 2004.

Index

AAFP 210, 235
AAMC 215–216, 224, 230, 235–236
ABCnews 236
ABIM 215, 219, 223
ABMS 116–118, 124
abortions 183
addiction 43, 92, 112, 115, 160, 217, 231, 235
adolescence 93, 159–160
aerospace 174
Aesop 211, 223
Aesthetic 33, 90, 215, 223
Aethena 22
Aetna 39, 212, 232
affective computing 183–184, 191, 198–199, 220, 234–235
Affordable Care Act 38, 91, 111–112, 114, 175, 217
afterlife 74, 214, 237
Agnew, Ernest 211–212, 223
alcoholics 107
Alibaba 172, 228
allergy 29, 50
altruistic 76, 124, 158
Alzheimer 67, 168
AMA 10, 21, 55, 113–114, 217–218, 223, 231, 233
Amazon 14, 55–56, 168, 175, 220, 236, 238
Americans 7, 26, 91
amnesia 167
amputations 74, 85
AMSA 215, 233
anaphylaxis 66
anatomy 16, 42
ancestor 14, 70, 131, 184, 187, 190
android 188
anemia 206
anesthesia 35, 41
angiogram 129
Annals of Family Medicine 7, 209, 216, 224, 235
antiaging 77
antibiotics 35, 55, 60, 64, 66, 149, 180, 205
antidepressant 27, 146
antidote 140, 154
antiseptic 61, 211, 232
antitrust 117–118, 121, 123–124, 218, 224
AOL 221, 228

apothecaries 42
appendicitis 41
arbitration 88, 90, 94
Aristotle 36, 45
Armageddon 210, 234
ARRA 10, 209, 223
arrhythmia 51, 196
artificial intelligence 2, 14, 47, 57, 135, 162, 181–184, 187, 191, 210, 213, 220–221, 225, 229, 232, 238–239
aseptic 36
Asimov, Isaac 22, 210, 224
atelectasis 206
attending 164
attorney 78, 84, 90, 119, 215, 233
autism 184, 187, 199, 233

Babylon 12, 182, 210
Bach 172, 219, 224
bacteria 35–36, 180, 205
Bactrim 67
Bactroban 149
Bakalar, Nicholas 213, 224
bankruptcy 115
Barre 97
BBC 51, 168, 179, 183, 186, 210, 213–214, 219, 221, 225–226, 228, 230
bedside 40, 81, 147, 213, 239
Beowulf 80, 184, 221, 239
Bethlehem 37–38
Bill and Melinda Gates Foundation 176–177, 220, 223–224, 226, 235
biochemistry 35, 101, 187
biofeedback 171, 184
biohackers 73
biologic 131–132, 167, 182, 186–188
biology 15, 77, 101, 210, 218, 221, 235, 238–239
biomedical 179
biopsy 68, 148
biotech 46
bloggers 100
bloodletting 47
BMJ (*British Journal of Medicine*) 108, 214, 216, 218, 227–228, 239
Boston 19, 188, 215, 219, 221, 225, 231, 234

241

Index

botfly 66
bowel 5, 36, 43, 46, 208
Brill, Eric 91, 215, 219, 225
Brynjolfsson, Erik 219
Buddhists 76
Buffett, Warren 176, 220, 223
bureaucracy 52, 189
burnout 3, 9, 12, 22, 98, 101, 108, 123, 193, 209–210, 215–216, 227, 235, 237

cadavers 36, 42
calculator 28, 30, 166–167
calculi 203
California 27, 38, 79, 106, 122, 175, 178, 189, 214, 216, 218, 220, 224, 227–228
Cambridge Analytica 56, 59, 211, 213, 218, 220, 226, 231, 234, 239
Campbell, Joseph 5, 209, 225
camphor 43, 66
cancer 13, 18, 29, 33, 37, 51–53, 58, 62–65, 72–73, 83, 89, 92–93, 100, 113, 115, 117, 148, 153, 155, 171, 174, 177–179, 181, 189, 203, 213–215, 223, 228, 231–232, 235
candidate 26, 51, 86, 93, 106
cannabis 215, 223
capitalist 10, 39, 70, 113, 175, 180, 197
carcinogens 92
Card, Orson Scott 211, 225
cardiac 50, 71, 120, 142, 212, 225
cardiologist 58, 99, 169
cardiovascular 65, 99
cardioversion 51
career 1, 3–4, 45, 82, 84, 101, 107, 109, 112, 135, 194
caregivers 112, 198
carotid 67, 203
Carr, Nicholas 9, 159, 168, 209, 218–219, 224–225
cataract 43
Cave, Stephen 12, 76, 86, 189–190, 214, 225
CBS 83, 212–215, 220, 227, 231, 238–239
cellulitis 66, 68
Census Bureau 151, 209, 229
CEO 10, 39, 83, 114–115, 120, 124, 149, 188–189, 209, 212, 217, 227, 230, 232
charlatans 85
chemotherapy 119, 179, 203
cigarette 92–93, 202–203, 206, 215, 227, 232
CIGNA 39
Cline, Ernest 190, 211, 221, 226
clinic 9, 12, 40, 44, 59, 97, 104, 121, 173, 198, 209–211, 217–218, 226, 232, 234–237
CME 103
CNBC 211, 221, 229, 235
CNN 119, 211, 217, 232, 235
CNNMoney 232, 235
cochlear 188
Cochrane Report 213, 231
colleges 12, 33, 110, 118, 230, 236
Collins, Suzanne 211, 220, 226
colonics 36

colonoscopy 29
computers 5, 9, 21, 23–24, 32, 51, 73, 113, 133, 155, 161–164, 166–168, 172, 183–184, 187–188, 198, 209, 218–219
concierge medicine 175, 220, 226
congress 9, 23, 27, 36, 44, 109, 114, 209, 212, 217, 229–231, 236
connectome 14, 210, 227
consciousness 14, 128, 132, 185
conspiracy 56, 121
consumer 10, 23, 43, 49–50, 104, 111, 158, 184, 212, 224–225, 230, 235
COPD 93, 205
corporation 9, 14, 120, 122, 175, 182, 194, 228, 230
cortex 157, 159, 161, 165, 167, 184, 189–190, 218–219, 221, 235, 238
Costandi, Moheb 159, 218, 226
coverage 88, 102, 111, 171
cowboy 31, 48
CPR 70, 196
craft 1–2, 33, 40, 46–47, 52, 57, 100, 118, 171
creatine 142, 150
credentials 39, 216
Crichton, Michael 201, 222, 226
cryotherapy 148
Cummings, Mary 28, 211, 226
curriculum 26, 102
cyberattack 50
Cyberdyne 198
cybersecurity 50–51, 212–213, 223, 225–226
CyberWeird Stories 233

DARPA 16
Darwin, Charles 15, 41, 176, 186, 221, 226
Dary, David 212, 226
dataharvesting 27
dataism 130–131, 134–135, 137–138
DEA 102–103
deathbed 81
deaths 41, 43, 50, 57–59, 81, 146, 188
decoded 14
Deepmind 182–183, 220, 226–227, 239
dehydrated 97
Dell 215, 238
delusional 162
democracy 91, 114
Democrat 115
Democritus 134
dentists 122
depression 197
dermatologist 52–53, 99, 213, 228
Descartes, Rene 45, 128–129, 131, 163–164, 218–219
deskilling 219, 230
devaluation 163
diabetes 10, 73, 89, 149–150, 153
diagnosis 5, 11, 29, 32–34, 47, 49, 51, 53, 61, 68–69, 75, 83, 88, 96, 114, 133–134, 139–141, 156, 169–170, 189, 195, 203, 211, 213, 226, 235, 239

Index

digital 1, 7–8, 10, 14–15, 17, 29, 45, 47, 51–52, 55, 110, 113, 133, 157, 159, 166–168, 171, 177, 200, 211, 213, 219–220, 224, 239
Digoxin 143
dilemma 161
diploma 39, 111
diplomacy 177
disease 11, 13–14, 27, 33–35, 37–40, 45, 61, 63, 65, 67–69, 73, 75, 80, 96, 99, 132, 140–141, 158, 164–165, 174, 176–180, 207, 212, 229, 231, 236
Disney 183, 226
dissection 42, 87
diuretic 142–143, 150
divine 134
DMV 200
DNA 13, 15, 18, 27, 49, 63, 76–77, 135, 149, 178–180, 188, 201–202, 220–221, 227, 237
Doctors' Bill of Rights 2, 10, 89, 109, 111–112, 120, 124, 177, 216–217, 223–224, 230, 236
Doctors Without Borders 177, 220, 224, 230
Dodgson, Charles 18
dodo bird 18, 202, 210, 222, 226, 239
doublethink 20
drowning 58, 142
DrWes.blogspot.com 215, 239
dualist 129, 131, 134, 137
DVT 68
dyslexia 116
dystopia 20–21, 23, 25, 27, 29, 194

earache 165
ebola 176–177, 220, 227
ECG 5, 62, 67, 129
ecosystem 18, 23, 145
educational 60, 97–98, 110–111, 199, 213
EEG 51, 62
EHR 8, 21, 27, 209–210, 216, 223–224, 226, 233, 235–236, 239
electrocardiogram 62
elixir 43–44, 77, 212, 224
Eliza 44, 162–163, 172, 192
email 34, 49, 59, 63, 110, 136, 165
Emboli 144
emergency 9, 21, 26, 36, 39, 51, 63, 70, 97–98, 100, 171, 209–210, 225, 230
emeritus 64, 165
EMG 51
emphysema 93
EMR 7–11, 21–23, 34, 49–50, 94, 102–103, 109, 123, 158–159, 161–162, 164, 168
enema 36, 211, 232
England 8, 24, 58, 83, 85, 105, 178, 211, 216, 220, 224, 231, 235
entrepreneur 51, 113–114
Epictetus 140
Epicurianism 137
epidemic 38, 163, 176–178
epidemiologic 9
epigenetic 185, 187, 221, 224, 236
ethics 69, 78, 86, 113, 115, 119, 188, 214, 217, 220–221, 223, 225–226, 228, 230–231, 237–238
exoskeleton 16, 198
experimental 15
experts 99
explicit knowledge 4–5, 43, 106, 165, 167, 172
extinction 17, 27, 178, 210, 239

Facebook 13, 16, 53, 55–56, 189, 213, 221, 234, 238–239
facetime 59
factory 52, 54, 57, 144, 148–151
faculty 37, 102
fate 74–75, 84
FBI 119
FCC 25–26, 211, 233
FDA 43–44, 50–51, 92–93, 119, 212–213, 223–226, 232
fecal 36
federally 93, 124, 178
fellowship 102
fertility 16
fibrillation 51, 143
film 20
firewalls 56
Fitbit 51, 200
fluxing 80
FMRI 137
Foer, Franklin 55–56, 213, 228
Forbes 210–211, 216, 219–220, 224, 228, 232, 234, 237
foundation 22, 122, 137, 162, 176, 209–210, 213, 220–221, 223–224, 231–232, 237
four humors 228
foxglove 43
Frankenstein 49, 162–163
Franklin, Benjamin 38, 211–212
fraud 1, 86–87, 119, 214, 217, 227, 229–230, 232
FTC 224

Gaiman, Neil 127–128, 218, 228
gallbladder 97
gastric 70
gatekeepers 4, 25, 56
gene 13, 52, 76–77, 179, 181, 186–187, 216, 221, 227–228, 236
genetic 15, 17, 35, 49, 52, 77, 88, 132, 135, 138, 149, 178–180, 186–187, 202–203
genome 14
genotype 178
genus 135
geriatric 219, 221, 232, 237
Gilgamesh 72–73, 201, 214, 234
GlaxoSmithKline 119, 217, 229, 234
global health 229
glucose 16, 210, 232
Gonzalez-Crussi 211, 229
Google 33, 47, 55–56, 73, 81, 158, 172, 182–183, 191, 211, 219–220, 224, 227, 229–230, 232, 235, 237
government 10, 13, 25, 40, 50, 52, 54, 56, 87,

89, 111, 114, 119–120, 124, 134, 151, 154, 174–178, 197, 199, 217, 220, 232, 237
granulomas 205–206
grief 105, 197, 214, 232
grieving 58, 214, 232
The Guardian 225, 229, 234, 238
gunshot 202
gynecologist 100

habitualization 29
hacked 27, 74
hallucinating 97
haptic 195
HarperCollins 218
Harvard 105, 159, 181
Hawking, Stephen 51, 57, 213, 225, 235–236
Health Affairs 107, 183, 209, 213, 215–217, 229–230, 237
healthcare 7, 38, 51, 89, 125, 209–210, 212–213, 215–221, 224–225, 227–236, 238
hearts 111, 170, 194, 197
heaven 72, 74, 138
hedonism 134–135
hemoglobin 16, 153
hemorrhoids 43
heroin 43
herpes 208
hi-tech 27, 211, 223, 230
HIPAA 27, 211, 216, 230
hippocampus 136–137, 157, 167
Hippocrates 35–36, 61, 99, 138, 217–218, 228, 238
HIV 58, 141, 177, 183
HMO 121, 174, 217, 229
holistic 85
homicide 105
homunculus 208
hormone 36, 64, 149, 151–152, 154, 199, 211
hospice 78, 81
hospitals 8, 16, 25, 37–38, 40, 44, 57, 59, 115, 117, 122, 124, 174, 182, 212, 224
HSV 208
Huffington Post 234
humanism 128, 131, 134, 137–138
humanoid 188, 233–234
hybrid 220, 229
hyperplasia 208
hyperthyroidism 151
hypocrisy 103
hypothesis 195

IBM 133, 171, 181, 219–220, 228, 233, 237
IBS 208
ICU 180
idealist 3, 18, 24
immunization 13, 15, 45, 174, 220, 229
implantable cardiac devices 50, 190, 212
industrialization 180
infection 36, 43, 66–67, 149, 177
infertile 135
infusion pumps 50, 212

inhalants 93
innovation 6, 12, 16, 18, 50–51, 53, 57–58, 124, 127, 171, 176, 182, 191, 219, 230, 234
inotrope 143
internet 24–26, 33, 57, 64, 72, 100, 131, 136, 138–139, 145, 159–161, 166, 172, 210, 212, 218–219, 227, 237
intersubjective 127–131, 134, 137
interventional 53, 68
intestines 208
intoxicated 105
inventor 192, 195, 226
investors 70, 182
ischemic 145
Italy 173
ITunes 226
IV 16, 70, 77, 166

JAMA (Journal of the American Medical Association) 21, 84, 108, 140, 209–211, 214, 216–218, 227, 233–234, 236–237
Japan 174, 197–198, 219, 221, 228–229, 231, 238
JIBO 198, 221, 224
Johns Hopkins 40, 179, 212, 231, 238
Journal of the American Medical Association 8, 108, 118, 209–210, 213, 215–216, 219–220, 223, 235–239
journalism 56
JPMorgan 175, 236
The Juncture 80, 132
Jurassic 201, 222, 226

Kant, Immanuel 4, 209, 231
keloids 148
keratosis 148, 203
Kevinmd.com 100, 215–216, 235
keystroke 9, 51, 196
Kubler-Ross, Elisabeth 75–76, 214, 232
Kurzweil, Ray 72–73, 214, 224, 239

laboratory 154, 187, 195, 213, 239
Lacks, Henrietta 178–179, 220, 225, 237, 239
Laicifitra 202–203
Lancet 83, 108, 214, 216, 234–235
laptops 73
Larson, Eric 87, 214, 232
laser 16, 196, 203
lawsuit 82–83, 85, 88–90, 94–95, 100, 102, 118, 121, 214–215, 223, 233, 238
Laxosmith 234
legislation 22, 93, 117, 120
liability 29, 89, 92, 124
librarian 139–141, 143, 145, 147, 149, 151–153, 155–156
lifespan 14–15, 135, 173
limbic 184
Lincoln, Abraham 84, 214, 237
Lister, Joseph 36, 211, 232
litigation 83, 85, 88, 90, 110, 214
lobbyist 82–83, 85, 87, 89, 91, 93–95, 115, 124
lobotomies 36

Index

Locke, John 114–115, 217, 232
longevity 15
Lozar, D.C. 31, 233
luddite 1, 49, 52, 58, 191, 224
lumbar 89
lunacy 211, 236
lymphoma 68, 133

machine breaking 52
mainframe 55
malpractice 82–85, 87–90, 94–95, 100, 102, 110, 124, 214–215, 227, 231, 233–234, 237–238
mammograms 29
management 53–54, 110, 161, 165, 194, 211, 213, 219, 230, 236–238
Mannix, Kathryn 73, 214, 233
marijuana 93, 215, 225, 228, 233, 238
Matrix 128
Mayo Clinic Proceedings 9, 12, 209–211, 217, 226, 235, 237
mayor 42
McAfee 172, 219, 225, 231
MCAT 101, 215, 229
McFarland & Company, Inc., Publishing 211–212, 223
Medicaid 8, 10, 217, 223, 234
Medical economics 21, 24, 113, 115, 117, 119, 121, 123, 125, 210, 233
Medicare 8, 10, 87, 114–115, 118–119, 214, 217, 223, 227, 232–234, 239
Medscape 8, 87, 89, 106, 108, 209, 212, 214–216, 223, 225–226, 229, 232–233, 235
menopause 37, 149, 152
metaphysical 127
metastasis 52, 93, 148
methamphetamine 93, 104
Michelangelo 72, 214, 234
micromanagement 199
Microsoft 176, 210, 234
mimicry 156, 170
minion 145–146, 148, 205
MIT 28, 172, 183, 187, 189, 198, 214, 218, 220–221, 224, 226, 235–236
mitochondrial 77
mitral 196
MOC 116–118, 164, 217, 223, 227, 229
Mohs 148
molecular 15, 63, 213, 217, 223, 239
Monty Python 74, 214, 229
Morgan, Richard 185, 220–221
morphine 50
mortality 44, 80, 175, 184, 213, 221, 231, 233
MRA 67
MRI 14, 52, 63, 67–68, 84, 159, 174, 176, 219, 231, 239
MRSA 148–149
multidrug 176
Musk, Elon 16, 30, 51–52, 213, 228–229

nannybot 199–200
nanobiotech 191

Napoleon 62
narcotic 147
nares 149
NASA 28, 211, 236
Nature 228–229
NBC 220
NBC News 225
NEJM (New England Journal of Medicine) 105, 108, 215, 219, 223–224, 237
nematode 14
neocortex 132, 184
neolithic 130
nephropathy 10
nerves 52, 160
neurology 99, 225
neuromatrix 46–47, 131, 199
neuromuscular 189
neuron 128, 146, 167, 184, 186–188
neuropathic 147
neuroplasticity 137, 159–160, 165, 168, 186, 218, 226
neuroscience 218–219, 225–226, 237
neurosurgeon 171
neurotransmitters 146
nevermind 184, 220, 234
New York Times (NYT) 92, 106, 131, 158, 211, 213–215, 217–218, 220, 224–225, 229, 231–234
New Yorker Magazine 228, 232
Newsweek 117, 217, 219–220, 227, 237
NHS 182–183, 209, 220, 225, 230, 232
Nietzsche, Friedrich 131, 218, 234
nightingale 44
NIH 14, 78, 108, 179, 220, 223, 225, 228–229, 236–239
noncompliance 152, 155
noninvasiveness 52, 168
nonprofit 38, 79, 115–116, 124
Northwestern Medical School 4, 118, 236
Nowlan, Philip Francis 12, 210, 234
NPR 212, 216, 219, 224, 233
NRMP 212, 215, 235, 239
nystagmus 129
NYU 212, 214, 237

Obama, Barack 25, 111, 115, 211, 214, 228, 233
Obamacare 175
obstetrics 231
Odin 201
oligarchic 25
Olympics 230
oncology 99, 181
Opensecrets.com 91, 215, 227, 232
operations 8, 41, 123
ophthalmoscope 62
opioid 120, 216, 218, 228, 238
optics 191
Orwell, George 20–21, 23, 25, 27, 29, 210, 234
osteoporosis 151
otolaryngology 223
ovaries 152

Oxford 226
oxycodone 87
oxygenated 165
ozone 135

pacemakers 50, 143
pagans 218, 238
palliative 73, 78
palpitations 143
panacea 6
pantheon 30
paradox 24, 46, 210–211, 223, 227, 235
paraplegics 188
parasite 7, 35
The Pareto Chart 125, 218, 235
Parkinson 52, 64
Pascale, Carayon 168, 219, 225
patented 43, 56, 124, 171, 179
paternalist 63
pathognomonic 34
pathology 35, 52–53, 68–69
pathophysiology 96
paxil 119
peacemakers 130
pediatric 217, 231
penicillin 29, 35, 67
peristalsis 46, 208
peritonsillar 36
peroxide 236
pharmaceutical 16, 44, 115, 119–120, 124, 154, 171, 174
phenylketonuria 178
philosopher 79, 134, 140, 218, 238
phlegm 61
phobias 31
physicals 11
Picard, Rosalind W. 183, 185, 191, 220, 235
PKU 178
placebo 42
plague 135
Plato 160–161, 219, 235
PMR 216
pneumonia 53, 173, 176, 206, 213, 232
Polak, Petr 210, 235
Polanyi, Michael 4, 209, 235
The Polar Express 37, 221, 239
policymakers 8–9
polio 179
politician 13, 43, 91, 93–94, 124, 133
postgraduate 124
prescient 188
prescribed 29, 31, 36, 43, 202
president 25, 44, 56, 111, 115, 211, 233
prevention 43, 64, 106–107, 119, 126, 197–198, 216, 229, 231, 234
pricefixing 121
Princeton 209, 225
prolapse 196
propagation 187
propecia 86
prostate 99, 203

psoriasis 148
psychiatry 36, 38, 96, 99, 101, 122, 161, 219, 225, 237
PubMed 223, 235, 237–238
pulmonary 17, 34, 63, 73, 144

quacksalver 36
quadriplegia 64
Quiko 80
quinine 43
quirks 185

radar 199
radiation 119, 174, 179
radicular 89
radiologist 29, 52–53, 99, 213
rales 62
Rand Health 8–9, 58, 94, 209–210, 228, 230, 236
Rapael Smart Glove 16, 210, 236
rash 29, 34, 129, 193
Reagan, Ronald 27, 211, 236
rebooting 13, 137
reengineered 201
referral 32, 68, 108, 114, 195
reflux 34
regeneration 210, 218, 238
rehabilitation 216, 237
reimbursement 9–10, 55, 86, 109, 114, 158
relationship 1, 7–8, 10, 12, 14, 16–19, 22, 24, 26, 28, 30–32, 34, 36, 38, 40, 42, 44–46, 48, 50, 52, 54–56, 58, 60, 62, 64, 66, 68–70, 74, 76, 78, 80, 84, 86–88, 90, 92, 94, 98, 100, 102, 104, 106, 108, 110, 112–116, 118, 120, 122–124, 126–128, 130, 132–134, 136–138, 140, 142, 144, 146, 148, 150, 152–154, 156, 158, 160, 162, 164, 166, 168, 170, 172, 174, 176, 178, 180, 182, 184–186, 188, 190, 192, 194, 196, 198, 200, 202, 207, 211, 236
renal 203, 227
repayment 110
representatives 37, 106
residency 4, 23, 40–41, 96–97, 101–102, 110–111, 114, 124, 212, 215, 217, 231, 235–236
retinopathy 10
retirement 12, 14, 103, 146, 149, 152
Reuters 105, 216, 227
rheumatology 99
robocall 153
robotic 2, 14, 22, 50, 135, 170, 184, 198, 212, 221, 224, 226, 229, 234
Rosenthal, Elisabeth 10, 38, 40, 209, 212–213, 236
rotation 202–203
rounds 40, 96–98
RPR 67
Rush, Benjamin 38, 212, 236

sadist 57
Sanders, Bernie 120, 218, 228
Sanger, Margaret 44, 212, 237

sanitation 15, 174
sawbones 41, 47
scar 206
Scholastic 211, 226
Schrödinger 46
Scientific America 15, 76, 210, 213–214, 227, 236–238
sclerosis 64, 236
screenwriter 201
scut 40
sedation 41
senator 93, 120, 229
senescence 77
senility 31
seniors 197–198
sentiment 144
Septra 29
Sequel 96
serotonin 132, 146
Shakespeare, William 72, 213–214, 228, 237
Shem, Samuel 96, 215, 231, 237
Shermer, Michael 77, 214, 237
singularity 52, 73, 233, 239
SIRI 47
skeletons 87
slaughterbots 188, 221, 237
smartphone 49, 53
Smithsonian Magazine 212, 222, 233
smoker 89, 92
snakebites 36
socialization 165–166
socioeconomic 125, 174, 199
Socrates 160–161, 215, 218, 238
Solow paradox 24, 210, 223, 227
Soylent Green 79, 214, 228
specialty 8, 40, 55, 58, 108, 112, 115–116, 217, 223, 227
species 15, 18, 80, 135, 180, 184, 187
sphygmomanometer 62
spinal 160
spiritualism 174
sputum 63
spyware 188
SSRI 146
Stanford 15, 43, 53, 210, 213, 226, 232
Staphylococcus 148
Star Trek 20–21, 30, 210, 238
statin 150–151
statistical 160, 218, 225
statistics 16, 57, 112, 160, 176, 218, 225, 227, 232, 234
STD 27, 35
stenosis 67, 143
Stephenson, Neal 211, 238
sterile 35, 107, 157, 159, 202
steroid 148–149
stethoscope 3, 59, 62, 195
stockholders 120
stoic 129, 134
strategies 198, 211, 226
streptococcal 43

subdural 16
suicide 70, 79, 98, 106–107, 109, 112, 125, 146, 189, 194, 197–198, 216, 221, 223, 230, 234, 238–239
superhero 3
supernatural 5
surgeon 16, 41–42, 111, 118, 210–212, 215, 223, 227, 232, 234–235
Sweden 89
synaptic 132, 160, 167
syndrome 188, 190, 193, 208
syphilis 67–68
systolic 142

tacit knowledge 4–6, 165–167, 171–172
tacitus gloves 196, 203
tattoo 39
taxpayer 8, 115, 175
Taylorism 53–55
technology 1, 6–14, 16, 18–24, 26–32, 34–36, 38, 40, 42, 44–60, 62–64, 66, 68, 70, 72–74, 76–78, 80–81, 84, 86, 88, 90, 92, 94, 98, 100, 102, 104, 106–108, 110, 112–116, 118, 120–124, 126–128, 130, 132, 134, 136–138, 140, 142, 144–146, 148, 150, 152, 154, 156, 158–160, 162, 164, 166–172, 174, 176–178, 180, 182, 184, 186–192, 194–198, 200, 202, 210–211, 213–214, 217–221, 224–225, 228–229, 231, 233–236, 238–239
telecommunication 25
teleconference 64
telehealth 64
telemarketer 7
telemedicine 49–51, 53, 55, 57, 59, 63, 110
teleportation 136–137
televisit 50
telomere 15, 77–78, 138, 210, 226–227, 236
template 1, 8, 11, 24, 32–33, 45, 47, 64, 158, 161, 170
tenants 113, 124, 137, 201
tendon 208
tenets 4, 111, 128
terabytes 14
teratology 223
testosterone 89, 154–155
thalidomide 44
thermometer 129
Thomas, Dylan 75, 214, 238
thoracic 212
thyroid 149, 151
tic 188, 221, 237
tincture 43, 47
tissue 66, 179, 206
Tokyo 198
tomography 52, 62–63
tonsillectomies 41
toothaches 43
Topol, Eric 58–60, 213, 238
tort 83, 85, 89, 215, 223
torture 96
toxicology 212, 229

transgenerational 187
transhumanism 73, 81, 210, 237
transplant 52, 78, 186, 221, 226
tricyclics 147
truisms 5
Trump, Donald 56, 85–86, 214, 228
tuberculosis 176
tumor 16, 84, 195
typewriter 167

UCLA 64, 161, 186
ultrasound 62, 68, 151, 195
Ulysses 44
uncanny valley 184–185, 198, 221, 233–234
unethical 113
uninsured 39, 115
unions 55, 120–122, 124–125, 193
United Health 39, 212, 217, 232
uploads 231, 235–236
ureter 196
urethra 208
urinary 67
USA 87, 214, 224, 230
USC 218, 238
USMLE 215, 238–239
USNews 228
utopia 7, 9, 11–13, 15, 17, 19, 214, 237

vaccine 177, 179, 220
validation 17, 84
valve 17, 196
vampires 36
VDRL 67
vectors 180
venoscope 16
venous 68
venture 5, 70, 153, 221
vesicular 34
vessels 142
viruses 50
vitalism 45–47, 130

Vitalist 46, 129, 132, 201
Volney, Steel 212, 238

Wachter, Robert 29, 211, 213, 220, 239
The Wall Street Journal (WSJ) 213, 230
Washington Post 229
Watson 133, 169, 171–172, 181, 219–220, 228, 233
wayfinding 136
wealth 175
wearable 16, 49, 73, 189, 210, 228, 233
Webmd.com 25
WeirdBook 233
Weizenbaum, Joseph 162–164, 172, 192, 219, 221, 239
werewolves 36
wheelchair 119, 188, 190, 198
wheeze 64
Whitman, Walt 44
Wible, Pamela 106, 216, 239
Wikipedia 158
Wiley Act 43, 219, 225, 232–233
Wired Magazine 73, 159–160, 210, 214, 227, 239
witches 36
wrist 68, 125

xeroform 66
xerox 9, 186

Yale 78, 211
Yonck, Richard 184, 220, 239
Younker, Marin 38, 211–212, 239
Yuval, Harari 131, 135, 218, 229

Zarathustra 234
zealot 189
zika 176
zombies 16
Zuckerberg, Mark 189, 221, 238

www.ingramcontent.com/pod-product-compliance
Ingram Content Group UK Ltd.
Pitfield, Milton Keynes, MK11 3LW, UK
UKHW041936140426
5217IPUK00014B/500